The Society and Population Health Reader

The Society and Population Health Reader

Volume I: Income Inequality and Health
Edited by Ichiro Kawachi, Bruce P. Kennedy, and Richard G. Wilkinson

Volume II: A State and Community Perspective
Edited by Alvin R. Tarlov and Robert F. St. Peter

The Society and Population Health Reader

Volume II
A State and Community Perspective

2000

Edited by
ALVIN R. TARLOV AND
ROBERT F. ST. PETER

The New Press
New York

Published in the United States by The New Press, New York, 2000
Distributed by W. W. Norton & Company, Inc., New York

LIBRARY OF CONGRESS CATALOGING-IN-PUBLICATION DATA

The society and population health reader. Volume II : a state and community
perspective / edited by Alvin R. Tarlov and Robert F. St. Peter.
        p.   cm.
    Includes bibliographical references and index.
    ISBN 1–56584–527–7 (hc.)
    ISBN 1–56584–557–9 (pbk.)
    1. Public health — Social aspects.   2. Social medicine.
I. Tarlov, Alvin R. (Alvin Richard), 1929–   II. St. Peter,
Robert F.
RA418.S6725   2000
306.4′61 — dc21   99–23899

The New Press was established in 1990 as a not-for-profit alternative to the large, commercial publishing houses currently dominating the book publishing industry. The New Press operates in the public interest rather than for private gain, and is committed to publishing, in innovative ways, works of educational, cultural, and community value that are often deemed insufficiently profitable.

The New Press, 450 West 41st Street, 6th floor, New York, NY 10036

www.thenewpress.com

Printed in Canada

2 4 6 8 9 7 5 3 1

CONTENTS

Preface
  Robert F. St. Peter and Alvin R. Tarlov   vii

Introduction
  Alvin R. Tarlov and Robert F. St. Peter   ix

PART ONE. GENERAL FRAMEWORK
AND THE HEALTH OF THE COMMUNITY

---

1. Healthy Societies: An Overview
   J. Fraser Mustard   3

2. Socioeconomic and Behavioral Differences in Health, Morbidity,
   and Mortality in Kansas: Empirical Data, Models, and Analyses
   Gopal K. Singh   15

3. Social Cohesion and Health
   Ichiro Kawachi   57

4. Building Healthy Communities
   Stephen B. Fawcett et al.   75

PART TWO. CHILD DEVELOPMENT AND HEALTH

---

5. Social and Educational Indicators of Childhood Well-Being in Kansas
   Thanne Rose and Frank Song   97

6. Early Influences on Development and Social Inequalities:
   An Attachment Theory Perspective
   Peter Fonagy and Anna Higgitt   104

7. Early Development in Monkeys   131
   Stephen J. Suomi

8. Early Child Development in the Context of Population Health   143
   Clyde Hertzman

PART THREE. ADULT HEALTH AND FACTORS THAT INFLUENCE IT

9. The Social Context of Smoking, Nutrition, and Sedentary Health
   Behavior in Kansas   161
   Manuella Adrian and Anna Wilkinson

10. Labor Markets and Health: A Framework and Set of Applications   178
    Benjamin C. Amick III and John N. Lavis

11. Social Relations, Hierarchy, and Health   211
    Richard G. Wilkinson

12. Race and Health in Kansas: Data, Issues, and Directions   236
    David R. Williams

13. Social Networks and Health: The Bonds That Heal   259
    Lisa F. Berkman

14. Social Status, Stress, and Health in Female Monkeys   278
    Carol A. Shively

PART FOUR. PERSPECTIVES

15. Inequalities in Health: Causes and Policy Implications   293
    Michael Marmot

16. Public Policy Frameworks for Improving Population Health   310
    Alvin R. Tarlov

Appendix: 323
   What Kansans Recommend to Improve Health and Well-Being
   Bloomquist et al.

About the Contributors   338

About the Editors   340

PREFACE

IN April of 1998 a conference, whose participants included more than two hundred and
fifty leaders from the state of Kansas, was held to
examine the health status of the Kansas population, to explore the reasons why Kansas's health
ranks in the middle of the fifty states, to explore
why the United States' health status ranks in the
lowest quartile among the twenty-five industrialized nations of the world, and to place special
emphasis on social factors that have profound influence on health. The conference drew to the
American heartland leading experts from around
the world in the field of social determinants of
health, and it began a discussion of profound importance to the health of people not only in Kansas but throughout the nation and the world.

This volume presents a synthesis of the information presented at the conference, a summary
of the discussion that took place about the application of the new information in the participants'
own communities, and the reaction of political
and business leaders to the various topics raised.
This second volume of *The Society and Population
Health Reader* complements the first volume, *Income Inequality and Health,* edited by Ichiro
Kawachi, Bruce P. Kennedy and Richard F.
Wilkinson, by adding a state and community
perspective to the important work they have assembled.

While the pages that follow attempt to capture
the scientific knowledge that was disseminated
during the conference, they can only partially
convey the truly transformative thinking that

took place about the factors that make up a society's health. An awareness was developed of the
importance of social factors in determining a
population's health and this has been demonstrated in a number of subtle but important ways,
such as local philanthropies initiating grant programs which address social capital, and communities deciding to include social determinants in
their health assessment strategies.

The conference and its related activities are
only the beginning of a long-term process, but
the seeds have fallen on fertile ground. We hope
that this comprehensive and authoritative review
of information on the social factors that influence the health and well-being of people and
communities—together with community perspectives on its relevance and application—will
help others begin a similar process.

Support for the Kansas Conference on Health
and Its Determinants and for the publication of
this volume was generously provided by the Kansas Health Foundation, a philanthropic organization based in Wichita, Kansas, whose mission
is to improve the health of all Kansans. The vision and leadership of Marni Vliet, President
and Chief Executive Officer of the foundation,
enabled the initiation of this statewide process of
research into the social determinants of health in
Kansas.

Charles E. Gessert, M.D., president of the
Kansas Health Institute (KHI) until July, 1997,
led the initial effort to plan a statewide conference on the determinants of health. Alvin R.

Tarlov, M.D., interim president of KHI beginning in July 1997, then assumed responsibility for the conference. He had the benefit of a small group of advisors: Linda Aiken, Univeristy of Pennsylvania; Arnold Kaluzny, University of North Carolina; J. Fraser Mustard, Canadian Institute for Advanced Research; and Edward Perrin, University of Washington.

Staff of the Kansas Health Institute worked tirelessly in preparing for the conference and the subsequent compilation of information it produced. KHI research staff members Gopal Singh, Anna Wilkinson, Frank Song, Thanne Rose, Manuella Adrian, and Edwin Fonner, Jr., completed two publications under tight time constraints in anticipation of the conference. These volumes, entitled *Health and Social Factors in Kansas: A Data and Chartbook, 1997–98,* and *Health and Social Trends in Kansas,* together represent a unique compilation of comprehensive health and social data from a specific state in order to highlight the relationships between the health and social well-being of communities. Administrative staff of KHI, led by Cindy Pennington and assisted by Tami Akin and Stephanie Morrison, provided logistic and organizational support for the conference.

The board of directors of the Kansas Health Institute provided support and guidance for the conference and the preparation of this volume. Members of the Board at the time the conference was held included Jack Focht (Chairman), W. Kay Kent (Vice Chair), Frank Lowman (Secretary/Treasurer), the Honorable Karen Humphreys, Estela Martinez, and Tom Simpson.

The conference benefited immeasurably from an excellent planning committee, composed of leaders from around the state: W. Kay Kent, Lawrence-Douglas County Health Department (Chair); Leonard Bloomquist, Kansas State University; Gary Brunk, Kansas Action for Children; S. Edwards Dismuke, University of Kansas Medical Center; Stephen Fawcett, University of Kansas; J. Anthony Fernandez, Fort Hays State University; Robert C. Harder, independent consultant; Elaine Johannes, Kansas State University; Gary Mitchell, Kansas Department of Health and Environment; Richard Morrissey, Kansas Department of Health and Environment; Sandy Praeger, State Senator; and Wayne White, Kansas Legal Services.

Robert F. St. Peter
Alvin R. Tarlov

INTRODUCTION

Alvin R. Tarlov and Robert F. St. Peter

A Proposition Defined

THE proposition that social and societal characteristics exert a principal influence on population health is with increasing force being supported by research in the United Kingdom, in other centers in Western and Eastern Europe, in Canada and the United States, and elsewhere. Some of the terms of the proposition as used in this introduction should be clarified.

Social characteristics refer to the quality and dependability of the personal interactions that people experience in everyday living in their homes, neighborhoods, schools, and workplaces. The interactions include those with family, friends, teachers, co-workers, supervisors, retail clerks, private sector and government personnel on whom people depend for services, strangers, and so forth. The interactions can be emotionally and physically supportive, or they can be destructive of well-being.

Societal characteristics are those contextual and structural features that provide organization for people to manage living within the social order. These include laws, regulations, social norms and expectations, work wages, and systems for access to food, clothing, shelter, medical care, learning, transport and communication, physical and economic security, fair treatment, respect for self and others, and so on. For the most part, provision of our needs is mediated through institutions that have been built over time, such as governments, schools, religions, businesses, nonprofit associations, and the like. The purposes of these institutions are uniformly benevolent, but with passage of time and failure to revise or eliminate useless or even harmful components, these structures can evolve into forces that create distortions of social purposes. Although these distortions can appear benign, they can also do violence to the social order, and they can be detrimental to health.

Population health. Individual health and population health should be clearly distinguished. The health of a single individual is affected principally by genetic inheritance, health habits, and immediate social environment at home, in the community, and at work. Interventions to improve an individual's health take place largely through medical care, the individual adoption of healthy behaviors, and support provided by the family.

Population health, on the other hand, refers to the aggregate health of a collection of people grouped together because they share distinguishing features such as race, ethnicity, gender, age, social class, a common social environment, or residence in a neighborhood, city, county, state, or nation. Population health is not simply the health of a large number of individuals summed and averaged. Rather, population health is the average health as a reflection of the collective social experience of the entire group. It is measured in terms of the prevalence and incidence of disease, death rates, average life expectancy, functional capacity, disability rates, and economic productivity. Population health is influenced principally by social and societal characteristics of the large, macrosocial environment. Population health improvement is within the province of public health and public and private sector policies.

Influences on population health. There are five major categories of influence on population health: genes and associated biology; health behaviors such as dietary habits, tobacco use, alcohol and drug use, and physical fitness; medical care and public health services; the ecology of all living things; and social and societal characteristics (Figure 1). Note in the figure that dashed radial lines are intended to denote a very rough approximation of the relative influence of genes and biology, health behaviors, and medical care. No line demarcates total ecology from social/societal characteristics—not only because of the difficulty of separating them conceptually, but also because it is unclear whether the residual de-

terminants after the first three are attributable entirely to the fourth and fifth categories.

1. Genes and associated biology. This category includes the 4,000 mutant genes that cause diseases such as sickle-cell anemia, cystic fibrosis, and Huntington's disease. Although the number 4,000 is large, the frequency of occurrence of most inherited diseases is low, so that mutant genes account for only a small fraction of the total world burden of disease.

This category also includes polygenic inheritance: that is, the specific combination of multiple normal alleles (genes) that when present does not itself cause disease but confers on the holder a bias toward the development of one specific chronic disease rather than another when external circumstances (social and societal characteristics, certain health behaviors) favor the development of a chronic disease. Under the influence of unhealthy social/societal circum-

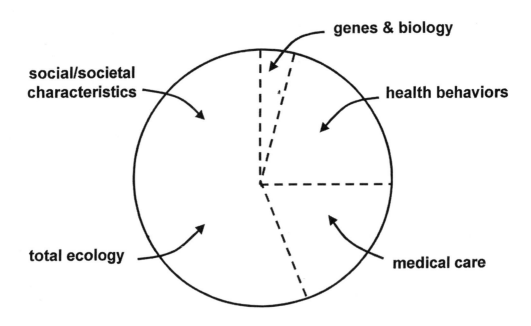

Figure 1

stances, some individuals have a specific multigene combination that favors the development of diabetes, while others may have a different multigene combination, one that confers a biological bias toward the development of heart disease. Polygenic inheritance is a relatively recently discovered phenomenon and is not yet fully understood. It might be reasonable to assume at this time that polygenic inheritance, while not itself a primary of disease, might influence specific types of diseases (and perhaps even their severity) in vulnerable individuals. In other terms, polygenic inheritance might not influence the prevalence of chronic disease overall but does affect the distribution of specific chronic diseases in a population.

2. Health behaviors. Evidence accumulated over the past 40 years incontrovertibly supports the causative role of diet, tobacco use, alcohol and illicit drug use, physical fitness, and reckless behavior in the genesis of most chronic diseases including cardiovascular disease, lung disease, diabetes, some cancers, some liver diseases, some brain deteriorations, disabilities secondary to injuries, and others. Drever[1] has published some analyses that appear to show that the relative proportion of chronic disease attributable to health behaviors was greater in the earlier part of the twentieth century but has progressively declined in the past 25 years. The influence of social inequality on health appears to have gained force and mitigated other influences. Marmot,[2] and Lantz[3] and collaborators, using multiple regression analyses of 1990s data, have reported that health behaviors, independent of other variables including class hierarchy and medical care, account for about one fifth of the disease burden of Britain and the United States.

3. Medical care and public health. There is little research on the effect of medical care and public health on population health. McKeown[4] thought the effect of medical care was small and that most of the improvement in life expectancy in the twentieth century was due to public health accomplishments such as improvements in sani-

tation. Fogel[5] attributed most of the health gain since 1700 to improved nutrition.

Bunker, Mosteller, and Frazier[6] used trends in twentieth-century disease-specific death rates as indicators of changes in population health. They also reviewed clinical studies of the effectiveness of medical interventions. By intersecting these two data sets, they derived estimates of the proportion of declining death rates and extension of life expectancy that could be attributable to medical care. They concluded that of the 40-year gain in life expectancy in the U.S. in the twentieth century, about one sixth can be fairly attributed to medical care. Bunker[7] also presented some evidence that, with improvements in medical diagnosis and treatment in the past three decades, the proportion of the gain in life expectancy due to medical care in the recent 30-year period has become greater than one sixth. He speculated that if functional capacity and well-being could be used as indicators of effectiveness rather than death, the value of medical care might be shown to be substantially higher.

4. The ecology of all living things. The determinants of population health extend far beyond the above three categories of influence to include the interdependence of all plant and animal life and the natural environment. Human health, individual and population, will be affected by assaults on the physical environment; the stress of population size on air, water, and soil quality; agricultural production; depletion of energy sources; limitations of the earth's capacity to adapt to temperature swings; and so forth. Conceptualization and measurement of the complete ecology of population health confront serious limitations both analytically and in reference to the development of practical programs to improve population health. A more complete approach to understanding the determinants of population health that includes total ecology has not as yet been undertaken by the scientists working in the field of society and health. Richard Levins, however, an agricultural ecologist, made a useful start in his 1998 Robert E. Ebert

Lecture titled "Looking at the Whole: Toward a Social Ecology of Health,"[8] sponsored by the Kansas Health Foundation, and in a subsequent manuscript.[9]

5. Social and societal factors. The influence of social and societal characteristics on population health is discussed at other places in this introduction and is the topic of each chapter in this book. To minimize redundancy, it will not be discussed further at this point. A rough statement that would probably gain support from most authors of this book's chapters is that social and societal characteristics impose a major influence on population health.

Conclusion (for 1999): Proportional Influence of Determinants

The question, "What is the relative proportional influence on population health of genes, behaviors, medical care, social/societal factors, and the total ecology?" might be unanswerable in a quantitative way. Figure 1 should be interpreted only as a crude approximation. The dashed radii are intended to convey rough estimates, as well as the interactiveness/interdependence of the influences. The absence of a radial line separating total ecology from social/societal characteristics reflects the lack of quantitative knowledge on these two categories of determinants at the present time. Even if the influence of the first three categories were known with high certainty, it would not be reasonable to attribute all of the residual unknown to social and societal factors and ignore the influence of the total ecology. There are likely to be categories and subcategories of influence that have not even been thought of, far less studied. Further, all of the influences are interactive with each other. Changes in one induce responses in the others. New medical therapies might be helpful for a specific purpose—lowering high blood pressure, for example—but might also evoke an unwanted response in the genome's production of selected proteins and in the microchemical environment in which bodily adaptations are made. New technology has sharply enhanced the survivability of small babies, but one consequence has been to increase the prevalence of several disorders of childhood and adolescence, congenital heart disease and mental retardation being examples. Evolution of social norms is accompanied by changes in health behaviors, and so forth. There are positive and negative feedback interactions among the influences, as well as cancellation and synergistic effects. A graphic depiction of the hundreds of variables that influence population health might look like an intertwined tangle, with each variable connected to all other variables in reciprocating directions.

The unanswerability of the question posed might require that we be satisfied with a general formulation, as follows. Genes, behaviors, medical care, social/societal characteristics, and the larger ecological systems make up a big, complex, and dynamic network of interactive variables that influence population health. Attempts to derive estimates of relative proportional influence are likely to yield unreliable information at this time. At some later time, rough but nonnumerical approximations might be derived. These approximations might be of some practical usefulness in designing interventions to improve health, but only after a more complete understanding of population health ecology has been attained and a theory of population health improvement has been developed and tested.

The Proposition

Meanwhile, the proposition that social and societal characteristics exert a principal influence on population health is supported by much of the research evidence. The proposition can be accepted tentatively to facilitate research, provide a hypothesis upon which to construct interventions to improve population health, and evaluate the interventions' effectiveness.

KNOWLEDGE DEVELOPMENT: 10,000 B.C. TO A.D. 1900

E VIDENCE for the proposition that social and societal characteristics exert major influences on population health has been accumulating over the past 12 millennia.

Ice Age: Natural Food Sources

Earlier in human history, during the last ice age—say before 9,000–10,000 B.C.—our human ancestors were largely migratory hunters and gatherers in search of meat, fruits, and nuts. They organized themselves on principles of cooperation and sharing. Their small societies were egalitarian. The principal threat to health was from exposure to low temperatures and from inadequate natural food supplies.

Domestication of Food Sources: Weather

With the end of the last ice age and the melting of glaciers, beginning approximately 9,000 B.C., fertile valleys and ample water supplies were uncovered, allowing the development of agriculture (planting of grain seeds) and the domestication of animals (mountain goats and wild boar, at first). Thus, reliable food supplies permitted the development of geographically stable residential arrangements. During this period of relatively low population density, the principal threats to health and life came from drought and crop failure.

Copper Age: The Building of Settlements

During the Chalcolithic Period, 4,500 B.C. to 3,500 B.C., from the Balkans to the tip of the Sinai Peninsula, it was discovered that chunks of blue rocks containing copper ore, when heated to high temperatures (2000 degrees Fahrenheit), yielded a shiny metal that was malleable and stronger than stone. The copper could be used for making tools such as axes, awls, and chisels and ritual objects such as mace heads, ornamental standards, and crowns.

Metal-crafting industries from that period have been discovered. A description of the early copper industry was described by Katherine Ozment in the April 1999 issue of *National Geographic*.[10] Ore, mined in the Wadi Faynan mountain region of western Jordan, was carried by donkey 100 miles or more to metalworking settlements in the Beersheba Valley of Israel, where fertile valleys and ample stream water supported the development of villages with 1,000 or more residents. One such village, Shiqmim, was excavated in the late 1970s. The dwellings had been built into hillsides and contained extensive networks of underground rooms for storage of grain. The remains of copper smelting were found, including furnace pits and clay crucibles and molds for casting. The extensiveness of the social organization at Shiqmim is evidenced by the presence of structures larger than dwellings, where meetings were held for religious, economic, and social activities. This period might mark the early shift from health hazards secondary to drought and famine toward health hazards related to population growth, crowding, and social organization.

Bronze Age: Crowding and Sanitation

Beginning around 2,500 B.C. the principal health threat evolved due to the unforeseen consequences of higher levels of social organization.[11] At about that time it was discovered that when a combination of lead and tin was smelted, the resultant alloy, bronze, could be forged or molded easily and economically into vessels and tools that were hard and durable. Thus arose a manufacturing and trade industry in Mesopotamia for bronze pots, pans, liquid and grain storage vessels, cooking tools, farm implements, and weapons for hunting and war. There was a large market for these products, especially in the Far East. Trade routes were busily traveled, with bronze products headed east, while cloth and spices headed west.

Workers migrated into the manufacturing centers in Mesopotamia. Soon large urban concentrations arose, some with populations of 500,000 people. Sanitary systems for disposal of human and other waste were primitive or nonexistent. Clean water supplies were exhausted. Pestilence, plagues, and epidemics supervened. Soon an entire civilization in Mesopotamia was destroyed, overcome by the consequences of social and societal organization that, though developed for good reason, created mortally unhealthy circumstances.

Modern Age of Epidemics and Pandemics: Infectious Diseases

From the Bronze Age to roughly A.D. 1900, a period of about 4,500 years, bacterial and viral infections were the principal threat to individual and population health.[12] Plagues and epidemics erupted from population crowding, poor sanitary conditions, and malnutrition. Transoceanic expeditions for trade and conquest bore critical health consequences. Pathogens were introduced into previously unexposed and therefore nonimmunized indigenous populations by soldiers of war seeking conquest of land and natural resources for the gain of their imperialistic nation sponsors.[13]

Thus, it can be assumed in a general sense that before the metallic ages, population health was influenced in major ways by man's battle with natural phenomena, primarily the climate, weather, and food supply. Since the Bronze Age, however, the major threats to population health have come not from natural phenomena but from man-made social and societal inventions that provided arrangements for organizing living that, unwittingly, were unhealthful. Infections, plagues, epidemics, and pandemics emerged and reigned as the principal threat to population health for almost 5,000 years.

THE TWENTIETH CENTURY

THE man-made social and societal inventions of the twentieth century appear to have resulted in two major transitions in population health in the industrialized nations, one gradually becoming evident around the end of the nineteenth and the beginning of the twentieth century, and the other gradually becoming more evident since the mid-twentieth century.

The first transition, becoming complete around the turn of this century, was the replacement of infectious disease by chronic disease as the leading cause of death. Tuberculosis, pneumonia, and sepsis have been replaced in population significance by coronary heart disease, high blood pressure, stroke, diabetes, cancer, emphysema, cirrhosis, and so forth. The decline in infectious deaths can be ascribed mostly to improvements in sanitation, nutrition, and other public health measures. The introduction of both mass vaccination and antibiotics came much later.

The rising preponderance of chronic disease appears to have been related to rising affluence, which placed within economic reach of larger fractions of populations the adoption of high-fat (meat) diets, rising consumption of alcohol, and widespread tobacco smoking. The invention of machines and the power to run them led to reductions in strenuous work and the adoption of sedentary lifestyles generally. These habits are the antecedent, predisposing factors for most of the chronic diseases. In the late nineteenth and early twentieth centuries these negative health behaviors came within the financial reach of progressively increasing proportions of the population.

The second transition, of greater significance to the theme of this book, has been the change since the mid-twentieth century in the factors that explain the genesis of most chronic disease. In the first half of this century health behaviors explained more than half the prevalence of chronic disease. The explanatory power of health behaviors in the second half of the twentieth century appears to have progressively declined, while social/societal factors (social inequalities—that is, hierarchical social structures as measured by education, income, total assets, or job class) have progressively risen.[14]

While the declining influence of health behaviors can be accounted for partially by the adoption of healthier lifestyles, the rising significance to health of social/societal factors independent of health behaviors establishes them as major influences on population health. Regardless of the shift of prevalence from infectious disease to chronic disease, and the shift of influence from health behaviors to social hierarchical structures, the socioeconomic gradient in health is duplicated in both periods and for almost all diseases. Heightened vulnerability to diseases in general appears to be conferred by social stratification.

Current State of Knowledge

REVIEWS of the development in the past 30 years of knowledge relating social/societal factors to population health appear in many places.[15-30] In this introduction it might be useful to reduce the research results to five central, robust, and confirmed findings that define the field in 1999 and to add a speculation.

First, disease prevalence and death rates (population health) *vary nonrandomly* within a nation or within a state, city, or neighborhood. Health varies systematically with socioeconomic class, whether defined by differences in education, job classification, income or net assets, with progressively higher levels of social position associated with better levels of health.

Second, the *health/social gradient is continuous* throughout the socioeconomic spectrum. This is evident in comparing health across the lower classes, middle classes, and upper classes. The gradient is not due simply to differences between the poor and the rich. It is likely, although it has not been specifically studied to our knowledge, that the contribution to the aggregate health deficit of the entire nation is greatest for the middle classes because of the greater number of people in those categories.

Third, related to the direction of influence (the chicken or egg problem): Does social position influence health, or does health influence social position? Although ill health can affect socioeconomic position, the bulk of the research evidence indicates that the predominant force is in the direction of socioeconomic position influencing population health.

Fourth, within a population in economically developed nations, *the gradient of health with class is not ascribable to material deprivation*—of food, clothing, shelter, or access to medical care. The weight of the evidence supports a hypothesis that social inequality itself, independent of material availability, is responsible for a large share of the variance in health across the class structure. Relative social position, rather than absolute material deprivation, appears to be central to the social/health gradient.

Fifth, when comparing member nations of the Organization for Economic Cooperation and Development (OECD), the rank order of average life expectancy of each nation is in reverse order to the steepness of the gradient in social inequality.[31] The steeper the gradient of income inequality across the population, the shorter the nation's life expectancy. Sweden and Japan, with relatively flat social hierarchies, enjoy the longest life expectancies, whereas the U.S., with a relatively steep hierarchical organization, ranks in the bottom third of health indicators within the OECD group of 25 industrialized nations.

A Speculative Formulation of Mechanisms

THIS section is more speculative and not yet fully illuminated by research results. The relationship of social class to health might be more complex, textured, and embedded in societal structures than the more easily measured income and job class, which are used in most research. Relevant societal structures might include governments, laws, regulations, social norms, work arrangements, wages, business and banking policies, systems for access to food, housing, medical care, learning, transport and communication, physical and economic security, fairness, and respect for self and others. Taken as a whole, the functioning of these societal structures might have contributed importantly to the development, reinforcement, and growth of social inequality. Perhaps people become consciously aware of and responsive to differential limitations of opportunity, privilege, and influence. Restraints on socioeconomic mobility, made real in reference to providing the fruits of life, such as housing and education for one's family, might increasingly become regarded as gross unfairness. Cynicism with respect to the intent of societal structures, such as the functioning of government, to serve the general well-being might overcome increasingly larger fractions of the public. Participation in civic organizations and in voting for elected officials declines. Cohesion and shared purposes within communities become eroded. The rates of social pathology rise—that is, disruption of family structure and function, truancy, delinquency, drug abuse, crime, violence, homicide, and organizational corruption. During periods of accelerated growth of social inequality and its consequences, the state of the world that people live in every day, and their position in it, is processed in the mind. Adaptation mechanisms to the imposed limitations of socioeconomic position are triggered, perhaps in the hypothalamic-pituitary-adrenal hormonal axis, in the autonomic nervous system, and in the immune system. These metabolic adaptations, when sustained over long periods of time, might themselves inflict cellular injury, or might trigger other processes that are the antecedents of chronic disease. The magnitude of social and metabolic effects are in inverse relationship to the individual's position in the socioeconomic hierarchical structure. Over years, an interactive and interdependent social-health gradient is fed. As social inequality grows, so also grows the inequality of health across a population. When comparing nations, the rank order of population health is in close concordance with the degree of social inequality within that nation. That is, flatter hierarchical structures are associated with better population health, proportionally.

THIS BOOK

THIS book is intended as a general reference source for the growing numbers of Americans concerned about rising inequality in our nation and elsewhere. These include the reading public, intellectuals, policy specialists, politicians, public health officials, journalists, researchers, teachers, and students. Most of this audience is already conversant with the alarming growth of income inequality. But few are aware that social inequality has serious consequences for the health and well-being of the entire spectrum of the American public, including the poor, the middle classes, and the upper classes.

Since 1989, as previously referenced, sixteen complete volumes on the relationship of social/societal factors and population health have been published. This book is somewhat different in that it attempts to focus attention when appropriate on a single defined population group, the 2.6 million citizens of the state of Kansas. The planning committee for the conference that was the predecessor of this book sought to have an impact on Kansas. Nonetheless, the committee and we editors believed that the general principles of society and health as illustrated in Kansas are applicable to all populations, at least in the economically developed nations.

The focus on Kansas and the generalizability of the Kansas data were facilitated through two mechanisms. First, the lead chapters in Part One, on the Community; Part Two, on Child Development; and Part Three, on Adult Health, present comprehensive charts and tables of data on the social and health status of Kansas and Kansans. Second, each chapter's author was given a copy of *Health and Social Factors in Kansas: A Data and Chartbook 1997–98*[32] and asked whenever feasible to integrate into his or her manuscript data and other information of pertinence to social circumstances and health in Kansas. Considering that of the lead authors of the sixteen chapters four are Kansans, seven are Americans from elsewhere than Kansas, two are Canadian, and three are British, the effectiveness of this book's focus on Kansas is notable.

Part One.
General Framework and the Health
of the Community

Chapter 1. Healthy Societies: An Overview, by J. Fraser Mustard. After providing a review of the knowledge of the socioeconomic gradient in population health, Mustard turns to early childhood cognitive development as a mediating mechanism between socioeconomic class and adult health. He presents a powerful and wide-sweeping hypothesis that excellent nutrition, optimal brain stimulation, and a supportive environment during early childhood result in strengthened cognitive capacity (learning, math, IQ) in children and fewer behavioral problems (truancy, violence, crime), higher rates of school completion in adolescents, greater success in adult life (jobs, marriage, children), better adult health, and strengthened economic growth for the nation.

Chapter 2. Socioeconomic and Behavioral Differences in Health, Morbidity, and Mortality in Kansas: Empirical Data, Models, and Analyses, by Gopal K. Singh. Dr. Singh is the principal author of the 1998 Kansas Health Institute publication *Health and Social Factors in Kansas: A Data and Chartbook 1997–98*. Singh, using health measures from that publication, including life expectancy from birth, infant mortality, disease prevalence, self-assessed health status, and self-assessed vitality, discovered that of all the socio-demographic-economic factors that describe the people of Kansas, education and income provide the most consistent and strong correlations with health. Relative social position (defined by edu-

cation and income) did not simply describe the health differences between the poor and everyone else but defined the relationship of health to social position throughout the entire social hierarchy. That is, starting with the poor in Kansas progressively better health is experienced by the lower middle class, middle class, upper middle class, and upper class.

Chapter 3. Social Cohesion and Health, by Ichiro Kawachi. Kawachi continues to push forward with leading work on the community context in which life is played out and health and disease are shaped. While not minimizing the influence on health of individual variables such as education, income, and health behaviors, these analyses (and the data of Singh) lend strong support to the determinant role in health of the community context, including associational relationships, interpersonal trust, mutual respect, norms of reciprocity, social integration, social cohesion, community cohesion, collective efficacy, and civil society.

Chapter 4. Building Healthy Communities, by Stephen B. Fawcett and colleagues. Fawcett and associates at the University of Kansas have had vast experience in 30 communities in Kansas in facilitating and evaluating community development for healthful purposes. The parables of Prairie Center and Sunflower with which they begin their chapter are startling. The authors provide principles for action, a conceptual framework, and practical recommendations for community and health improvement. Their focus is on the social-ecological context in which population health is produced, and their model emphasizes the importance of strengthening social capital, including associational networks, mutuality and trust, and community efficacy. Special attention is given to reinforcing the opportunity for successful child development in the community.

Taken together, the first four chapters present a bold and panoramic sweep of the social and societal landscape in which gradations in health in different populations can be explained. Factors specific to individuals, such as early childhood development and variations in education and income, as well as community and socio-structural contextual characteristics, such as social capital and community coherence, are important to health production. But is there a common denominator that ties these seemingly disparate variables of life together? Is it inequality, on many levels? There are individual variables and social and societal characteristics on the input side of the equation, and health on the output side. What processes of the mind and physiology mediate the connection between the two? Subsequent chapters provide some clues.

Part Two.
Child Development and Health

Chapter 5. Social and Educational Indicators of Childhood Well-Being in Kansas, by Thanne Rose and Frank Song. The authors, although they do not have complete research analyses, do have interesting preliminary results suggesting that a child's immediate social environment does influence their ability to attain educational goals. Using Kansas data they showed that low high school graduation rates were associated with divorce, single-parent households, poverty, unemployment, out-of-home placement, high student-teacher ratios, and urban settings. Higher high school completion rates were associated with high parental education and income, high rates of adults over 60 years old in the environment, and the availability of child care.

Chapter 6. Early Influences on Development and Social Inequalities: An Attachment Theory Perspective, by Peter Fonagy and Anna Higgitt. Dr. Fonagy, a scientist and practicing psychiatrist, works both in London and at the Menninger Clinic in Topeka, Kansas. In this chapter he reviews the major risk and protective factors in the emotional and cognitive development of the child, and he summarizes critically, and usefully, the results achieved by numerous programs intended to foster successful child development.

Dr. Fonagy emphasizes the importance to the child of "relationship building," especially the attachment between child and mother. Drawing on his wide experience, he favors approaches that are parent centered and have been supported by either experimental data or common sense and experience. He recommends home visits by professionals to provide advice to parents, parent training in child behavior management and parent sensitivity enhancement, parenting education for low-income mothers and fathers, adoption of preschool performance standards for cognitive and emotional development, explicit affective training of the child in preschool, and programs for children and their parents who are negotiating divorce.

Chapter 7. Early Development in Monkeys, by Stephen J. Suomi. Principally at the National Institutes of Health, Dr. Suomi has led several decades of research on early cognitive, emotional, and behavioral development in rhesus monkeys. In this chapter he highlights two broad principles that have been learned. First, the early social experiences of rhesus monkeys, especially with primary attachment figures (mothers), have profound lifelong consequences for both physiological and psychological functioning. Second, both physiological and psychological responses to specific events in young as well as in adult monkeys are predictable in individual monkeys but highly variable among monkeys. The non-uniformity of responsiveness among monkeys, Suomi hypothesizes, is probably due to the interaction of specific genetic and experiential differences.

The knowledge derived from work with monkeys by Suomi, and by Shively (Chapter 14), provides opportunities for experimentation in human populations with innovations at both the individual and the sociostructural levels to improve population health, although the degree of homology of the dynamic interactions of genes, child development, adult experiences, social structures, and health between the two species is not fully known.

Chapter 8. Early Child Development in the Context of Population Health, by Clyde Hertzman. Dr. Hertzman, director of the Population Health Program of the Canadian Institute for Advanced Research, uses data from a British study that has followed continuously a cohort of 17,000 individuals from their birth in 1958 in England, Scotland, and Wales to the present time. The *British Birth Cohort Study* has accumulated detailed information on each individual regarding early childhood experiences, signposts of child development, adolescent behavior, adult health, and other characteristics. Hertzman and colleagues draw two main conclusions.

First, from their "latency model," early childhood experiences such as being read to by parents and some behavioral characteristics contribute importantly to health outcomes later in life.

Second, from their "pathways model," continuing experiences over a lifetime also influence health substantially. These experiences include those related to social position, educational attainment, material circumstances, job control and security, control over one's life generally, and trust in others.

An interesting development in Canada, described by Hertzman, is the formulation by national, provincial, and territorial government representatives of a National Strategy on Healthy Child Development based on both the latency and pathways models. The strategy recommends that government, nongovernmental social organizations, and the private sector work together to implement several policies: *1)* strengthen prenatal services, assure adequate nutrition, and foster the development of secure relationships (targeted at preconception to age five), *2)* improve opportunities for family strengthening, *3)* diminish socioeconomic inequities that deprive the child of wholesome material and social environments, *4)* mobilize crosssectoral collaborations for child development, and *5)* improve the monitoring systems and research related to the progress of child development and health.

The four chapters in Part Two illustrate the importance of early childhood experiences, including relationship building (attachment), to a variety of outcomes, including adolescent behaviors and success in school, adult reactivity, and adult health. But in addition to early childhood experiences, adult health is also importantly influenced by genetic makeup, medical care, and a wide variety of continuing experiences with family in the home, friends and acquaintances in the neighborhood, and colleagues at work and by structural features of society that affect opportunities differently for different social groups.

Given that the ultimate social purpose of research on society and health is to provide guidelines for the construction of policies and programs to improve population health, these four chapters provide ample justification for developing programs to strengthen child development, as well as for other programs to strengthen the family as an institution, improve work experiences, build the community, and work toward creating sociostructural features that are more healthful.

Part Three.
Adult Health and Factors That Influence It

Chapter 9. The Social Context of Smoking, Nutrition, and Sedentary Health Behavior in Kansas, by Manuella Adrian and Anna Wilkinson. The authors used Kansas data at the individual county level to construct statistical models to help understand the influence of individualperson factors (already known to influence health behaviors) and community-level characteristics on smoking rates, sedentary lifestyle, and low fruit and vegetable consumption, known risk factors for cardiovascular disease. They discovered that, indeed, even with limited measures of community context (population density and average education, income, and unemployment), these community features did have an independent influence on tobacco smoking in men, and on diet in both men and women, in Kansas counties. Their study is one of the first attempts to understand the influence of specific community characteristics on health behaviors, behaviors heretofore considered by many to be primarily a matter of individual choice.

Chapter 10. Labor Markets and Health: A Framework and Set of Applications, by Benjamin C. Amick III and John N. Lavis. In a sweeping and bold conceptual integration of social context, work policies, governmental labor policies, job characteristics, worker variables, worker experience at work, worker health and productivity, and company profitability, Amick and Lavis have reopened and widened the research and policy opportunities related to work. The breadth and comprehensiveness of their concepts are breathtaking. They conclude with three general recommendations supported by their research as a start to elevate health and productivity: maintain high rates of employment; enlarge workers' authority to make decisions on the job; and structure the labor market to increase the proportion of high-skill jobs.

Chapter 11. Social Relations, Hierarchy, and Health, by Richard G. Wilkinson. Wilkinson, with persistence, critical assessment, and profundity, has over the past decade examined diverse sources of data from Eastern Europe, Western Europe, and North America in search of the causal mechanisms that connect greater social inequality with worse health. In this chapter, focused on developed nations, he synthesizes a broad range of observational and experimental data on men, monkeys, apes, and rats. Wilkinson continues to reject explanations of intrasociety health gradients based on the absolute distribution of material products such as income, clothing, housing, and medical care. Rather, he posits, with empiric support for most of his points, that social inequality is based principally on income inequalities and that the psychosocial consequences of inequality yield chronic states of humiliation and disrespect, continuous overactivation of stress mechanisms in the brain, and morbid states of hostility, violence, disintegration of social cohesiveness, and general heightened susceptibility to disease. (Wilkinson's formulations are congruent with the research results of Shively, Chapter 14.)

Wilkinson ends his well-argued and energetic essay with three general conclusions to guide social restructuring for a more healthful society. First, an improved or more egalitarian social environment is more important to health than improved material resources. Second, income inequality, Wilkinson advances, is the predominant force that builds and sustains social environments that are harmful to dignity and respect, increase the rates of violent behavior, destroy social cohesiveness, and are harmful to health. Third, without specifying in detail the actions to be taken, Wilkinson advises that the social institutions that have been built and that provide frameworks for living be systematically assessed and revised to provide people with a greater sense of belonging and self-worth and to thereby strengthen social cohesion.

Chapter 12. Race and Health in Kansas: Data, Issues, and Directions, by David R. Williams. Using data on Kansans and comparing Kansans with the U.S. population overall, Williams shows that although the largest fraction of the low health status of black Americans is explained by low socioeconomic status (SES), a substantial fraction is also ascribable to pervasive racism, and racism contributes substantially to maintaining low socioeconomic status.

Racism's effect on health, Williams argues, is mediated by the psychological impact of being considered inferior, by differential application of medical technology and care, and by systematic segregation in housing, which sharply lowers purchasing power per dollar and limits access to education, transportation, and jobs. Racism, therefore, institutionalizes and assures continuity of SES subordination.

Williams, examining the high rates of tobacco

smoking and alcohol use among many minority groups, argues that these habits are not reflective of a willful desire to pursue poor health. Rather, smoking and drinking are among the only avenues that some chronically oppressed people have for relief of tension. These habits are encouraged by commercial practices of targeting marketing and advertising specifically to the black population. Additionally, local government regulatory agencies issue permits that allow alcoholic beverage sales in neighborhoods already oversupplied with beverage stores. To summarize, Williams emphasizes the social and structural context that initiates, encourages, reinforces, and sustains racial prejudice, socioeconomic subjugation, racially biased medical care, and substandard health.

In this chapter Williams covers a wide range of technical and interpretive issues—that is, race as a social as opposed to a biological category, the interaction of SES and racism, the importance of distinguishing wealth from income, the broad consequences of housing segregation, and the root fundamental influences on tobacco and alcohol use. He concludes with these sentences, "The larger social environment plays a large role in the generation of racial disparities in health. Changes in the social environment must be a critical part of any effective strategy to reduce socially induced health inequalities."

Chapter 13. Social Networks and Health: The Bonds That Heal, by Lisa F. Berkman. *Social support* stems from the interactions that an individual has with family, friends, neighbors, colleagues, and the community's institutions that provide intimacy, love, trust, meaning to life, sense of belonging, dependency when needed, and a sense of self-worth. *Social networks* refer to the interconnected web of social relationships in which a person is embedded. Berkman reviews the evidence, results from her own research and that of others, which is plentiful and compelling, that the extent of social networks and social support is related inversely to the prevalence of most diseases, to the severity of the disease, to the dis-

eases' responsiveness to treatment, and to the ultimate outcomes of disease, including disability and death. The outcomes may vary, astonishingly, up to sevenfold depending on the degree of social support. We, the authors of this introduction, believe that the startling facts related to social support have received too little attention from our society and the health research community and from public health professionals interested in interventions to improve population health.

Berkman provides a useful review of the literature and concludes that the evidence shows that the salutary effect of social support on health is biologically plausible, and she offers a physiological conceptualization of how it may work (see also Shively, Chapter 14).

Finally, Berkman offers general suggestions for building social support to improve population health. She aims at work and welfare policies to strengthen families and child development, urban development that considers housing, transportation, and job creation together, and organizational arrangements for family and nonfamily support of children, the chronically ill, and the elderly. This is a compelling chapter.

Chapter 14. Social Status, Stress, and Health in Female Monkeys, by Carol A. Shively. Shively, at Wake Forest University, in remarkable experiments studying the development of coronary atherosclerosis and depression in female monkeys living in captivity provides notable confirmation in nonhuman primates of the results in humans given by Wilkinson and Berkman in their chapters.

Shively's monkeys organize themselves naturally into social status hierarchical relationships ranging from degrees of dominance to degrees of subordination. Shively correlates over time *a*) *position* in the hierarchical structure, *b*) *behavior* related to social support, including receipt of hostility, time in affiliative behavior such as grooming, time in vigilant scanning, and time spent alone in isolation, *c*) *physiological* features such as rate of cortisol secretion, ovarian function, and hypothalamic-pituitary-adrenal (HPA) axis activity, and *d*) *disease* state related to coronary artery atherosclerosis and function and mental health. Shively reports that the stress of social subordination in monkeys leads impressively to HPA overactivity, ovarian dysfunction related to ovulation, higher levels of suppressed aggression, observable postural signs of depression, and more severe coronary artery disease. These results in monkeys lend weight to sociopsycho-physiological mechanisms in humans that have been hypothesized to explain the gradient of health with socioeconomic status.

Together, the six chapters in Part Three emphasize the importance of the fundamental sociostructural context in producing the gradient in adult health, and the possible psychological states that might mediate the connection of context to the health gradient.

Invoked as important contextual characteristics are community factors that include population density, average education, income, and unemployment rates; labor market qualities, the structure of work, and the work environment, including firm policies and profitability; the steepness of the slope of income inequality across a population; racism and business, housing, and governmental policies that sustain subjugation; and social networks that build interconnections among physical, social, and emotional support structures. Finally, the experiments in monkeys support the observations in humans of the importance to the gradient in health of hierarchical positioning in social organizations and the association of social position with variations in physiological states and disease prevalence.

The authors of the six chapters on adult health speculate on the psychological states that result from contextual social inequality and offer a rich inventory of policy options intended to reduce social inequality and improve population health.

Part Four.
Perspectives

Chapter 15. Inequalities in Health: Causes and Policy Implications, by Michael Marmot. A premier scientist and leader in the social-health gradients field, Marmot was the first Kansas Health Foundation Distinguished Lecturer at the Kansas Conference on Health and Its Determinants. His chapter is adapted from that lecture, given in Wichita on April 20, 1998.

Drawing broad perspectives from his and others' 25 years of scientific discoveries in society and population health, Marmot states that inequalities in health, running from the most to the least advantaged members of society, are predominantly manifestations of social inequalities and that policies to reduce social inequalities are likely to reduce health inequalities and to improve population health.

Minimizing material deprivation and individual-level risk factors such as serum cholesterol levels and tobacco smoking as explanations for the health gradient, Marmot discusses his own and others' data to point to the causative factors for the gradient, which he argues are psychological (editors' footnote). These include early life experiences, such as the quality of parenting, social support and social integration, the work environment, sense of self-control over health, and level of hostility, all of which vary with social position. A later, or "downstream" (editors' term), element in Marmot's model (Figure 4, Chapter 15), triggered by psychosocial factors, is chronic activation of the neuro-endocrine-immune systems, leading to the pathophysiological processes that are the antecedents to chronic disease.

Chapter 16. Public Policy Frameworks for Improving Population Health, by Alvin R. Tarlov. The author believes that the mediating pathways by which hundreds of social and societal factors influence health and illness make up a complex

---

Editors' footnote. Marmot, Wilkinson, and others use "psychosocial" to connote the interactive effect of a person's distinctive psychological makeup with specific features of the social environment.

system that cannot be understood or quantified by knowledge of the system's individual component parts. Feedbacks, synergistic effects, cancellation effects, and uncountable numbers of adaptations and interactions render linear-effect models and other multivariate models unhelpful when applied to health production systems. The author posits, therefore, that guidance for selection of interventions to improve population health will not rise from statistical treatments that use regression methods applied to social epidemiologic survey data. Yet, he argues, approximations can be derived from existing data that are adequate for formulating policies and designing interventions that could affect population health importantly. Awaiting more certain information that might be derived from future advances in analytical methods for studying complex systems will delay by several decades or longer attempts to improve population health.

Two frameworks are presented as guides to developing strategies to improve population health. The Intervention Framework, on its vertical dimension, identifies five broad targets for intervention that are likely to be substantially salutary for population health: improve child development, strengthen community cohesion, enhance opportunities for self-actualization, increase socioeconomic well-being, and modulate hierarchical structuring. On the horizontal dimension, interventions are classified as either ameliorative or fundamentally corrective. For example, approval of a city ordinance to allow surplus space in public school buildings to be used for preschool activities and to reinvigorate YMCAs and YWCAs so that after-school supervised recreational activities become generally available would be ameliorative interventions to improve child development. Fundamentally corrective interventions would be programs to train fathers and mothers in parenting skills and in establishing home environments conducive to positive cognitive and behavioral development and the development of day-care programs having high standards, well-trained and culturally

diverse professionals who earn professional wages, transportation that makes the programs within practical reach of families, and financial foundations that make the programs affordable to all. The Intervention Framework could help a community or organization develop short-range and long-range planning, select objectives most appropriate to their needs and capacities, and identify specifically whether their proposed implementation will be helpful in the short term or fundamentally corrective and permanent over the long range.

The second framework, Public Policy Development Process, separates the process into two phases. The first phase builds on culture, problem identification, research, and public awareness to reach a majority public consensus and establish a national agenda. The second phase, authorized by the public consensus, initiates political processes that establish public policies. Political activity is the endgame of the public policy development process. Once a public interest organization has chosen a particular public policy for attention, the framework for Public Policy Development can help select the specific arena that will be appropriate for initiation of their strategy. Efforts to establish public policies related to society and population health will have to start at the public awareness stage because public knowledge and media attention to the subject have been insufficient for establishment of a national agenda and activation of the political process. Different policy development topics will enter the process at different places.

Many authors in this volume make specific recommendations in their special areas of interest to improve population health: Fawcett and colleagues in Chapter 4, Fonagy and Higgitt in Chapter 6, Hertzman in Chapter 8, Amick and Lavis in Chapter 10, Wilkinson in Chapter 11, Williams in Chapter 12, and Berkman in Chapter 13. Each of the recommendations is supported, although indirectly in some cases, by research results. But in a complex system an intervention in one specific domain is likely to influence many, or even all, other domains. Future policy frameworks should advance from individual recommendations in one domain to more comprehensive sets of recommendations across a wide span of restructuring to improve population health. The 39 recommendations advanced in the *Independent Inquiry into Inequalities in Health*,[33] the Sir Donald Acheron Report from the United Kingdom, are the most ambitious attempt to date to develop a comprehensive plan to improve population health.

Marni Vliet is president of the Kansas Health Foundation and now also chair of Grantmakers in Health, the umbrella organization of nearly 150 philanthropies active in health. Some six years ago Vliet was the first, or among the first, leaders in philanthropy to understand the real significance of social and societal factors for population health improvement and to seize the concept as a major opportunity for the foundation. Her leadership of the foundation's board and staff led to the creation of the Kansas Health Institute, the Kansas Conference on Health and Its Determinants, and the publication of this book.

Vliet's consistent and visible attention to the social determinants of health has sparked a broad engagement throughout Kansas in the search for practical means by which the health and well-being of all Kansans can be elevated. This is not easy, the subject is complex, and there are no precedent programs to draw upon. The search continues.

At the Kansas Conference in April 1998, Vliet addressed the audience of Kansans near the end. The title of her presentation was "How Do We Get There From Here?" With inspiring encouragement, she urged the assembled to undertake the search for practical methods to improve population health through adjustments in social and societal factors. She urged that the definition of health be broadened beyond the conventional bounds of medical care and said that restructuring for more healthful circumstances will require a broad coalition of interests and common vision among the general public, community organizations, the educational community, religious organizations, business, governments, the media, philanthropy, and more. Further, she encouraged all sectors to accept the risks and take some steps into the adequately, but not completely, understood territory of the social determinants of health. Building on the subjects of the conference, Vliet suggested that efforts be made to build community social capital to elevate the probability of successful child development, to enhance the opportunities for families to succeed and attain their goals, and to optimize everyone's chances to improve their economic and social standing.

NOTES

1. Drever, F., Whitehead, M., and Roden, M. "Current Patterns and Trends in MALE Mortality by Social Class (based on occupation)." Population Trends 1996: 86:15–20.

2. Marmot, M. G. "Inequalities in Health: Causes and Policy Implications." *Society and Population Health Reader,* vol. II, *A State and Community Perspective.* (New York: The New Press, 2000), Chapter 15, Figure 5.

3. Lantz, Paula, House, James, Lepkowski, David, et al. "Socioeconomic Factors, Health Behaviors, and Mortality." Journal of the American Medical Association 279 no. 21 (1998): 1703–1746.

4. McKeown, Thomas. *The Modern Rise of Population.* (London: Edward Arnold Ltd., 1976).

5. Fogel, Robert W. "Nutrition and the Decline in Mortality Since 1700. Some Preliminary Findings." In Stanley L. Engerman and Robert E. Gallman, eds. *Long-Term Factors in American Economic Growth.* (Chicago: University of Chicago Press, 1986), 439–555.

6. Bunker, John P., Frazier, Howard S., and Mosteller, Frederick. "Improving Health: Measuring Effects of Medical Care." *The Milbank Quarterly* 72, no. 2 (1994): 225–258.

7. Bunker, John P. "Medicine Matters After All." *Journal of the Royal College of Physicians* 29, no. 2 (1995): pp. 105–112.

8. Levins, Richard. "Looking at the Whole: Toward a Social Ecology of Health." The 1998 Robert H. Ebert Health of the Future Lecture. (Wichita, Kansas: The Kansas Health Foundation, 1998).

9. Levins, Richard. "An Ecologist Looks at Health." Typescript, Harvard School of Public Health, May 1999.

10. Ozment, Katherine. "Journey to the Copper Age." *National Geographic* 195, no. 4 (April 1999): 70–79.

11. Weiss, H., Courty, M.-A., Wetterstrom, W., Guichard, F., Senior, L., Meadow, R., and Curnow, A. "The Genesis and Collapse of Third Millennium North Mesopotamia Civilization." *Science* 261 (August 10, 1993): 995–1,004.

12. McNeill, William H. *Plagues and Peoples.* (Garden City, New York: Anchor Press/Doubleday, 1976).

13. Verano, John W. and Ubelaker, Douglas H., eds. *Disease and Demography in the Americas.* (Washington and London: Smithsonian Institution Press, 1992).

14. Marmot, M. G. "Inequalities in Health: Causes and Policy Implications." *Society and Population Health Reader,* vol. II, *A State and Community Perspective.* (New York: The New Press, 2000), Chapter 15.

15. Bunker, John P., Gomby, D. A., and Kehrer, B. H., eds. *Pathways to Health: The Role of Social Factors.* The Henry J. Kaiser Family Foundation, Menlo Park, California, 1989.

16. *Prosperity, Health and Well-Being.* Proceedings of the 11th Honda Foundation Discoveries Symposium, October 16–18, 1993, Toronto, The Canadian Institute for Advanced Research.

17. Evans, R. G., Barer, M. L., and Marmor, T. R., eds. *Why Are Some People Healthy and Others Not?* (New York: Aldine De Gruyter, 1994).

18. "Health and Wealth," *Daedalus,* Journal of the American Academy of Arts and Sciences (Fall 1994).

19. Mielck, Andreas, and Giraldes, Maria Do Rosario, eds. *Health Inequalities: Discussion in Western European Countries.* (Munster, New York: Waxmann, 1994).

20. Amick, B. C., Levine, S., Tarlov, A. R., and Walsh, D. C., eds. *Society and Health.* (New York: Oxford University Press, 1995).

21. Blane, D., Brunner, E. J., and Wilkinson, R. G., eds. *Health and Social Organization.* (London: Routledge, 1996).

22. Wilkinson, Richard G. *Unhealthy Societies: The Afflictions of Inequality.* (London: Routledge, 1996).

23. Hertzman C., Kelly, S., and Bobak, M., eds. *East-West Life Expectancy Gap in Europe: Environmental and Non-Environmental Determinants.* (Norwell, Mass.: Kluwer Academic Publishers, 1996).

24. Kuh, D., and Ben-Shlomo, Y., eds. *A Life Course Approach to Chronic Disease Epidemiology.* (New York: Oxford University Press, 1997).

25. *The Milbank Quarterly: A Journal of Public Health and Health Care Policy* 76, no. 3. (Boston: Blackwell Publishers, 1998).

26. Bartley, M., Blane, D., and Davey Smith, G., eds. *The Sociology of Health Inequalities.* (Malden, Mass.: Blackwell Publishers, 1998).

27. Keating, Daniel P., and Hertzman, Clyde, eds. *Developmental Health and the Wealth of Nations: Social, Biological and Educational Dynamics.* (New York: Guilford Publications, 1999).

28. Marmot, Michael G., and Wilkinson, Richard G., eds. *Social Determinants of Health.* (London: Oxford University Press, 1999).

29. Kawachi, Ichiro, Kennedy, Bruce P., and Wilkinson, Richard G., eds. *The Society and Population Health Reader,* vol. I, *Income Inequality and Health.* (New York: The New Press, 1999).

30. Tarlov, Alvin R., and St. Peter, Robert F., eds. *The Society and Population Health Reader,* vol. II, *A State and Community Perspective.* (New York: The New Press, 2000).

31. *World Development Report 1993, Investing in Health.* (New York: Oxford University Press, 1993).

32. Singh, Gopal, Wilkinson, Anna V., Song, Frank F., Adrian, Manuella, Fonner, Jr., Edwin, and Tarlov, Alvin R. *Health and Social Factors in Kansas: A Data and Chartbook 1997–98.* (Topeka, Kansas: Kansas Health Institute, 1998).

33. *Independent Inquiry into Inequalities in Health:* Report. Sir Donald Acheson, Chair. (London: Her Majesty's Stationery Office, with the permission of the Department of Health, 1998).

Part One

GENERAL FRAMEWORK
AND THE HEALTH OF THE COMMUNITY

One

HEALTHY SOCIETIES: AN OVERVIEW

*J. Fraser Mustard**

THERE has always been an appreciation that the society in which individuals live and work has a powerful influence on the health and well-being of individuals and populations.[1][2][3][4] It has been difficult until recently for this subject to be an area of extensive research. As a result, our knowledge has been constrained as to how the environment in which individuals live and work determines their health and it has not been a major field of teaching in schools and universities and for public policy. In the last twenty years, there has been a substantial increase in our understanding of this subject particularly in the possible biological pathways by which the social environment contributes to the development of disease problems.[5][6] Ten years ago investigations showed that in some population groups the biggest risk factor for coronary heart disease is not cholesterol or smoking, but the nature of an individual's work, the control they have over their job, and their social support.[7][8] Even more interesting is the increasing body of knowledge that the risks for many of the chronic diseases in adult life are set in utero[9] and during the first 4 to 5 years of early life.[10]

Until recently, health and life expectancy were considered by many to be a matter of chance.[11] For example, some individuals living in desperate circumstances live long and healthy lives while others in privileged circumstances die early and have children with serious health problems. Although there is randomness about the health of individuals, there is now a better appreciation that how well individuals cope with the changing environments in which they live and work throughout the life cycle strongly influences their health and well-being. Throughout recorded history it has been recognized that individuals or populations that are less prosperous do not do as well as the more prosperous. Understanding and applying this knowledge in society is undoubtedly one of the major public health challenges today.

Medicine, until this century, was not thought to be important in the curing of disease. The vast increase in our knowledge about human biology and disease in this century has led to a substantial improvement in the role of medicine in the diagnosis and treatment of disease. The belief that diseases have specific causes, in part based on our understanding of the causes of infectious diseases, has led to a focus on trying to identify the causes of the chronic diseases of life from a similar perspective, leading to an emphasis on life style factors such as diet, exercise, and smoking, with little emphasis on the social environment. Most medical research controls for factors such as age, social class, education, work conditions,

*Founders' Network, Canadian Institute for Advanced Research

and sex, because these factors are strongly correlated with health and health-related behavior. The emphasis on the role of medicine and life style factors as major determinants of health has caused most investigators to ignore the social factors and focus on areas of current fashion such as health care, smoking, high fat diets, exercise, etc.[12]

The historical evidence indicates that the improved prosperity of societies working through better water supplies, sanitation, and nutrition has been of crucial importance in improved health and well-being.

SOCIETY AND HEALTH— A HISTORICAL NOTE

ONE of the dramatic events in the history of the human race has been the substantial decline in mortality and the exponential growth of the world's population over the last 500 years, particularly following the Industrial Revolution which began in the United Kingdom about 250 years ago.[13] [14] McKeown[13] examined why the mortality rates for the British population declined following the start of the Industrial Revolution. By a process of exclusion, he came to the conclusion that despite all the socio-economic turmoil associated with the Industrial Revolution, the decline in mortality was a consequence of improved overall nutrition of the population. He concluded that the contribution of medicine was very small and that public health measures, including better water sanitation and vaccination, accounted for about 25% of the decline in mortality. In essence, the gradually improving prosperity of the United Kingdom led to better production, importation, and distribution of food to the population. Although controversial, this landmark historical analysis affected one country's approach to health policy. In the 1970's, the government of Canada released the Lalonde report,[15] which was largely based on McKeown's research. This Canadian government document stated that the key determinant of health was

where people lived and how they lived and that although valuable in caring for sick people, medicine was of less significance in improving the health of populations.

Fogel,[14] an economist, was also troubled by McKeown's conclusion and set out to do a detailed analysis from the historical records of many western countries to examine if there was better food production and distribution resulting in better nutrition, leading to a decline in the mortality rate. He found from his detailed analysis that McKeown's conclusion was basically correct and that one of the biggest effects was on children, as assessed by the improvement in the mean height of the populations. He noted that as the mean height of the populations increased, so did life expectancy. He concluded that the changes in height were a manifestation of a better early childhood and that there was an association between the conditions of early childhood and the risks of chronic diseases in adult life. Fogel's historical analysis has shown the importance of improved nutrition and the latency effect of conditions of early childhood affecting health risks in adult life and the health of the population.

An important conclusion of Fogel's was that 50% of the economic growth of the United Kingdom following the Industrial Revolution was due to the better quality of the population. He also found some evidence that when economies got into difficulty, mean height could decrease and that this was associated with a decline in the health status of the population as estimated by life expectancy. From this work, he came to two important conclusions. The conditions of early childhood set much of the risk for chronic diseases in adult life, and the better quality of the population produced by improved conditions for children is an important factor in economic growth.

Another set of historical observations in this century provides further insights into the relationship among the economy, the social environment, and the health and well-being of populations. The British recognized that health as measured by mortality was a gradient when analyzed against social class.[12] During the Second World War, many social planners wanted to have a more equitable society at the end of the war in view of the wartime hardships and sacrifices of the population. One of the goals was to reduce the inequalities in health across the social classes. This led to the concept of the National Health Service. One of the key arguments put forward in the Beveridge[16] documents was that if government removed the financial barriers to access to health care, the inequalities in health across social classes would be decreased. This was clearly based on the belief that medicine was an important factor determining the health of populations. To the surprise of many, the government found when they examined the health service 30 years after it was started, that the social class gradient in health as measured by mortality had widened substantially.[17] The life expectancy of the population had improved, but maximum effect was in the upper classes with little effect on the lower classes. This led to a substantial debate as to why this had taken place. One outcome was that the Labour government set up a committee under Douglas Black (the CMO of the Department of Health and Social Services) to examine why health inequalities had increased. This committee reported in 1980.[18] They concluded that a major factor was a changing socio-economic environment with, among other things, a negative effect on the well-being of mothers and children. They, therefore, recommended that the government introduce programs to create more equitable social conditions for mothers and children if they wished to reduce the inequalities in health. Since Thatcher's government was now in power and trying to rebuild institutions and the economy, they ignored the recommendations in the "Black Report" that involved social issues. It is of interest that the new Labour government has reactivated the "Black Report" and may well tackle the issues around mothers and children and inequalities in health. Today the evidence

about the conditions of early life and health risks throughout the life cycle from a broad base of research is extensive and reinforces the conclusions from the historical research.

SOCIO-ECONOMIC GRADIENTS IN HEALTH

THE historical evidence illustrates that to create more equity in health in a society, we have to improve our understanding of how the social environment determines health and well-being. An important clue appears to be that when health (death or sickness) is measured against socio-economic factors, (income, education, employment, etc.), it is a gradient.[2 13 19] There is now a wealth of information from many countries showing health gradients against socio-economic measures, and in some countries the gradients appear steeper than in others. While it has been accepted that the poor do not do well in rich and poor countries, it is widely believed in developed countries that those that are not poor are minimally affected by the social environment. This implies a threshold with a sharp division between the group deprived of the essentials for a quality life and the rest of the population. The fact that health is a gradient when measured against socio-economic factors means that there is no threshold and that the social environment affects all members of society with increasingly negative effects on health the further one is down the socio-economic scale. Thus, to address the inequalities in health issue, it is important to understand what causes these gradients and why the gradients are steeper in some societies than others. It is also important to appreciate that many at the lower end of the socio-economic gradient do well. Why are these groups, despite their social and economic circumstances, successful? The understanding from research in this area applies to all members of society.

The studies of Michael Marmot and his colleagues[20 21] on a middle class population in the

United Kingdom have provided some key insights. Examination of the Whitehall Civil Service over the last twenty years has shown a clear gradient in health (as measured by death or sickness absence from work against position in the job hierarchy) in a middle class population engaged in mainly non manual work. The lower individuals are in the job hierarchy, the higher the mortality and sickness absence rates. Most of the major causes of death, including smoking and non–smoking related cancers, strokes, myocardial infarction, gastrointestinal disease, suicides and accidents, are a gradient. A similar non–disease specific mortality gradient assessed against socio-economic factors has been described for the population of Scotland.[22] What are the factors in the UK civil service or in Scotland that can contribute to a non–disease specific mortality gradient in health? One of the explanations is that individuals lower in the hierarchy have a bad life style. In Marmot's work, he and his colleagues examined the explanatory power of life style factors for the gradient in death for coronary heart disease. They found that cholesterol, smoking and family history could account for only about 25% of the gradient. The biggest factor seemed to be some aspect of work conditions related to an individual's position in the job hierarchy. Controlling for this factor eliminates most of the gradient.

Swedish studies[23] had examined the relationship between the demands of work and the degree of control an individual has on health. They found that individuals in what were assessed to be high-demand jobs with poor control had a higher mortality rate than individuals in high-demand jobs with a high degree of control. This analytical technique was applied to the Whitehall Civil Service with similar findings.[24] The further down the job hierarchy individuals are, the greater the number that are in jobs perceived to be high demand with poor control. Thus, although the top civil servants have very demanding jobs, they have substantial control and better

health as measured by mortality rates and sickness absence from work. One physiological measure that indicates civil servants at the top cope better is blood pressure changes. While the blood pressure of all civil servants goes up when they come to work, the blood pressures of the top civil servants tend to go down when they leave work, while many of those who have jobs farther down the hierarchy do not show this. (Blood pressure is influenced by demand or stress.) While how hierarchies and work are structured is important in influencing these gradients, we again know that some do well despite where they are in the hierarchy.

One measure that relates to the coping skills and competence of individuals is level of education.[25] The top civil servants in the United Kingdom have a higher level of education than those farther down the hierarchy. This could mean that the competence and coping skills (assuming level of education reflects this) of individuals are important. We know that competence and coping skills are influenced by events throughout the life cycle, particularly events during childhood.[26][27] It is difficult to test whether the early life of the civil servants is a factor determining their competence and coping skills. One measurement of the civil service that can be used to examine if early life events are a possible factor is height. The mean height of the top level is greater than the next level which is greater than the level below it. Thus, mean height is a gradient in the civil service. If it is assumed that the genetic factors for height have the same distribution for all levels of the civil service then this implies (since height is a product of nutrition during early childhood and genes) that those at the top had, on average, a better early childhood than those at the bottom of the hierarchy. Recently a considerable body of evidence has emerged showing that the conditions of early childhood have a strong influence on behavior, learning, and health throughout the life cycle. A key component in this story is our improved understanding of factors influencing the development of the brain in early life and the relationship among the development of the brain, coping with the challenges of life, and the effects on the endocrine and immune systems.

Brain Development, Behavior, Learning, and Health

LIKE most organs in the body, brain development in early life is strongly influenced by the quality of nutrition and stimulation or use in early life.[28 29 30] We now know that the stimulation the brain receives in the early stages of life plays an important part in its differentiation and function. The basic structure and function established in this critical period of development have a significant effect on the competence and coping skills of individuals throughout their life cycle. Competence can be considered to include what we have learned and our ability to learn. Coping includes how we respond to challenges and how we handle stress. A key part of the story from developmental neurobiology is our understanding of the factors that influence how nerve cells differentiate and form their connections (the "wiring of the brain"). At birth, the brain has only established the initial connections and paths among its billions of neurons. The neural activity that stimulates the creation of the complex nerve circuits that are key for optimum function is driven by the flood of sensory experiences in early life received through the body's sensory pathways (touch, sound, vision, smell, and taste).

A critical period for the development of what some call the core function of the brain (the midbrain and the limbic system) is in the early years of life. Neglecting or abusing an infant during this period can produce neuron connections and functions in the core brain that can lead to dysfunctional behavior.[31] This part of the brain is important in our response to arousal, our emotions, appetite, and other basic responses. Thus, an infant brought up in circumstances where there is conflict and abuse between the care givers will pick this up through the developing sensory pathways, leading to poor development of the core functions of the brain. This appears to be associated with an increased risk of poor behavioral responses at later stages in the life cycle of children brought up in such circumstances. A significant number of women brought up in disruptive families are at risk for depression in adult life.

Although genetics determines the core architecture of the brain, it is the effect of adequate nutrition and the quality of the stimulation during these sensitive periods during early life that drives the wiring of the brain and creates the core capacity for functioning throughout the life cycle.

One of the pioneering studies of the relationship between sensory inputs and the development of the brain was for vision. In newborn animals, if the signals from the eye are prevented from transmission to the cortex of the brain until the animal matures, the region of the cortex responsible for vision does not develop.[31 32] If the block on optic nerve transmission to the cortex is released when the animal matures, the stimulus from the eye can no longer cause this region of the cortex to differentiate to see what the eye sees. In humans, it is known that the children with lens defects should have the defects corrected in early life if they are to develop normal vision. Experiments in rats have shown that if the mother cannot lick her pups during early life, the thickness of the cortex of these animals is about 50% of that of the animals licked by their mother.[33] The smaller cortex is not due to lack of neurons, but due to fewer connections among the neurons (synapses). Recently, it has been found through modern imaging techniques that children brought up in severely chaotic circumstances during their early years had a significantly smaller frontal cortex than a group of controls.[34] It is now clear that stimuli in the early period of life are crucial for the wiring of the brain and that this has long term effects.

We now have some understanding of the critical periods for the development of the core functions of the brain. These are abstract thought, concrete thought, affiliation, attachment, sexual behavior, emotional reactivity, motor regulation, arousal, appetite/satiety, sleep, blood pressure, heart rate, and body temperature. Perhaps one of the key new insights is that children who have an adverse early childhood will have difficulty coping with the school system when they enter kindergarten because of deficits in behavior and cognition. Some male children, because of inadequate development of their core brain function in very early life will, when they meet the challenge of school, show an abnormal arousal behavior.[35] Some of these children become antisocial and show disruptive and, in some cases, violent tendencies in the classroom. In one study, more than 29% of male children classified as antisocial when they entered the school system at age 5 were delinquent by the age of 13. An obvious question is, what can be done to help these children? The emerging evidence is that treatment, once the symptoms appear, is far less effective than prevention through good environments for early childhood development.[36] Although the brain has considerable adaptive capability, it would appear that the quality of the early period of development is more important than previously realized and that for many core functions, it is difficult to turn things around in the later stages of life. There are now a number of examples of the value of early supportive environments for children influencing behavior, learning, and health in later stages of the life cycle.[37 38 39]

In one study (High Scope), children in poor economic circumstances who were given a high-quality early childhood development program between the ages of 3 and 5, developed far better than the control group.[40] By the age of 27, those from the intervention group completed more schooling, were more likely to be married with children, had far fewer mental health problems, fewer criminal problems, and had jobs. It has been estimated that for every dollar this program cost, the return to society after more than 20 years is at least 7 dollars. Although there are no equivalent longitudinal studies of the effects of supportive interventions in high-risk populations earlier in life, there are some that show the effect of early intervention on development in the first years of life. Grantham-McGregor[39] and colleagues found that the development of a high-risk group of children during the first two years of life was substantially enhanced by either better nutrition or stimulation. When both interventions were given together, these high-risk children performed as well as the normal control group by the age of two. One suspects, in view of what we now know, that if the High Scope study had been started earlier, the results would be even more impressive. It has been found that the cognitive ability of children is influenced by the quality of stimulation they receive in these early years. In the Carolina study,[40] an early intervention substantially improved the IQ of children in poor socio-economic circumstances. Key cognitive functions in mathematics are acquired between the ages of 4 and 7. A preschool intervention was found to create superior achievement[41] in mathematics for a group of children from a low socio-economic background when compared with a control group from similar circumstances. By age 9, the performance of the children from the intervention group surpassed that of children from middle class backgrounds in magnet schools.

The evidence from neuroscience, animal experiments, and studies in humans has established that the quality of brain stimulation in early life has substantial effects on competence and coping skills throughout life. This clearly affects learning and behavior and health throughout the life cycle.

The effects of early childhood on health in later life also are beginning to be seen from longitudinal studies of children born more than 30 years ago.[42] There is a substantial body of evidence from animal studies showing that the conditions of early life affect health and well-being in adult life.[43] In humans, the gradient in health in the United Kingdom by social class is found to be directly related to the social class at birth. Similarly, the gradient in school performance is also related to the social class at birth. Since the longitudinal studies in respect to health are also affected by events in later years, it is not possible to conclude that the health gradients in adult life are solely due to the conditions of early childhood. However, studies of the 1958 British birth cohort indicate that early life is important and that by age 33, self-rated health, mental health, and obesity are all gradients when assessed against the social class at birth.[44] Barker[45] and colleagues have shown that events in utero and in early life set risks for conditions such as heart disease, high blood pressure, and diabetes in later life.

The biological pathways by which the brain affects health are now being clarified. More than 60 years ago, Selye[46] observed that stress could not only protect the body but could also damage it. Acute stress (in the sense of the "fight or flight" response or major life events) and chronic stress (the accumulation of continuous day-to-day stresses) can have long-term consequences. The pathways are through the hypothalamic-pituitary-adrenal axis and the response of the cardiovascular, metabolic, and immune systems.[47] [48] These pathways are sometimes described as psychoneuroendocrinology and psychoneuroimmunology. How well an individual copes with challenges will influence the activity of these pathways. We now know that repeated stress in early life can increase the incidence of diabetes. Children brought up in circumstances of family instability have an increased incidence of insulin-dependent diabetes.[49] These pathways have been shown to increase athersclerosis[50] and coronary artery disease in nonhuman primates under chronic stress. These pathways also affect the brain and can influence its function, including mental health problems. It is not surprising that we now recognize that adverse childhood experience is associated with both acute and chronic psychosocial problems in adult life.[51] [52] Children brought up in broken homes or subject to maltreatment in early life are at increased risk of behavior problems and depression in adult life.

All of this evidence indicates that factors influencing the development of the brain when it is most plastic in the early stages of life have a long reach throughout the life cycle. While it is possible to compensate for individuals with disabilities in the later stages of life, it is obvious that prevention is the best route. We now understand how the environment in which we live and work throughout the life cycle influences our capacity to learn, our behavior, and our health. We also have an improved appreciation of what needs to be done in communities where there are major problems.

SOCIAL ENVIRONMENTS AND HEALTH

THERE is a substantial body of knowledge showing that the support individuals have in society influences their health status.[53] [54] [55] Those who have the least support appear to be vulnerable to a variety of disorders. Individuals may be more isolated in their communities for personal or social reasons. Some of the factors influencing this may be related to their early childhood (behavior and personality) and the structure of social support. The quality of social support appears to be important during all stages of the life cycle, including the elderly. One of the compelling pieces of evidence about social support comes from the social-economic turmoil in eastern Europe following the breakup of the Communist block. There was a sharp rise in mortality rates in these populations.[56] Many have attributed this to the stresses affecting behavior, leading to more alcohol consumption, increased smoking, poorer diets, and other negative lifestyle behaviors. Others believe that the changes were too rapid to be mainly explained by changes in life style behavior. In Poland, it was found that the groups most affected by the changes were single men and women.[57] They appeared to be the most vulnerable and would tend to be the groups with the least social support to help them cope with the changes. This implies that major socio-economic change will affect the health of populations and hit the most vulnerable groups hardest.

The fact that gradients in health exist in wealthy societies indicates that whatever is creating inequalities in health has to be in some way related to the biological pathways of individuals being influenced by their social environment.

The social capital of a society is recognized to affect the quality of the social environment.[58 59] This term includes measures of trust, helpfulness, and group membership. There are a number of studies showing a relationship between income inequality and mortality in developed countries.[60 61] Kawachi and colleagues[62] have recently provided some insight into how income inequality might affect trust in a society and health. Studying the relationship between measures of trust within states in the United States, they observed a strong correlation between measures of trust and income inequality. Those states with the greatest income inequality had the least trust. A very strong correlation was found between measures of trust in a state and mortality rates. Those states with the least trust had the highest mortality rates. This presents an important clue as to how the dynamics of a society in which individuals live and work can affect their health status.

Since we now have a better understanding of how the brain develops in early life and its strong influence on key biological pathways, we have to consider how much of the social environment effect on human beings is set in early childhood. Certainly the conditions of early childhood could leave individuals with poor coping skills to handle the changing socio-economic circumstances and demands in adult life. The evidence

supports the concept of an early life embedding characteristics that interact with forces throughout the life cycle. This is not just related to the wealth of a region but to how its resources are distributed. Countries in the developing world that provide support for mothers and children in the early stages of a child's life have much better health statistics than countries of the same per capita wealth that do not provide the same support for mothers and children.[63] Thus, regions that can, despite their economic circumstances, invest resources to support mothers and children, will have a healthier population.

The quality of social environments is strongly influenced by how regions or countries create and distribute wealth. As countries such as Canada and the United States have been coping with the deep and broad effects of the present technological revolution, they have created increasing stresses in their societies. What may be described as the "chips for neurons revolution" is changing the way our societies do things and the way wealth is created and distributed.[64] Unfortunately, there is no good measure of how societies are coping with the change, but one economic measure gives an approximate estimate. This is called total factor productivity. When the United States went through the transition from steam power to electricity, total factor productivity went flat for more than two decades.[65] At present, this measure is flat in both Canada and the United States.[66] In the past when this occurred there was a decline in the income of some sectors in society. Today we are also seeing a decline in the income of the bottom half of the population and the population under 40 years of age. This has a major effect on the more vulnerable groups in society, such as mothers and children. It is not surprising, therefore, that we are seeing an increasing number of young children with poor cognitive development and antisocial behavior when they come into the school system.

When economies are undergoing major adjustments, those with resources try to protect their position, leading to a strong pressure to cut government expenditure and taxes. Thus the wealth distribution functions of governments are constrained, which in Canada has begun to cause growing income inequality, particularly for the population under 45 years of age.[67] These are the individuals with the responsibility of caring for young children.

In view of the evidence about the long-term effects of a poor early childhood on learning, behavior, and health, how can societies cope with these complex changes without damaging too many members of the next generation? Increasingly, there is a strong interest in communities organizing themselves to take the steps to provide the support for mothers and children by making use of their financial and nonfinancial resources to provide a more supportive environment for early childhood development. Many of these initiatives are led by what might be described as social entrepreneurs. The tough question is how to finance this entrepreneurship and sustain it. It may turn out that it is the societies with the strongest base and support for social capital that do best. Governments need to develop incentives to get the private sector to invest in social entrepreneurship and build social capital that will enhance the quality of early childhood. Failure to do this could lead to an increase in social problems that will undermine the economy and possibly the base for tolerant democratic states. Both the World Bank and the Inter-American Bank recognize the importance of this for the economies of the developing world.

Dahrendorf,[68] the former head of the London School of Economics, has written that western countries (the developed world) face a major challenge as they try to adjust to the economic change they are going through. If they focus on just the economic and ignore the social adjustments, they may find it increasingly difficult to sustain high-quality supportive populations and pluralistic tolerant democratic states. Fortunately, we now have a better understanding of the determinants of economic growth, human

development, and health to do a better job of handling this change than in the past. The challenge is to integrate this knowledge and apply it at the local and national level in both the public and private sectors of society to improve the health and well-being of all sectors of society.

The initiative of the Kansas Health Foundation with the Kansas Health Institute represents an extraordinary opportunity to do this. If this can be done in one region of the United States, it will show the rest of the country what can be done with our new knowledge in relation to the economy, human development, and health. Leadership at the community level has the best chance of showing the way forward.

NOTES

1. Wilkinson, R. G. *Class and Health*. London: Tavistock Publications, 1986.

2. Evans, R. G. *Why Are Some People Healthy and Others Not? The Determinants of Health of Populations*. New York: Aldine de Gruyter, 1994.

3. Amick, B. C., Levine, S., Tarlov., A. R., and Walsh, D. C. *Soceity and Health*. New York: Oxford Unidersity Press, 1995.

4. Blane, D., Brunner, E., and Wilkinson, R. *Health and Social Organization: Towards a Health Policy for the 21st Century*. London: Routledge, 1996.

5. McEwen, B. S. and Schmeck, H. M. *The Hostage Brain*. New York: The Rockefeller University Press, 1994.

6. Seeman, T. E. and McEwen, B. Impact of Social Environment Characteristics on Neuroendocrinology. *Psy. Med.* 58 (1996): 459.

7. Marmot, M., Bobak, M., and Davey Smith, G. Explanations for Social Inequalities in Health. In *Society and Health*. Amick, B. C., Levine, S., Tarlov, A. R., and Welsh, D. C., eds. New York: Oxford University Press, 1995.

8. Marmot, M., Ben-Shlomo, Y., and White, I. Does the Variation in the Socioeconomic Characteristics of an Area Affect Mortality. *British Medical Journal* 312 (1996): 1013–1014.

9. Barker, D. J. P. Fetal and Infant Origins of Adult Disease. Papers written by the Medical Research Council. Environmental Epidemiology Unit. *British Medical Journal* (1992).

10. Power, C. and Hertzman, C. Social and Biological Pathways Linking Early Life and Adult Disease. *British Medical Bulletin* 53, no. 1 (1997): 210–221.

11. MacIntyre, S. Understanding the Social Patterning of Health: The Role of the Social Sciences. *Journal of Public Health Medicine* 16 (1994): 53.

12. MacIntyre, S. The Black Report and Beyond: What Are the Issues? *Social Science and Medicine* 44, no. 6 (1997): 723–745.

13. McKeown, T. *The Origins of Human Disease*. New York: Basil Blackwell, 1988.

14. Fogel, R. W. *Economic Growth, Population Theory, and Physiology: The Bearing of Long-Term Processes on the Making of Economic Policy*. Cambridge, Mass: National Bureau of Economic Research, 1994.

15. Lalonde, M. *A New Perspective on the Health of Canadians*. Ottawa: Government of Canada, 1974.

16. Beveridge, W. Lord. *Social Insurance and Allied Services*. London: HMSO. Cmnd. 6404, 1942.

17. Merrison, Sir Alec. *Royal Commission on the National Health Service*. London: Her Majesty's Stationery Office, 1979.

18. Black, D. *The Black Report*. London: Penguin Books, 1982.

19. MacIntyre, S. Area, Class and Health: Should We Be Focusing on Places or People? *Journal of Social Policy* 22, no. 2 (1993): 213–214.

20. Marmot, M. Sickness Absence as a Measure of Health Status and Functioning: From the United Kingdom Whitehall II Study. *Journal of Epidemiology and Community Health* 49 (1995): 124–130.

21. Marmot, M. Improvement of Social Environment to Improve Health. *The Lancet* 351, no. 9095 (January 3, 1998): 57–60.

22. Carstairs, V. and Morris, R. *Deprivation and Health in Scotland*. Aberdeen: Aberdeen University Press, 1991.

23. Karasek, R. and Theorell, T. *Healthy Work: Stress, Productivity and the Reconstruction of Working Life*. New York: Basic Books, 1990.

24. Marmot, M., Bosma, H., Hemingway, H., Brunner, E., and Stansfeld, S. Contribution to Job Control and Other Risk Factors to Social Variations in Coronary Heart Disease Incidence. *The Lancet* 350, no. 9073 (July 26, 1997): 235–239.

25. Marmot, M., Bobak, M., and Davey Smith, G. Explanations for Social Inequalities in Health. In *Society and Health*. Amick, B. C., Levine, S., Tarlov, A. R., and Welsh, D. C., eds. New York: Oxford University Press, 1995.

26. Hertzman, C. and Wiens, M. Child Development and Long-Term Outcomes: A Population Health Perspective and Summary of Successful Interventions. *Social Science and Medicine* 43, no. 7 (1996): 1083–1095.

27. Mustard, J. F. Achieving Health for All: Implications for Canadian Health and Social Policies. *Canadian Medical Association Journal* 136 (1987): 471–473.

28. Huttenlochere, P. R. Synapse Elimination and Plasticity in Developing Human Cerebral Cortex. *American Journal of Mental Deficiency* 88 (1984): 488–496.

29. Rakic, P., Bourgeois, J.-P., and Goldman-Rakic, P. S. Synaptic Development of the Cerebral Cortex: Implications for Learning, Memory, and Mental Illness. In Van Pelt, J., Corna, M. A., Uylings, H. B. M., and Lopes da Silva., P. H., eds. *The Self-Organizing Brain: From Growth Cones to Functional Networks*. Amsterdam and New York: Elsevier, 1994.

30. Kolb, B. Brain Development, Plasticity, and Behavior. *American Psychologist* (1989): 1203–1212.

31. Hubel, H. D. and Wiesel, T.N.J. *Physiology* 160 (1962): 106–154.

32. Cynader, M. S. Mechanisms of Brain Development and Their Role in Health and Well-Being. *Daedalus, Journal of the American Academy of Arts and Sciences* 123, no. 4 (Fall 1994).

33. Sapolsky, R. M. The Importance of a Well-Groomed Child. *Science* 277, no. 5332 (1997): 1620–1621.

34. Perry, B. and Pollard, R. Altered Brain Development Following Global Neglect in Early Childhood. CIVITAS Child Trauma Programs, Baylor College of Medicine, Houston, Texas. Society for Neuroscience Abstract (1997).

35. Tremblay, R. E. Early Disruptive Behaviour, Poor School Achievement, Delinquent Behaviour, and Delinquent Personality. *Journal of Consulting and Clinical Psychology* 60, no. 1 (1992): 64–72.

36. Tremblay, R. E. Kindergarten Behavioral Patterns, Parental Practices, and Early Adolescent Antisocial Behavior. In *Coercion and Punishment in Long-Term Perspectives*. New York: Cambridge University Press, 1995.

37. Sen, A. The Economics of Life and Death. *Scientific American* (May 1, 1993): 40–47.

38. Young, M. E. *Early Childhood Development.* Washington: The World Bank Development Department, 1997.

39. Grantham-McGregor, S. M. et al. Nutritional Supplementation, Psychological Stimulation and Mental Development of Stunted Children: The Jamaican Study. *The lancet* 338, no. 8758 (July 6, 1991): 1–5.

40. Campbell, F. A. and Ramey, C. T. Effects of Early Intervention on Intellectual and Academic Achievement: A Follow-Up Study of Children from Low Income Families. *Child Development* 65 (1994): 684–698.

41. Case, R. Socioeconomic Gradients in Mathematical Ability and Their Responsiveness to Compensatory Education. In *Tomorrow's Children* New York: Guilford, 1998.

42. Power, C. Longitudinal Data: The 1958 Birth Cohort. Chapter 2 of *Health and Class: The Early Years* by Power, Manor, and Fox. London: Chapman and Hall, 1991.

43. Suomi, S. J. Early Determinants of Behaviour: Evidence from Primate Studies. *British Medical Bulletin* 53, no. 1 (1997): 12–15.

44. Power, C., Hertzman, C., Matthews, S., and Manor, O. Social Differences in Health: Life-Cycle Effects Between Ages 23 and 33 in the 1958 British Birth Cohort. *American Journal of Public Health* 87, no. 9 (1997): 1499–1503.

45. Barker, D. J. P. Growth in Utero, Blood Pressure in Childhood and Adult Life, and Mortality from Cardiovascular Disease. *British Medical Journal* 298 (1989): 564–567.

46. Selye, H. *The Stress of Life* (rev. ed.) New York: McGraw-Hill, 1976.

47. McEwen, B. S. et al. The Role of Adrenocorticoids as Modulators of Immune Function in Health and Disease: Neural, Endocrine and Immune Interactions. *Brain Research Reviews* 23, (1997): 79–133.

48. McEwen, B. S. and Schmeck, H. M. *The Hostage Brain.* New York: The Rockefeller University Press, 1994.

49. Hales, C. N. Non-Insulin-Dependent Diabetes Mellitus. *British Medical Bulletin* 53, no. 1 (1997): 109–122.

50. Shively, C. A. and Clarkson, T. B. Social Status and Coronary Artery Atherosclerosis in Female Monkeys. *Arteriosclerosis and Thrombosis* 14, no. 5 (1994): 721–726.

51. Chase-Lansdale, P. L., Cherlin, A. J., and Kiernan, K. E. The Long-Term Effects of Parental Divorce on the Mental Health of Young Adults: A Developmental Perspective. *Child Development* 66 (1995): 1614–1634.

52. Maughan, B. and McCarthy, G. Childhood Adversities and Psychosocial Disorders. *British Medical Bulletin* 53, no. 1 (1997): 156–169.

53. Cassel, J. The Contribution of the Social Environmental to Host Resistance: The Fourth Wade Hampton Frost Lecture. *American Journal of Epidemiology* 104, no. 2 (1976): 107–123.

54. Kaplan, G. A. Social Connections and Mortality from All Causes and from Cardiovascular Disease: Prospective Evidence from Eastern Finland. *American Journal of Epidemiology* 128, no. 21 (1988).

55. Berkman, L. F. and Syme, S. L. Social Networks, Host Resistance and Mortality: A Nine-Year Follow-Up Study of Alameda County Residents. *American Journal of Epidemiology* 109 (1979): 186–204.

56. Hertzman, C. Czechoslovakia and the East-West Life Expectancy Gap. Working Paper no. 16. (Toronto: Canadian Institute for Advanced Research, 1992).

57. Watson, P. Explaining Rising Mortality Among Men in Eastern Europe. Paper presented at ESRC Research Seminar on "Gender, Class and Ethnicity in Post-Communist States," June 30, 1994.

58. Putnam, R. D. *Making Democracy Work: Civic Traditions in Modern Italy.* Princeton: Princeton University Press, 1993.

59. Fukuyama, F. *Trust.* London: Penguin Books, 1995.

60. Wilkinson, R. G. *Unhealthy Societies: From Inequality to Well-Being.* New York: Routledge, 1996.

61. Kaplan, G. A. *Income Inequality and Mortality in the United States.* (1995).

62. Kawachi, I., Kennedy, B. P., and Prothrow-Stith, D. Income Distribution and Mortality: Cross Sectional Ecological Study of the Robin Hood Index in the United States. *British Medical Journal* 312 (1996): 1004–1007.

63. Caldwell, J. C. Routes to Low Mortality in Poor Countries. *Population and Development Review* 12 (1986): 171–200.

64. Mustard, J. F. Policy Frameworks for a Knowledge Economy. (Queen's University. John Deutsch Institute for the Study of Economic Policy, 1996).

65. David, P. Computer and Dynamo: The Modern Productivity Paradox in a Not-Too-Distant Mirror. *Technology and Productivity: The Challenge for Economic Policy* (1991): 315–347.

66. The Technology/Economy Programme. *Technology and the Economy: The Key Relationships.* (Organization for Economic Co-operation and Development [OECD], 1992).

67. Noreau, N. et al. *Statistics Canada. Crossing the Low Income Line.* (1997).

68. Dahrendorf, R., Precarious Balance: Economic Opportunity, Civil Society, and Political Liberty. *Responsive Community* 5, no. 3 (1995).

❦

Two

SOCIOECONOMIC AND BEHAVIORAL DIFFERENCES IN HEALTH, MORBIDITY, AND MORTALITY IN KANSAS: EMPIRICAL DATA, MODELS, AND ANALYSES

*Gopal K. Singh**

INTRODUCTION

IN 1990, the U.S. Department of Health and Human Services introduced a national initiative in disease prevention and health promotion called *Healthy People 2000*. This health initiative presents a national strategy for increasing the span of healthy life among Americans, reducing health disparities among Americans, and providing access to preventive health services for all Americans. Since the launching of this national effort, states and other geopolitical areas in the United States, such as counties, cities, and metropolitan areas, have become increasingly interested in population health monitoring and in providing background data needed to understand a population's health issues.

Population health monitoring should not be restricted to simply documenting health-related data for various communities and subgroups of the population. It should also include an analysis of health differentials according to important personal and societal characteristics that are amenable to change through social and public policy interventions. However, health statistics in the United States are rarely presented in conjunction with data on relevant social and economic characteristics. As a result, we have not been able to substantially enhance our understanding of the most fundamental reasons for shifts in population health and widening health disparities among various societal groups.

Despite the remarkable achievements made in improving the overall health of the population during the course of the twentieth century, particularly with respect to increases in life expectancy and reductions in overall mortality, substantial variations in health among various social groups continue to exist, and in many instances the health disparities appear to be widening (Singh 1997; Singh and Yu 1995; Pappas, Queen, Hadden, and Fisher 1993). Social factors, whether expressed in terms of education, occupation, income, wealth, social class, ethnicity,

Prepared as a background paper for the Kansas Conference on Health and Its Determinants held in Wichita, Kansas, April 20–21, 1998.

*At the time of the preparation of this manuscript, the author was affiliated with the Kansas Health Institute, Topeka, Kansas.

family structure, or living arrangements, remain underlying and fundamental determinants of health and disease. While these social characteristics themselves may not be direct determinants of health, they can certainly create conditions or circumstances that give rise to risk factors (e.g., smoking, alcohol and drug use, fatty diet, lack of physical activity, and hypertension) that cause disease, ill health, and death. The social determinants involve such resources as "knowledge, money, power, prestige, and social connections that strongly influence people's ability to avoid risks and to minimize the consequences of disease once it occurs" (Link and Phelan 1996). Inequalities in health are closely linked to social inequalities through several intervening mechanisms, including health behaviors, medical care, working conditions, environmental exposure, personality, and early life conditions (Williams and Collins 1995). To reduce health disparities, we must address inequalities in access to social and economic resources that reflect for different social groups differential opportunities with respect to education, income, employment, housing, social connection, and medical care. For a more detailed discussion of social inequalities in health, please refer to the recent works by Amick, Levine, Tarlov, and Walsh (1995); Blane, Brunner, and Wilkinson (1996); Evans, Barer, and Marmor (1994); Hertzman, Kelly, and Bobak (1996); Townsend, Davidson, and Whitehead (1988); Wilkinson (1986 and 1996); and Social Science and Medicine (1997).

Emphasizing the role of social factors in determining health is important for at least three reasons (Blane 1995). First, estimating the health disparities between the least and most advantaged social groups can tell us about the extent to which a society's health can be improved. Second, documenting health statistics according to social factors can help identify social groups who are at greatest risk of poor health and who are therefore in need of social and medical services. Third, considering social factors along with be-

havioral and health care factors can help us understand the mechanisms through which social factors affect health. A better understanding of the pathways through which social variations in health occur should help us develop and implement more effective social and public health interventions for population health improvement.

Although the data on various health measures in Kansas, especially those based on vital statistics, have been available for several decades, no systematic analysis of health status and health disparities among Kansans has yet been carried out. The aim of this chapter is to examine current differentials in health, morbidity, and mortality of Kansans by socioeconomic, behavioral, and geographic factors within a multivariate framework and to present comparative time trends in such health measures as mortality and life expectancy, empirical data on which are readily available or derivable. Specifically, gross and adjusted differentials in health, morbidity, and mortality in Kansas are analyzed according to such social and behavioral characteristics as age, sex, race and ethnicity, marital status, household composition, education, occupation, employment status, income, place (county) of residence, smoking, drinking, obesity, sedentary lifestyle, and health care coverage. Social and behavioral differences in survival, all-cause and cause-specific mortality, and disability derived from census and vital statistics are analyzed at the population (macro) level using aggregate zip-code and county-level data, whereas individual mortality risks as well as survey-based non-mortality health measures for the adult population, such as self-assessed health, vitality, and risk of diabetes, are analyzed at the micro-level according to a host of social and behavioral characteristics using individual-level data.

MATERIALS AND METHODS

Data Sources

To analyze current social differentials as well as historical trends in health and mortality, a variety of federal and state data sources were used. Data on infant, child, and maternal mortality, general mortality, and cause-specific mortality were derived from the National and State Vital Statistics Systems and the National Longitudinal Mortality Study, whereas those on self-assessed health status, vitality, diabetes, and health-risk behaviors were drawn from the Kansas Behavioral Risk Factor Surveillance Survey. Each of these data sources is described in some detail below.

NATIONAL AND STATE VITAL STATISTICS MORTALITY FILES

The national vital statistics mortality data, compiled and maintained by the National Center for Health Statistics (NCHS), are available on an annual basis in published form from 1900 to the present and on public-use micro-data computer tapes from 1968 to the present. This data source allows the examination of mortality differentials by cause of death according to individual characteristics and such geographic areas as state, metropolitan/non-metropolitan areas, county, zip code, and other sub-national geographic areas. The national mortality data system is one of the very few administrative sources of health statistics in the United States that is routinely available, that covers all events, and that is comparable at the international, national, state, and local levels.

The national mortality files are based on information from death certificates of every death occurring in the United States each year. In 1996, 2.32 million deaths occurred in the U.S. The *U.S. Standard Certificate of Death,* revised most recently in 1989 by the U.S. Department of Health and Human Services, is the basis for the national mortality data. The *Standard Death Certificate* serves as the model for state death certificates in an effort to establish uniform certificates. Most state certificates conform closely to the standard, with modifications to meet particular state needs or legislation. Although the principal responsibility for data collection, data processing, data quality maintenance and improvement rests with

the states, the federal government is required to collect and publish national vital statistics data (see Hoyert, Singh, and Rosenberg 1995; Singh, Kochanek, and MacDorman 1996).

For the study of mortality differentials, the following variables on the death certificate are available: sex, race and ethnicity, age at death, place or country of birth of decedent (US- or foreign-born), place of residence (state, county, city, metropolitan/non-metropolitan area, zip code, etc.), educational attainment, occupation, industry, and marital status of decedent, underlying and multiple causes of death (coded according to the *International Classification of Diseases*), autopsy status, place of death (hospital, clinic, nursing home, residence, etc.), and injury at work.

The most current national mortality data available in electronic form are for the 1995 calendar year (Anderson, Kochanek, and Murphy 1997). For Kansas, however, information on individual death records is available in electronic form for 1996 through the state vital statistics system (Sommer 1998). Race-, sex-, state-, and county-specific population data from the decennial censuses and intercensal population estimates prepared by the U.S. Census Bureau serve as the denominators in computing mortality rates. For pericensal years (i.e., those centering around the census years), it is also possible to estimate mortality by such socioeconomic characteristics as education, occupation, industry, and marital status using vital statistics data. Relevant population (denominator) data on socioeconomic characteristics can be obtained from the Public Use Microdata Samples derived from the decennial censuses.

The major advantages of the national mortality file are its size, geographic detail, and the fact that the information on individual death records is available electronically since 1968. Moreover, the availability of published information since 1900 on an annual basis makes it especially useful for analyzing long-term national and state trends in mortality, survival, and life expectancy (Hoyert, Singh, and Rosenberg 1995).

NATIONAL LONGITUDINAL MORTALITY STUDY

To examine socioeconomic differentials in mortality, I analyzed micro-data from the National Longitudinal Mortality Study (NLMS), which is a longitudinal data set for examining socioeconomic, occupational, and demographic factors associated with all-cause and cause-specific mortality in the United States. The NLMS was conducted by the National Heart, Lung, and Blood Institute in collaboration with the U.S. Bureau of the Census and the National Center for Health Statistics (Rogot, Sorlie, Johnson, and Schmitt 1992; Sorlie, Backlund, and Keller 1995). The public-use NLMS file consisted of five Current Population Survey (CPS) cohorts between 1979 and 1981 whose survival (mortality) experiences were studied for 9 years (National Heart, Lung, and Blood Institute 1995). The CPS is a sample household and telephone interview survey of the civilian noninstitutionalized population in the United States and is conducted by the U.S. Bureau of the Census to produce monthly national statistics on unemployment and the labor force. Data from death certificates on the fact of death and the cause of death were combined with the socioeconomic and demographic characteristics of the 1979–1981 CPS cohorts by means of the National Death Index. Detailed descriptions of the NLMS have been provided elsewhere (Rogot, Sorlie, Johnson, and Schmitt 1992; Sorlie, Backlund, and Keller 1995; Hoyert, Singh, and Rosenberg 1995; Kposowa and Singh 1994).

The NLMS consisted of 2,622 and 2,830 Kansas-born men and women (respectively) aged 25 years and older at the baseline. The number of deaths during the 9-year follow-up was 390 for men and 307 for women. The individual-level analyses of mortality were conducted separately for men and women and included such covariates as age, race/ethnicity, marital status, rural/urban residence, education, occupation/employment status, and family income.

AREA RESOURCE FILE

Most of the census data and some vital records data used in this chapter were derived from the Area Resource File. The Area Resource File, developed and maintained by the U.S. Health Resources and Services Administration, is a computerized county-based data set that contains time series information on a variety of socioeconomic and health characteristics for every county in the United States (Singh and Yu 1996). The data set, in fact, pools together health and socioeconomic data from more than 200 different data sources and combines them into a single computerized data base (Stambler 1988). The Area Resource File is currently updated and distributed once a year. The latest data file available for analysis is 1997 (Bureau of Health Professions 1997). The Area Resource File is especially useful for analyzing ecological relationships among socioeconomic, demographic, health services variables, and health outcomes. The file can also be used to prepare socioeconomic and health resource profiles of various counties and communities in the United States.

KANSAS BEHAVIORAL RISK FACTOR SURVEILLANCE SYSTEM

Individual-level data on self-assessed health status, recent vitality, diabetes, as well as health-risk behaviors were drawn from the Behavioral Risk Factor Surveillance System (BRFSS). This data set is a state-based surveillance system that is coordinated by the Centers for Disease Control and Prevention (CDC). The survey, conducted annually in almost all states, collects sociodemographic, behavioral, and attitudinal data on quality of life, modifiable risk factors for chronic diseases, injuries, and premature death, lack of health care coverage and preventive health services, and on awareness of certain medical conditions such as hypertension, diabetes, and high blood cholesterol (see Singh, Wilkinson, Song et al. 1998; Powell-Griner, Anderson, and Murphy 1997). The high-risk behaviors for which data are routinely collected include cigarette smoking, heavy and binge drinking, physical inactivity, obesity, and non-use of seat belts. Preventive health services for which information is generally available in the survey include mammography, Pap smear tests, colorectal cancer screening, and pneumonia and influenza vaccinations.

The Kansas Department of Health and Environment (KDHE), which has conducted the behavioral risk surveys in Kansas annually since 1992, uses a simple random sampling design to select samples of adults in households with telephones. The samples consist of civilian non-institutionalized persons aged 18 years and older (KDHE 1997) who have an equal chance of being selected in the survey. Most of the data presented in this paper include cumulative data from the years 1993 through 1995. The sample size was 1,440 for the 1993 survey, 1,441 for the 1994 survey, and 2,009 for the 1995 survey (KDHE 1997). The behavioral risk survey data presented here may underestimate the prevalence of certain social, behavioral, and medical risk factors to the extent that telephone ownership is associated with income and other socioeconomic characteristics.

The behavioral risk survey includes a core set of questions that are asked in every state on an annual basis, a rotating set of core questions that are asked every other year, as well as state-specific questions. The core questions asked in Kansas cover topics including health care coverage, preventive health behaviors such as screening for cancers and hypertension, potential health risk behaviors such as drinking, smoking, eating, and exercising, as well as injury control, and attitudes toward HIV/AIDS. The rotating core questions cover a given topic in more detail. For example, with eating behaviors one rotating core set of questions may cover fat consumption, while a second may deal with the daily consumption of fruits and vegetables (Singh, Wilkinson, Song et al. 1998).

Statistical Techniques

In order to make comparisons of relative mortality risks across groups, geographic areas, or over time, all-cause and cause-specific death rates were computed by adjusting for age compositional differences by the direct method. The age-adjusted death rate, a summary index of mortality, is the weighted average of the age-specific death rates, with the weights (for this particular study) being the age-specific proportions of the 1940 U.S. population. The age-adjusted death rates were calculated using the following age groups: <1 year, 1–4, 5–14, 15–24, 25–34, 35–44, 45–54, 55–64, 65–74, 75–84, and 85 years and over. The following equations algebraically represent the calculation of age-adjusted death rate and its variance:

$$ADDR = \Sigma_x W_x^S M_x$$
$$Var\,(ADDR) = \Sigma_x (W_x^S)^2\,[\,(M_x/P_x) \cdot (100000 - M_x)]$$

where $ADDR$ = age-adjusted death rate (directly standardized) per 100,000 population.

$Var\,(ADDR)$ = variance of the age-adjusted death rate.

W_x^S = age-composition of the standard population $\Rightarrow \Sigma_x W_x^S = 1$.

x = age group (<1, 1–4, ...,75–84, $\geq$ 85 years).

M_x = age-specific death rate per 100,000 population for the given demographic group.

P_x = age-specific population for the given demographic group.

Age-specific life expectancy estimates for Kansas for the periods 1900, 1990, and 1995 were calculated by the standard life table methodology using published mortality and population statistics. Observed age-specific death rates ($_nM_x$) for age groups x to x+n were converted into life-table probabilities of dying ($_nq_x$) by the formula: $_nq_x = 2 \cdot n\,(_nM_x)/[1 + n(1 - _na_x) \cdot (_nM_x)]$. The quantity, $_na_x$, is the fraction of the interval between x^{th} and $(x+n)^{th}$ birthdays lived on average by those dying within that interval (see Namboodiri and Suchindran 1987; Namboodiri 1991). Except for the first year of life, those dying within an age interval are assumed to have died around the mid-point of that interval. Life expectancies for Kansas for the other time periods and for the U.S. came directly from the National Vital Statistics System.

Exponential and arithmetic rates of change were used to describe time trends in all-cause and cause-specific death rates (Singh and Yu 1995; 1996). Specifically, the death rate was modeled as a log-linear function of time:

$$\text{Log}_e\, Y_t = \alpha + \beta\, t \qquad (1)$$

where $\text{Log}_e\, Y_t$ is the natural logarithm of the death rate for a specific age group (e.g., infant mortality rate) in year t, α is the intercept, and β is the slope to be estimated. Note that 100 $(e^\beta - 1)$ measures the annual percent change in the death rate (e.g., infant mortality rate). Furthermore, whenever appropriate, differences in death rates and rate-ratios were tested for statistical significance (Singh and Kposowa 1996).

Multivariate regression models were used to estimate socio-behavioral differences in health, morbidity, and mortality, after adjusting for the effects of other covariates. When the dependent variable (Y) was a continuous variable (e.g., the number of days feeling very healthy and full of energy during the past month or the county-level age-adjusted cause-specific death rate), it was regressed on socioeconomic and behavioral covariates using the following ordinary least squares (OLS) regression model:

$$Y = \alpha + \Sigma_j \beta_j X_j + e \qquad (2)$$

where α is the intercept, e is the random disturbance term, X_j's (j = 1,2,...,K) are the K covariates and β_j's are the unknown parameters associated with the K covariates.

When the dependent variable was a discrete (dichotomous) variable (e.g., self-assessed health status measured as fair/poor vs. good/excellent; presence or absence of diabetes or some other chronic disease), the following logistic regression model was used to estimate the effects of covariates:

$$P = \exp\,(\alpha + \Sigma_j \beta_j X_j)\, /\, [1 + \exp\,(\alpha + \Sigma_j \beta_j X_j)] \quad (3)$$

Equation (3) can also be rewritten so that the logits or log-odds are a linear function of X_j's.

$$\text{Log}_e\,[(P/(1-P)] = \alpha + \Sigma_j \beta_j X_j \qquad (4)$$

where P is the probability of fair/poor health or diabetes, Log_e is the natural logarithm to the base e, α is the intercept, β_j's are a set a unknown logistic parameters to be estimated, and X_j's are the K covariates as mentioned above. The coefficient β_j represents the effect of the jth covariate X_j, controlling for the effects of the other covariates. The parameters in the above model were estimated by maximum likelihood method using the LOGISTIC procedure of SAS (SAS Institute 1989).

Estimated odds ratios (OR) were obtained by exponentiating the logistic coefficients (β_j's). Thus, OR=exp(β_j). An OR > 1 indicates that the relative risk of poor health outcome is higher for the covariate category (included in the model), compared to the reference group. An OR < 1 has the opposite interpretation. The 95% confidence interval (CI) was estimated by $\exp[(\beta_j) \pm 1.96\text{SE}(\beta_j)]$, where $\text{SE}(\beta_j)$ is the estimated standard error of the parameter estimate, β_j.

When the dependent variable was the individual mortality risk measured longitudinally, Cox proportional hazards regression models were used to estimate the adjusted effects of socioeconomic and demographic covariates on mortality (Cox 1972; Namboodiri and Suchindran 1987; Singh and Kposowa 1996). A general form of the Cox regression model may be specified as:

$$h(t) = h_0(t)\exp(\Sigma_j \beta_j X_j) \qquad (5)$$

where h(t) is the hazard or risk of overall or cause-specific mortality at time t, β_j's are a set of unknown parameters to be estimated, and X_j's are the K covariates measured at the baseline (i.e., at the time of the CPS interview). The function, $h_0(t)$, is a baseline hazard function and is defined when all the covariates in the model are set to zero.

In the Cox model, the survival distribution function, defined as the probability of surviving from follow-up to at least time t, is given by

$$S(t) = [S_0(t)]^{\exp(\Sigma_j \beta_j X_j)} \qquad (6)$$

where $S_0(t)$ is the baseline survivor function representing the reference categories of the covariates. The proportionality of hazards was tested by inspecting the plots of $\ln[-\ln\{S(t)\}]$ against survival time t for the various covariate categories, including those for age and socioeconomic variables. The plots were found to be approximately parallel, and hence the proportionality assumption was taken to be satisfied by the data. The parameters in the Cox model were estimated by the maximum likelihood method using the PHREG procedure of SAS (SAS Institute 1991). The results are presented in terms of estimated hazard ratios or relative risks (obtained by exponentiating the hazard coefficients (β_j's)) and their 95% confidence intervals.

Measurement of Variables

At the population level, years of potential life lost rate, all-cause mortality, and mortality from major causes of death in Kansas were estimated as a function of selected socioeconomic and behavioral factors. Average annual age-adjusted death rates from all causes combined and from cardiovascular diseases, cancer, diabetes, liver cirrhosis, respiratory, and infectious diseases were computed using cumulative data for 1988 through 1995. The years of potential life lost rate was computed for the period 1989–1993 for persons under 75 years of age.

County-level covariates included percent of population below poverty level, percent of population aged 25 years or older with a college degree, unemployment rate, percent of population living in urban areas, percent of population aged 18 years and older which currently smokes cigarettes, percent of population aged 18 years and older which is obese, and percent of population without health care coverage. It is important to note that while the county-level socioeconomic indicators are based on complete-count census data, the smoking, obesity, and health care coverage rates are based on the 1992–1996 behav-

ioral risk survey data. For a number of small rural counties in Kansas, the estimates of smoking, obesity, and health-care coverage rates may be highly unstable as they are based on a few observations.

CONSTRUCTING AN INDEX OF SOCIAL DISADVANTAGE

The effects of social factors on mortality and disability at the community level were also estimated using aggregate data for 155 zip-code areas in metropolitan Kansas. Since the socioeconomic covariates of health and mortality at the zip-code level are highly correlated, an index of social disadvantage was created so as to minimize the problem of multicollinearity. The index construction was performed by applying factor and principal components analysis methods to the eight social indicators used as covariates. Factor analysis is a powerful tool for data reduction and scale construction. It is a statistical technique for grouping a set of variables into linear combinations of variables or principal components which are orthogonal (independent) to each other (Kim and Mueller 1978). The factor analysis yielded a one-factor solution. The factor thus obtained makes substantive sense and provides a theoretically and empirically meaningful clustering of the given social and economic indicators. The indicators defining the index were weighted using the factor score coefficients derived from the factor analysis. Specifically, the factor (index) scores are calculated as shown below by multiplying the standardized values of observed variables by the corresponding factor score coefficients.

$$\hat{F}_k = \Sigma_i W_i Z_{ik}$$

where $\hat{F}_k$ = the estimated factor score for the kth observation.

W_i = the factor score coefficient for the ith variable.

Z_{ik} = the standardized value of the ith variable for the kth observation.

The Social Disadvantage Index consists of eight social indicators that may be viewed as roughly approximating the living conditions as well as more extreme aspects of the social and economic disadvantage in a metropolitan community. Such indicators as educational distribution, per capita income, unemployment rate, poverty rate, 200% of poverty rate, minority concentration, and percent of households without a motor vehicle constituted the input to the index. Racial heterogeneity or minority concentration has been shown to be a strong correlate of racial segregation and serves here as a proxy for ethnic discrimination, inequality, and economic deprivation (Jiobu 1990). The factor loadings (correlations of indicators with the index) ranged from 0.89 for poverty rate to 0.66 for per capita income (see Table 1). Since the original factor scale was a standard normal variate with a mean of 0 and a standard deviation of 1, the factor was transformed into a standardized index by arbitrarily setting the mean of the index to be 50 and the standard deviation equal to 10. The reliability coefficient, Cronbach's alpha (α), for the index was 0.93.

MEASURING INDIVIDUAL-LEVEL DEPENDENT
VARIABLES AND COVARIATES

In the NLMS analysis, the dependent variables were risks of all-cause mortality and mortality from cardiovascular diseases, cancer, and injuries. In estimating the risk of mortality, all those surviving beyond the 9-year follow-up were treated as right-censored observations. The causes of death were coded according to the International Classification of Diseases, *Ninth Revision* (ICD-9). Except for age, all covariates of individual-level mortality were measured as categorical variables as shown in Table 2.

In the analyses based on behavioral risk data, the covariates included age, sex, race/ethnicity, marital status, household size and composition, educational attainment, employment status, annual household income, mobility or self-care limitation, health care coverage, smoking, drinking, obesity, and sedentary lifestyle. Age was treated as a categorical variable, with 18–24, 25–34, 35–44, 45–54, 55–64, and ≥65 years being the

six categories. Age was also used as a continuous variable in the multivariate modeling of self-assessed health and diabetes. Marital status consisted of the following four categories: single (never married), currently married, divorced or separated, and widowed. Race/ethnicity consisted of five major groups, including non-Hispanic whites, non-Hispanic blacks, Hispanics, Asian Americans or Pacific Islanders, and American Indians. Educational attainment (years of schooling completed) included five categories: <9, 9–11, 12, 13–15, and 16 or more years of education. Employment status consisted of such categories as employed, unemployed, student or homemaker, retired, and unable to work. Annual household income consisted of six categories, including <$10,000, $10,000–$19,999, $20,000–$34,999, $35,000–$49,999, ≥$50,000, and unknown. A dummy vector representing the unknown income category was included in all analyses, because a substantial percentage of respondents did not report their annual household income.

Behavioral risk factors such as smoking, heavy or chronic drinking, obesity, and sedentary lifestyle were defined as dichotomous dummy variables with code 1 if the individual engaged in the negative health behavior and code 0 if the individual did not. Mobility or self-care limitation and health care coverage, considered as covariates in the analysis of self-assessed health, were also represented as dummy variables coded 1 for individuals with activity limitation or lacking health insurance and 0 for those without any activity limitation or those with health insurance.

RESULTS

Life Expectancy

Life expectancy at birth is defined as the number of years a newborn is expected to live given the current levels of mortality at various ages. According to the decennial life tables of 1989–91, Kansans are estimated to live at least a year longer than their national counterparts. Current

Table 1.

Factor Loadings and Factor Score Coefficients for the Items Comprising the Social Disadvantage Index (Factor)
(Principal Components Analysis of Aggregate Census Data for 155 Zip Code Areas in Metropolitan Kansas, 1990)

Variable	Factor Loadings	Factor Score Coefficients
Percent of population below poverty level, 1990	0.88640	0.18124
Percent of population below 200% poverty level, 1990	0.88165	0.18026
Percent of households without a motor vehicle, 1990	0.82236	0.16814
Percent unemployed, 1990	0.76861	0.15715
Percent minority population, 1990	0.71408	0.14600
Per capita income ($), 1990	− 0.65956	− 0.13486
Percent of population with at least a college degree, 1990	− 0.66196	− 0.13535
Percent of population with at least a high school diploma, 1990	− 0.82322	− 0.16832

Table 2.

Multivariate Hazards Regressions Estimates of the Effects of Socioeconomic and Demographic Covariates on All-Cause Mortality Among Men and Women Aged 25 Years or Older Born in Kansas: National Longitudinal Mortality Study, 1979 through 1989

Covariate	Total Population (Age 25–64)		Total Population (Age 25+)		Men (Age 25+)		Women (Age 25+)	
	Hazard Ratio	95% CI	Hazard Ratio	95% CI	Hazard Ratio	95% CI	Hazard Ratio	95% CI
Age (years)	1.09 *	(1.07,1.11)	1.08 *	(1.07,1.09)	1.08 *	(1.07,1.09)	1.08 *	(1.06,1.09)
Sex								
Male	2.29 *	(1.69,3.09)	2.44 *	(2.06,2.89)				
Female	1.00	Reference	1.00	Reference				
Race/ethnicity								
Non-Hispanic White	1.00	Reference	1.00	Reference	1.00	Reference	1.00	Reference
Non-Hispanic Black	1.54	(0.74,3.20)	1.61 *	(1.01,2.57)	1.55	(0.84,2.89)	1.65	(0.79,3.41)
Other	0.56	(0.18,1.76)	0.59	(0.19,1.83)	0.76	(0.19,3.07)	0.39	(0.06,2.83)
Marital status								
Married	1.00	Reference	1.00	Reference	1.00	Reference	1.00	Reference
Single	1.91 *	(1.08,3.37)	1.26	(0.90,1.76)	1.24	(0.78,1.97)	1.43	(0.87,2.35)
Divorced/separated	1.05	(0.63,1.75)	1.06	(0.76,1.49)	0.82	(0.51,1.31)	1.55	(0.95,2.54)
Widowed	1.61	(0.98,2.64)	1.30 *	(1.06,1.60)	1.24	(0.90,1.70)	1.45 *	(1.09,1.94)
Place of residence								
Urban	1.06	(0.80,1.42)	1.09	(0.93,1.28)	1.06	(0.85,1.31)	1.51	(0.89,1.49)
Rural	1.00	Reference	1.00	Reference	1.00	Reference	1.00	Reference
Education (years)								
<9	2.41 *	(1.28,4.56)	1.58 *	(1.15,2.16)	1.60 *	(1.05,2.44)	1.52	(0.94,2.46)
9–11	1.70	(0.88,3.29)	1.56 *	(1.11,2.19)	1.54 *	(0.97,2.44)	1.57	(0.95,2.60)
12	1.80 *	(1.02,3.19)	1.39 *	(1.03,1.88)	1.41	(0.94,2.11)	1.35	(0.85,2.15)
13–15	1.72	(0.94,3.17)	1.44 *	(1.02,2.01)	1.59 *	(1.02,2.48)	1.25	(0.75,2.11)
16+	1.00	Reference	1.00	Reference	1.00	Reference	1.00	Reference

Occupation/employment status								
Professional	1.00	Reference	1.00	Reference	1.00	Reference	1.00	Reference
Non-Professional	1.05	(0.69,1.59)	1.05	(0.76,1.45)	1.00	(0.69,1.46)	1.03	(0.53,2.02)
Unemployed/outside the labor force	1.58 *	(1.00,2.50)	1.32	(0.95,1.84)	1.19	(0.80,1.77)	1.45	(0.76,2.76)
Family income (dollars)								
<5,000	2.91 *	(1.57,5.04)	1.96 *	(1.39,2.76)	2.54 *	(1.58,4.09)	1.40	(0.85,2.30)
5,000–9,999	2.20 *	(1.35,3.59)	1.87 *	(1.37,2.55)	2.23 *	(1.48,3.35)	1.42	(0.88,2.27)
10,000–14,999	1.68 *	(1.05,2.66)	1.39 *	(1.01,1.91)	1.67 *	(1.10,2.53)	1.01	(0.61,1.69)
15,000–19,999	1.15	(0.68,1.95)	1.37	(0.95,1.99)	1.64 *	(1.04,2.60)	0.99	(0.52,1.88)
20,000–24,999	1.42	(0.89,2.28)	1.42	(0.98,2.07)	1.58 *	(1.00,2.52)	1.23	(0.65,2.34)
25,000+	1.00	Reference	1.00	Reference	1.00	Reference	1.00	Reference
Unknown	1.95 *	(1.08,3.54)	1.60 *	(1.10,2.34)	1.66 *	(0.99,2.79)	1.40	(0.81,2.44)
Model Chi-Square	320.17 *		1377.50 *		786.82 *		576.40 *	
Degrees of Freedom	20		20		19		19	
Number of Deaths	219		697		390		307	
Population at Risk	4,238		5,452		2,622		2,830	

Notes: CI=confidence interval; * p<0.05.

life expectancy at birth in Kansas is 76.8 years, 1.4 years longer than that for the U.S. as a whole. During 1989–91, Kansas had the 13th highest life expectancy in the United States, dropping from a rank of 6 in 1969–71. Most of the states in the North-Central or the Great Plains region (such as Minnesota, North and South Dakota, Nebraska, and Iowa) currently have higher life expectancies than Kansas. Hawaiians and Minnesotans live the longest in the U.S., with a life expectancy of about 78 years.

An examination of the long-term trends in life expectancy shows dramatic improvement in survival since the turn of the century. Life expectancy at birth in Kansas increased from 56 years in 1900 to about 77 years in 1995. Table 3 presents life expectancy estimates at birth and subsequent ages for Kansas and the U.S. at various time points: 1900-1902, 1959-61, 1969-71, 1979-81, 1990, and 1995. As can be seen from this table, at the turn of the century, Kansans enjoyed a longer life expectancy at each age than their national counterparts. The life expectancy at birth in 1900 was about 7 years longer for Kansas than for the U.S. as a whole. By 1960, the relative advantage of Kansans had narrowed to only 2 years. In 1995, Kansans were estimated to live one year longer than their national counterparts. Moreover, as compared with the national average, Kansans currently have a longer life expectancy throughout the entire life course, although the differences are minimal at advanced ages, especially at ages 70 years and beyond.

Between 1900 and 1960, the largest gains in life expectancy in Kansas and the U.S. occurred among infants and children under 5 years of age, although the relative gains were more substantial nationally. Also, Americans aged 65 years and older posted larger gains in life expectancy during this period than their Kansas counterparts. Between 1960 and 1995, the relative gains in life expectancy for infants, children, and adolescents in both Kansas and the U.S. were much more modest than those for the elderly at ages 70, 75, 80, and 85 years.

Life expectancy at birth varies substantially within Kansas—from a low of 73.0 years for Wyandotte county to a high of 79.1 years for Johnson county. Cherokee, Geary, Riley, Leavenworth, Montgomery, Shawnee, and Sedgwick counties all have lower life expectancies than the state average of 76.8 years. Life expectancy also varies considerably by race and sex. White females in the state have the highest life expectancy (80.3 years), followed by black females (74.8 years), white males (74.0 years), and black males (67.0 years) (see Figure 1).

All-Cause and Cause-Specific Mortality

In 1994, 23,328 deaths occurred among all Kansas residents. Table 4 shows the number of deaths and death rates from selected major causes of death in Kansas and the United States in 1979 and 1994. Taken together, these causes of death accounted for over 86 percent of all deaths in Kansas and the United States. Heart disease was the leading cause of death in Kansas, accounting for 32% of all deaths, followed by cancer (23%), stroke (7%), and chronic obstructive pulmonary diseases (COPD) (5%). The distribution of deaths by these major causes was similar to that for the United States (Singh, Kochanek, and MacDorman 1996).

The overall mortality (in terms of age-adjusted death rate) in 1994 was almost 10% lower in Kansas than the national average. For most of the leading causes of death, such as heart disease, all cancers as well as respiratory and digestive cancers, stroke, diabetes, pneumonia and influenza, HIV/AIDS, liver cirrhosis, homicide, and non-motor vehicle injuries, mortality is generally lower among Kansans than the nation as a whole. However, mortality from motor vehicle accidents was 15 percent higher and brain cancer mortality was 23 percent higher among Kansans than their national counterparts. Compared to the national average, atherosclerosis mortality was 35% higher in Kansas (see Table 4).

As for changes between 1979 and 1994, the largest reductions in mortality among Kansans

Table 3.

Life Expectancy by Age for Kansas and the United States, 1900–1995

Average number of years of life remaining at each age

Age (years)	Kansas 1900	U.S. 1900–1902	Kansas 1959–61	U.S. 1959–61	Kansas 1969–71	U.S. 1969–71	Kansas 1979–81	U.S. 1979–81	Kansas 1990	U.S. 1990	Kansas 1995	U.S. 1995
0	56.0	49.2	71.9	69.9	72.6	70.8	75.3	73.9	76.9	75.4	76.8	75.8
1	60.1	55.2	72.5	70.8	72.9	71.2	75.2	73.8	76.5	75.1	76.3	75.4
5	59.4	55.2	68.8	67.0	69.2	67.4	71.4	70.0	72.6	71.2	72.5	71.5
10	55.4	51.1	64.0	62.2	64.3	62.6	66.5	65.0	67.7	66.3	67.5	66.6
15	51.2	46.8	59.1	57.3	59.4	57.7	61.5	60.2	62.8	61.3	62.6	61.6
20	47.2	42.8	54.4	52.6	54.8	53.0	56.8	55.5	58.1	56.6	57.8	56.9
25	43.5	39.1	49.7	47.9	50.1	48.4	52.1	50.8	53.3	51.9	53.1	52.2
30	39.7	35.5	45.0	43.2	45.4	43.7	47.5	46.1	48.5	47.2	48.3	47.5
35	35.8	31.9	40.3	38.5	40.7	39.1	42.7	41.4	43.8	42.6	43.6	42.8
40	32.0	28.3	35.6	33.9	36.0	34.5	38.1	36.8	39.0	38.0	39.0	38.3
45	28.1	24.8	31.1	29.5	31.6	30.1	33.5	32.3	34.3	33.4	34.3	33.8
50	24.3	21.3	26.8	25.3	27.2	25.9	29.1	27.9	29.8	29.0	29.8	29.3
55	20.5	17.9	22.7	21.4	23.2	22.0	24.8	23.9	25.5	24.8	25.5	25.1
60	17.0	14.8	18.8	17.7	19.3	18.3	20.9	20.0	21.5	20.8	21.4	21.1
65	13.7	11.9	15.3	14.4	15.8	15.0	17.3	16.5	17.8	17.2	17.6	17.4
70	10.7	9.3	12.0	11.4	12.6	12.0	13.9	13.3	14.3	13.9	14.2	14.1
75	8.2	7.1	9.1	8.7	9.7	9.3	10.9	10.5	11.2	10.9	11.1	11.0
80	6.3	5.3	6.6	6.4	7.3	7.1	8.2	8.0	8.5	8.3	8.4	8.3
85	4.8	4.0	4.6	4.6	5.3	5.3	6.1	6.0	6.2	6.1	5.9	6.0

Source: National State and Vital Statistics Systems. Life expectancies for Kansas in 1900, 1990, and 1995 were computed using published mortality and population statistics.

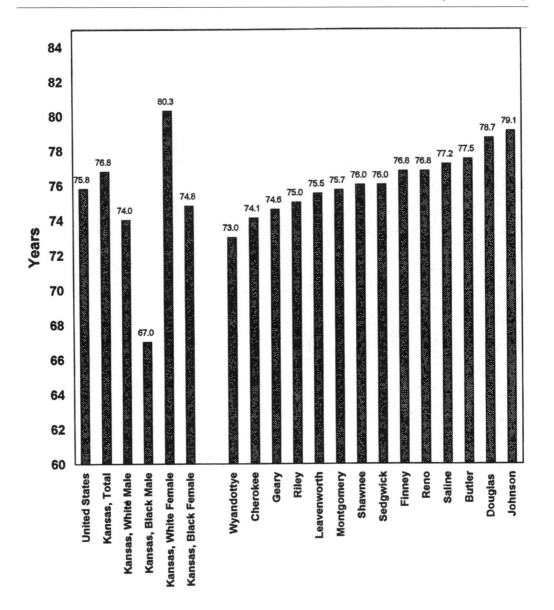

Figure 1
Life Expectancy at Birth (Average Lifetime in Years)
for the United States, Kansas, and Selected Kansas Counties, 1990–1994

Table 4.

Percent of Total Deaths, Age-Adjusted Death Rates per 100,000 Population for 1994, and Percent Change in Age-Adjusted Rates Between 1979 and 1994 for Selected Major Causes of Death: Kansas and the United States, 1994

Cause of Death (ICD-9 Codes)	Percent of All Deaths		Age-Adjusted Death Rate		Black/White Ratio		%Difference in Mortality Between Kansas and U.S.	%Change, 1979–94	
	Kansas	U.S.	Kansas	U.S.	Kansas	U.S.		Kansas	U.S.
All Causes	100.0	100.0	459.4	507.4	1.6	1.6	– 9.5	– 11.0	– 12.1
Heart disease (309–398, 402, 404–429)	31.8	32.1	121.7	140.4	1.5	1.5	– 13.3	– 29.8	– 29.6
Cancer (140–208)	23.0	23.4	126.3	131.5	1.3	1.4	– 4.0	6.7	0.5
Digestive System (150–159)	5.1	5.5	26.7	29.3	1.6	1.6	– 8.9	– 7.9	– 11.5
Respiratory System (160–165)	6.5	6.8	38.4	40.1	1.5	1.3	– 4.2	19.6	13.9
Skin (172–173)	0.4	0.4	2.2	2.5	0.2	0.4	– 12.0	4.8	13.6
Breast (174–175)	2.0	1.9	21.3	21.3	1.3	1.3	0.0	2.9	– 4.7
Genital organs (179–187)	2.8	2.7	12.8	13.2	1.2	1.8	– 3.0	6.7	– 2.9
Urinary organs (188–189)	1.0	1.0	5.3	5.1	1.0	1.0	3.9	– 10.2	– 1.9
Brain/nervous system (191–192)	0.1	0.5	4.3	3.5	0.5	0.5	22.9	30.3	2.9
Stroke (430–438)	7.3	6.7	23.2	26.5	1.7	1.9	– 12.5	– 34.3	– 36.3
Chronic obstructive pulmonary diseases (490–496)	4.7	4.5	21.0	21.0	0.8	0.8	0.0	34.6	43.8
Unintentional injuries (E800–E949)	4.1	4.0	31.6	30.3	1.3	1.3	4.3	– 27.7	– 29.4
Motor vehicle crashes (E810–E825)	2.0	1.9	18.5	16.1	1.0	0.1	14.9	– 30.3	30.6
All other injuries (E800–E807, E826–E949)	2.1	2.1	13.0	14.2	1.7	1.6	– 8.5	– 33.7	– 27.6
Pneumonia and influenza (480–487)	4.1	3.6	12.4	13.0	1.2	1.4	– 4.6	– 17.0	16.1
Diabetes mellitus (250)	2.2	2.5	10.8	12.9	2.3	2.4	– 16.3	25.6	31.6
Infectious diseases (001–139)	1.6	3.3	9.6	23.2	2.6	3.7	– 58.6	166.7	354.9
HIV/AIDS infection (*042–*044)	0.5	1.8	4.2	15.4	2.4	4.4	– 72.7	—	—
Atherosclerosis (440)	1.3	0.8	3.1	2.3	0.8	1.3	34.8	– 46.6	– 59.6
Suicide (E950–E959)	1.3	1.4	10.9	11.2	0.5	0.6	– 2.7	– 8.4	– 4.3
Nephritis, nephrotic syndrome, and nephrosis (580–589)	1.2	1.0	4.5	4.3	3.0	2.7	4.7	7.1	0.0
Homicide and legal intervention (E960–E978)	0.8	1.1	8.1	10.3	12.1	6.6	– 21.4	37.2	1.0
Chronic liver disease and cirrhosis (571)	0.8	1.1	5.7	7.9	2.7	1.4	– 27.8	– 20.8	– 34.2
Alzheimer's disease (331.0)	0.9	0.8	2.5	2.5	0.8	0.7	0.0	733.3	1150.0

Note: Age-adjusted death rates are computed by the direct method using the 1940 U.S. population as the standard.
Source: National Center for Health Statistics, National Vital Statistics System, 1979–94.

occurred for atherosclerosis (47%), stroke (34%), heart disease (30%), unintentional injuries (28%), and liver cirrhosis (21%), while the largest increases occurred for infectious diseases (167%) (because of the rise in HIV/AIDS mortality), homicide (37%), COPD (35%), diabetes (26%), brain cancer (30%), and respiratory cancer (20%). The considerable increase in Alzheimer's disease mortality likely reflects improvements in reporting and diagnosis of the disease rather than increases in actual prevalence.

Although all-cause mortality and mortality from several major causes of death is lower in Kansas than the national average, a number of states perform better than Kansas. For example, the state-specific cumulative mortality data for 1988-1992 indicate that Kansas has the 25th highest COPD mortality rate, 65% higher than the rate for Hawaii. Kansas ranks 17th in the nation in suicide mortality, and has a rate that is almost twice as high as the rates for the District of Columbia and New Jersey. Mortality from motor-vehicle related crashes in Kansas is the 26th lowest in the nation but it is almost double the rates of Rhode Island and Massachusetts. Furthermore, interstate comparisons of major causes of death for adolescents and youth indicate that the Kansas youth do not fare as well as the overall Kansas population. The teen homicide rate in Kansas (9.4 homicides for every 100,000 youth aged 15-19 years), ranked 21st in the nation, is almost three times the corresponding rates in Utah and Iowa. The teen suicide rate (15.2 suicides per 100,000 teens aged 15-19 years in Kansas), the 15th highest in the nation, is 3.4 times the rate for New Jersey. Motor vehicle crashes claim relatively more lives of teenagers in Kansas than in 39 other states; the Kansas rate of 41 motor vehicle deaths per 100,000 teens during 1990-1992 was more than twice the rates for Rhode Island, New Jersey, and New York. Each year Kansas teens, with an average annual firearm death rate of 22.5 per 100,000, are 2 and 3 times as likely to be killed by guns as their Iowa and Hawaiian counterparts, respectively.

COUNTY VARIATIONS

Age-adjusted mortality from all causes combined varies considerably within Kansas. During 1988–1994, Rawlins and Gove counties had the lowest mortality, while Wyandotte, Cherokee, and Geary counties had the highest mortality. The rates for the latter counties were 73, 59, and 55 percent higher than the rate for Rawlins, respectively. Between 1979 and 1994, most of the Kansas counties experienced a decline in mortality. However, mortality increased significantly for Stanton (17%), Decatur (17%), Smith (12%), and Marion (10%) counties.

Cardiovascular disease mortality is highest in Comanche and Cherokee counties—over two times greater than the rates for Hodgeman and Gove counties, 40 to 50 percent higher than the state average, and 25 to 35 percent higher than the national average. Wyandotte, Phillips, Elk, and Geary counties have the highest cancer mortality rates in the state—2 times higher than the rates for Stevens, Wichita, and Haskell counties. There is a striking spatial clustering, with counties in eastern and southeastern Kansas showing the highest levels of cardiovascular and cancer mortality.

Infant, Child, and Maternal Mortality

Historically, infant mortality in Kansas has generally been lower than that for the U.S. as a whole, and the rates for both Kansas and the U.S. have declined fairly consistently (in an exponential fashion) over the past 9 decades. However, the average annual rate of decline in infant mortality between 1915 and 1995 has been somewhat faster for the U.S. than for Kansas (3.1% vs. 2.9%). The latest figures indicate the 1995 infant mortality rate to be 7.0 infant deaths per 1,000 live births for Kansas, 8% lower than the U.S. rate of 7.6. A state-wise comparison of the 1995 data shows that 16 states, including Massachusetts, Utah, New Hampshire, Nevada, Hawaii, and Washington, reported considerably lower

(4% to 26% lower) infant mortality rates than Kansas.

The racial disparity in infant mortality has generally been higher in Kansas than in the U.S. Nationally, the infant mortality rate in 1995 was 2.40 times larger for blacks than for whites, whereas in Kansas, the rate was 2.84 times higher for blacks than for whites. In 1964, the corresponding black/white ratio was 1.96 for the U.S. and 2.18 for Kansas.

The maternal mortality rate in Kansas, generally lower than the national rate, has shown a remarkable decline over the past 8 decades, falling from a rate of over 600 maternal deaths per 100,000 live births in 1920 to a rate of only 5 in 1995. The downward national trend also has been equally dramatic, with the maternal mortality rate dropping from over 700 in 1920 to a rate of 7.1 in 1995.

COUNTY VARIATIONS

As for geographic variations within Kansas, among the counties with at least 10 infant deaths during 1989–1993, Lyon, Douglas, and Johnson counties had the lowest infant mortality rates (≤ 6 infant deaths per 1,000 live births), while Rice (16.9), Wilson (16.6), Bourbon (13.3), and Wyandotte counties (12.9) had the highest infant mortality rates. Other child mortality indicators also show considerable geographic disparities. The mortality rate for children under 15 years of age varies from a low of under 20 child deaths (per 100,000 children) for Woodson, Rush, and Chase counties to a rate of over 150 deaths per 100,000 children for Hodgeman, Geary, Hamilton, and Gove counties. Mortality among adolescents and young adults aged 15–24 years is lowest in Douglas and Riley counties and is highest among Rush, Chautauqua, and Comanche counties. The injury mortality rate among teens and children varies from a low of 10 or fewer deaths per 100,000 children and teens for Wabaunsee, Wallace, Scott, and Meade counties to a high of 90 deaths per 100,000 children and teens for Hodgeman, Kearny, and Gove counties.

Racial, Socioeconomic, and Behavioral Differences in Cause-Specific Mortality

Substantial racial differentials in mortality exist. Overall, black Kansans experience a 60% higher risk of mortality than their white counterparts (see Table 4). They also experience significantly increased mortality from heart disease, stroke, cancer, diabetes, liver cirrhosis, pneumonia and influenza, HIV/AIDS, homicide, and unintentional injuries. Racial disparities are particularly marked for homicide: blacks experience 12 times higher risk of homicide than whites in Kansas. Black Kansans have 2 to 3 times higher mortality from diabetes, cirrhosis, kidney, and infectious diseases than white Kansans.

ECOLOGICAL MODELS OF MORTALITY

Tables 5 through 7 present the results of the regression models that examine the relationship between socioeconomic factors and mortality using ecological or areal data gathered at the zip code and county levels. In Table 5, crude death rates and crude disability rates for 155 zip-code areas in metropolitan Kansas are regressed on the social disadvantage index and percent of population aged ≥65 years. After adjusting for age composition, social disadvantage is strongly associated with disability rate but not with mortality. Age composition and social disadvantage together account for 69% of the variance in the crude disability rate.

Tables 6 and 7 contain bivariate and multivariate models, showing associations between socioeconomic and behavioral factors and age-adjusted mortality measured at the county level. In Table 6, the percentage of population with at least a college degree, poverty rate, and unemployment rate as well as behavioral factors such as smoking and obesity rates, are all significantly associated with years of potential life lost (YPLL) rate, all-

Table 5.

Ordinary Least Squares Regressions of Crude Death Rate per 1,000 Population and Crude Disability Rate (Percent) on Index of Social Disadvantage: Based on 155 Zip Code Areas for Kansas City, Lawrence, Topeka, and Wichita Metropolitan Statistical Areas (MSAs), 1990

Independent Variable	Crude Death Rate			Crude Disability Rate		
	b	SE(b)	β	b	SE(b)	β
Bivariate Models						
Percent population aged >=65 years, 1990	0.384 **	0.069	0.407	0.381 **	0.028	0.735
Index of social disadvantage	0.152 **	0.054	0.221	0.216 **	0.025	0.570
Multivariate Models						
Percent population aged >=65 years, 1990	0.353 **	0.072	0.375	0.324 **	0.025	0.625
Index of social disadvantage	0.080	0.053	0.116	0.150 **	0.018	0.396
Intercept	− 0.500	2.580		− 5.853 **	0.878	
R^2	0.178 **			0.685 **		
df	152			152		

Source: Based on census and state vital statistics data.
Notes: b=unstandardized regression coefficient; SE=standard error; β=standardized regression coefficient.
  * p<0.05; **p<0.01.

Table 6.

Ordinary Least Squares Regressions of Years of Potential Life Lost (YPLL) Rate, All-Cause Mortality,
Cardiovascular Disease and Cancer Mortality on Socioeconomic and Behavioral Characteristics: Based on Aggregate Data for 105 Kansas Counties, 1988–94

Independent Variable	YPLL Rate 1989–1993			All-Cause Mortality 1988–1994			Cardiovascular Mortality 1988–1994			Cancer Mortality 1988–1994		
	b	SE(b)	β	b	SE(b)	β	b	SE(b)	β	b	SE(b)	β
Bivariate Models												
Percent below poverty level, 1989	1.207 **	0.343	0.327	6.317 **	1.179	0.467	2.090 **	0.360	0.496	0.853 **	0.275	0.292
Percent with a college degree, 1990	−1.171 **	0.123	−0.683	−4.108 **	0.470	−0.653	−1.354 **	0.139	−0.692	−0.546 **	0.123	−0.402
Percent unemployed, 1990	9.596 **	0.798	0.764	38.786 **	2.454	0.842	10.373 **	0.976	0.723	7.356 **	0.660	0.740
Percent urban population, 1990	0.024	0.061	0.039	0.194	0.222	0.086	−0.041	0.069	−0.058	0.092 *	1.047	0.189
Percent smokers, 1992–96	1.628 **	0.228	0.575	6.479 **	0.801	0.623	1.739 **	0.269	0.538	1.288 **	0.181	0.574
Percent obese, 1992–96	1.187 **	0.226	0.460	4.194 **	0.838	0.442	1.329 **	0.259	0.451	0.597 **	0.193	0.292
Multivariate Models												
Percent below poverty level, 1989	−0.119	0.219	−0.032	2.177 **	0.755	0.161	0.809 **	0.274	0.192	0.253	0.241	0.087
Percent with a college degree, 1990	−1.392 **	0.147	−0.812	−4.170 **	0.505	−0.663	−1.240 **	0.183	−0.633	−0.534 **	0.161	−0.393
Percent urban population, 1990	0.288 **	0.042	0.468	1.047 **	0.145	0.463	0.223 **	0.053	0.317	0.190 **	0.046	0.391
Percent smokers, 1992–96	0.520 **	0.177	0.184	2.566 **	0.608	0.247	0.591 **	0.221	0.183	0.754 **	0.194	0.336
Percent obese, 1992–96	0.342 *	0.154	0.133	1.302 *	0.531	0.137	0.410 *	0.193	0.139	0.194	0.170	0.095
Intercept	61.046 **	7.881		368.269 **	27.111		146.75 **	9.837		98.039 **	8.661	
R²	0.729 **			0.762 **			0.676 **			0.478 **		
df	99			99			99			99		

Source: Based on census, national and state vital statistics, and Kansas behavioral risk data.

Notes: b=unstandardized regression coefficient; SE=standard error, β=standardized regression coefficient; * p<0.05; **p<0.01.
 In estimating regression models, counties were weighted and normalized proportional to their relative population size in 1990.
 All-cause, cardiovascular disease, and cancer mortality rates are average annual age-adjusted death rates per 100,000 U.S. standard million population in 1940.
 YPLL rate per 1,000 population is computed for persons under 75 years of age.
 Bivariate models are unadjusted while multivariate models are adjusted for the effects of other independent variables.

Table 7.

Ordinary Least Squares Regressions of Diabetes, Cirrhosis, Respiratory, and Infectious Disease Mortality on Socioeconomic and Behavioral Characteristics: Based on Aggregate Data for 105 Kansas Counties, 1988–95.

Independent Variable	Diabetes Mortality 1988–1995			Cirrhosis Mortality 1988–1995			Respiratory Mortality 1988–1995			Infectious Mortality 1988–1995		
	b	SE(b)	β	b	SE(b)	β	b	SE(b)	β	b	SE(b)	β
Bivariate Models												
Percent below poverty level, 1989	0.132 *	0.075	0.171	0.116 **	0.039	0.285	0.302 *	0.141	0.207	0.100	0.079	0.124
Percent with a college degree, 1990	− 0.153 **	0.032	− 0.425	− 0.071 **	0.017	− 0.374	− 0.231 **	0.063	− 0.341	− 0.018	0.037	− 0.048
Percent unemployed, 1990	1.475 **	0.216	0.558	0.643 **	0.121	0.463	2.374 **	0.430	0.478	1.653 **	0.216	0.602
Percent urban population, 1990	− 0.000	0.013	− 0.002	0.010	0.007	0.146	0.053 **	0.023	0.219	0.074 **	0.011	0.549
Percent smokers, 1992–96	0.221 **	0.055	0.371	0.101 **	0.029	0.323	0.421 **	0.102	0.376	0.282 **	0.054	0.454
Percent obese, 1992–96	0.142 **	0.052	0.261	0.034	0.028	0.140	0.308 **	0.096	0.301	0.106 **	0.055	0.188
Multivariate Models												
Percent below poverty level, 1989	− 0.048	0.076	− 0.062	0.029	0.039	0.072	0.028	0.134	0.019	0.046	0.067	0.057
Percent with a college degree, 1990	− 0.181 **	0.051	− 0.502	− 0.089 **	0.026	− 0.471	− 0.337 **	0.089	− 0.497	− 0.166 **	0.036	− 0.442
Percent unemployed, 1990				0.210	0.160	0.151						
Percent urban population, 1990	0.032 *	0.015	0.245	0.027 **	0.008	0.393	0.122 **	0.026	0.502	0.107 **	0.012	0.793
Percent smokers, 1992–96	0.090	0.061	0.144				0.100	0.108	0.089			
Percent obese, 1992–96	0.027	0.053	0.050				0.143	0.094	0.140			
Intercept	10.227 **	2.717		4.099 **	0.990		31.496 **	4.796		5.068 **	1.297	
R²	0.271 **			0.323 **			0.359 **			0.464 **		
df	99			100			99			101		

Source: Based on census, national and state vital statistics, and Kansas behavioral risk data.

Notes: b=unstandardized regression coefficient; SE=standard error; β=standardized regression coefficient; *p.<0.05; **p<0.01.

In estimating regression models, counties were weighted and normalized proportional to their relative population size in 1990.

Diabetes, cirrhosis, respiratory and infectious disease mortality rates are average annual age-adjusted death rates per 100,000 U.S. standard million population in 1940.

Bivariate models are unadjusted while multivariate models are adjusted for the effects of other independent variables.

cause mortality, and mortality from cardiovascular diseases (CVD) and cancer. In simple or bivariate regression models of Table 6, standardized regression coefficients, β, represent bivariate correlations, showing unemployment, education, and smoking rates to be most strongly associated with the four mortality measures. The unemployment rate alone explains at least 52% of the variance in the YPLL rate, all-cause, CVD, and cancer mortality rates at the county level. The multivariate models of Table 6 show the independent effects of poverty, education, urbanization, smoking, and obesity on each mortality measure. The unemployment rate was not included in the multivariate models because it was very highly correlated with the other independent variables. In each of the multivariate models, the percentage of population with at least a college degree was the most important determinant of mortality, followed by percent urban and smoking. Even after controlling for socioeconomic factors, both smoking and obesity were positively related to the YPLL rate, all-cause mortality rate, and CVD mortality rate. Smoking in particular was strongly related to cancer mortality. The proportion of variance explained by these five covariates ranged from 76% for all-cause mortality to 48% for cancer mortality.

Table 7 shows substantial ecological correlations between unemployment and diabetes, cirrhosis, respiratory, and infectious disease mortality. Education is also strongly related to diabetes, cirrhosis, and respiratory disease mortality. In the multivariate models, only education and urbanization show significant effects on diabetes mortality; smoking and obesity do not show significant associations, net of socioeconomic factors. Education and urbanization are the two most important determinants of cirrhosis mortality; poverty and unemployment rates do not show a significant relationship once the effects of education and urbanization are controlled for. A similar pattern is observed for respiratory and infectious disease mortality, with

mortality rising with increasing levels of urbanization and mortality decreasing with increasing proportions of people with a college education.

INDIVIDUAL-LEVEL MODELS OF MORTALITY

Analyses of adult mortality differentials using individual-level NLMS data confirm the substantial socioeconomic differences in mortality observed at the ecological level. Table 2 shows net differences in mortality risks among those aged ≥25 years born in Kansas, according to such individual social characteristics as sex, race/ethnicity, marital status, place of residence, education, occupation, and family income. For the total population aged ≥25 years, education and income are both inversely and independently related to all-cause mortality. Moreover, there is generally a consistent gradient in mortality associated with income; those with annual family incomes less than $10,000 have twice the mortality risk of those with incomes ≥50,000. Socioeconomic differences partly account for the excess mortality risk among blacks, although blacks still have a 61% higher mortality risk than their non-Hispanic white counterparts of equivalent socioeconomic background. Men have a 144% higher mortality risk than women, and widowed individuals have a 30% higher mortality than their married counterparts.

Socioeconomic differences in mortality tend to be greater for those aged 25–64 years than the overall adult population (see Table 2). Those with less than 9 years of education have a 141% higher mortality than those with a college degree, whereas those with incomes <$5,000 have almost three times the mortality risk of those with incomes ≥50,000. Unemployment and singlehood carry a substantially increased mortality risk among those aged 25–64 years. When sex-specific models in Table 2 are examined, educational and income variations in all-cause mortality are more pronounced for men than for women.

Besides all-cause mortality, socioeconomic

differences in mortality from major causes of death are also worth mentioning (data not shown). While education, income, sex, and racial differences in cardiovascular and cancer mortality are similar to those for all causes combined, sex and especially income variations in external-cause (injury) mortality (ICD-9 codes E800-E999) were considerably more pronounced. Net of other factors, men aged ≥25 years have a 5.2 times higher risk of injury mortality than women, and individuals with incomes <$5,000 have a 17.2 times higher risk of injury mortality than those with incomes ≥50,000.

Self-Assessed Health

National trend data from the General Social Survey suggest a consistent and significant improvement in self-assessed health status in the United States from 1972 to 1996 (Davis and Smith 1996). Although there are no such trend data for Kansas, current social differentials in self-perceived health can be described using the behavioral risk factor data (KDHE 1997). Because estimates derived from the behavioral risk data are based on a sample of the Kansas population, they are subject to sampling variability.

Most Kansans (87.1%) consider themselves to be in excellent or good health. During 1993–1995, 12.9 percent of Kansans aged 18 years and older assessed their health as fair or poor, whereas the corresponding figure for all Americans in 1994 was 12.8 percent. Compared to their national counterparts, white Kansans were somewhat more likely and black Kansans significantly less likely to assess their health as fair or poor. As for the racial disparity in perceived health, black Kansans were 28% more likely than white Kansans to perceive their health as fair or poor. It is important to note that the rates of fair or poor health presented here are underestimated. The Kansas Behavioral Risk Survey (with a combined sample size of 4,890 during 1993–1995), like the National Health Interview Survey, excludes people who are in institutions, such as

nursing homes and hospitals, who presumably would have poorer health than the non-institutionalized population (that the Kansas Survey represents) (Adams and Marano 1995).

Tables 8 and 9 show variations in self-reported health among Kansans according to selected socioeconomic, behavioral, functional, and physical characteristics. Age is negatively associated with subjective health status; the older the age, the greater the probability of assessing self health as fair or poor. Thirty percent of Kansans aged 65 years and over assess their health as fair or poor, compared to less than 6 percent of Kansans aged 18–24 years.

Table 8 shows that self-assessed health varies significantly by race/ethnicity and marital status. When adjusted for age differences, blacks are almost three times more likely than whites to perceive their health as fair or poor, while single, divorced, and widowed individuals are respectively 68%, 83%, and 47% more likely than their married counterparts to rate their health as fair or poor.

Figure 2 shows substantial education and income gradients in self-assessed health. The higher the education and income levels, the lower the probability of assessing self health as fair or poor. Thirty-nine percent of people with less than 9 years of education assess their health as fair or poor, compared to only 5 percent of people with a college degree. Those with a high school diploma are over 3 times more likely than their college-educated counterparts to rate their health as fair or poor. About 27 percent of people with annual household incomes less than $10,000 describe their health as fair or poor, compared with 11 percent of people with incomes between $20,000 and $35,000 and 4 percent of people with incomes over $50,000.

It is important to note that educational and income variations in self-assessed health differ between men and women (see Table 8). Both education and income gradients are steeper and more consistent for women than for men. In other words, educational attainment and income

Table 8.

Self-Assessed Health Status (Fair or Poor Health) among Adults Aged 18 Years and Older,
According to Selected Social, Behavioral, Functional, and Physical Characteristics: Kansas, 1993–1995

Characteristic	Both Sexes Combined (n=4,869)				Men (n=2,129)	Women (n=2,740)
	Number	Rate (Percent)	Crude Rate Ratio	Age-Adjusted Relative Risk	Age-Adjusted Relative Risk	Age-Adjusted Relative Risk
Total population	626	12.9	—	—	—	—
Age (years)						
18–24	26	5.5	1.00	1.00	1.00	1.00
25–34	61	6.1	1.11	1.10	0.77	1.37
35–44	74	6.7	1.22	1.21	1.08	1.34
45–64	166	12.9	2.35*	2.49*	3.00*	2.16*
65+	298	30.1	5.47*	7.27*	7.56*	6.98*
Sex						
Male	237	11.1	1.00	1.00	—	—
Female	389	14.2	1.28	1.10	—	—
Race/ethnicity						
Non-Hispanic White	553	12.5	1.00	1.00	1.00	1.00
Non-Hispanic Black	47	22.8	1.82*	2.88*	2.64*	2.94*
Hispanic	13	8.0	0.64	0.95	1.08	0.90
Asian	4	11.1	0.89	1.40	0.52	2.97
American Indian	8	21.6	1.73	2.29	3.03	1.81
Marital status						
Married	293	10.2	1.00	1.00	1.00	1.00
Single	66	8.3	0.81	1.68*	1.45	2.00*
Divorced/separated	93	14.7	1.44*	1.83*	2.16*	1.65*
Widowed	169	31.8	3.12*	1.47*	1.85*	1.50*
Education (years)						
<9	67	39.0	7.80*	5.34*	3.52*	7.38*
9–11	89	27.8	5.56*	5.19*	4.46*	6.07*
12	248	15.7	3.14*	2.90*	2.33*	3.50*
13–15	155	10.5	2.10*	2.25*	1.89*	2.65*
16+	66	5.0	1.00	1.00	1.00	1.00

	n	%				
Household income ($)						
<10,000	98	26.9	6.40 *	7.15 *	6.34 *	8.80 *
10,000–19,999	154	18.7	4.45 *	4.05 *	4.02 *	4.71 *
20,000–34,999	149	10.8	2.57 *	2.41 *	2.26 *	2.81 *
35,000–49,999	55	6.4	1.52 *	1.57 *	1.31 *	2.01 *
50,000+	33	4.2	1.00	1.00	1.00	1.00
Unknown	137	20.9	4.98 *	3.57 *	3.08 *	4.45 *
Employment Status						
Employed	200	6.2	1.00	1.00	1.00	1.00
Unemployed	21	18.1	2.92 *	3.77 *	4.07 *	3.64 *
Homemaker/student	49	10.6	1.71 *	1.78 *	1.71	1.93 *
Retired	292	30.5	4.92 *	2.49 *	1.80 *	3.05 *
Unable to work	64	58.2	9.39 *	16.98 *	11.02 *	21.50 *
Sedentary lifestyle						
Yes	465	16.6	2.13 *	2.03 *	2.34 *	1.89 *
No	161	7.8	1.00	1.00	1.00	1.00
Obesity (based on BMI)						
Yes	211	17.4	1.53 *	1.60 *	1.34	1.84 *
No	415	11.4	1.00	1.00	1.00	1.00
Current cigarette use						
Yes	172	16.0	1.33 *	2.14 *	2.71 *	1.84 *
No	454	12.0	1.00	1.00	1.00	1.00
Chronic drinking						
Yes	22	17.3	1.36 *	2.38 *	2.82 *	2.10 *
No	604	12.7	1.00	1.00	1.00	1.00
Health insurance						
Yes	549	12.5	1.00	1.00	1.00	1.00
No	77	15.7	1.26 *	2.57 *	2.94 *	2.34 *
Current activity limitation						
Yes	233	27.4	2.80 *	4.42 *	3.33 *	5.17 *
No	393	9.8	1.00	1.00	1.00	1.00
Diabetes						
Yes	99	41.6	3.66 *	3.93 *	4.05 *	3.79 *
No	527	11.4	1.00	1.00	1.00	1.00

Source: Kansas Behavioral Risk Factor Surveillance Systems, 1993–1995. * p<0.05.

Table 9.

Multivariate Logistic Regressions Showing Adjusted Differentials in Probability of
Self-Assessed Fair or Poor Health by Socioeconomic, Behavioral, Functional, and Physical Characteristics: Kansas, 1993–1995

Covariate	Total Population (n=4,869)		Men (n=2,129)		Women (n=2,740)	
	Odds Ratio	95% CI	Odds Ratio	95% CI	Odds Ratio	95% CI
Age (years)	1.04 *	(1.03,1.05)	1.05 *	(1.03,1.06)	1.04 *	(1.02,1.05)
Sex						
Male	1.10	(0.89,1.37)				
Female	1.00	Reference				
Race/ethnicity						
Non-Hispanic White	1.00	Reference	1.00	Reference	1.00	Reference
Non-Hispanic Black	2.00 *	(1.33,3.00)	2.27 *	(1.14,4.52)	1.75 *	(1.04,2.94)
Hispanic	0.64	(0.34,1.23)	0.74	(0.26,2.11)	0.60	(0.26,1.40)
Asian	1.84	(0.56,6.02)	0.99	(0.11,8.71)	2.74	(0.62,12.15)
American Indian	0.87	(0.34,2.23)	0.78	(0.18,3.45)	0.83	(0.23,2.98)
Other	0.49	(0.06,4.10)	4.07	(0.38,43.59)	—	—
Marital status						
Married	1.00	Reference	1.00	Reference	1.00	Reference
Single	1.29	(0.89,1.86)	1.09	(0.60,1.97)	1.72 *	(1.05,2.81)
Divorced/separated	1.41 *	(1.00,1.98)	1.75 *	(1.04,2.94)	1.31	(0.82,2.09)
Widowed	1.36	(0.98,1.89)	1.93 *	(1.04,3.60)	1.30	(0.86,1.96)
Unknown	3.29 *	(1.05,10.20)	2.54	(0.24,26.38)	3.94 *	(1.04,14.98)
Household size	1.26 *	(1.05,1.50)	1.32 *	(1.01,1.73)	1.27	(0.99,1.63)
Education (years)						
<9	2.88 *	(1.83,4.55)	1.70	(0.82,3.51)	4.40 *	(2.38,8.12)
9–11	2.41 *	(1.60,3.61)	1.69	(0.88,3.24)	3.20 *	(1.86,5.52)
12	1.87 *	(1.36,2.56)	1.41	(0.88,2.25)	2.39 *	(1.53,3.74)
13–15	1.63 *	(1.17,2.27)	1.36	(0.83,2.23)	1.98 *	(1.25,3.12)
16+	1.00	Reference	1.00	Reference	1.00	Reference

	OR	CI	OR	CI	OR	CI
Household income (dollars)						
<10,000	2.06 *	(1.23,3.46)	2.23	(0.98,5.07)	2.02	(0.95,4.29)
10,000–19,999	1.71 *	(1.08,2.69)	2.19 *	(1.16,4.10)	1.55	(0.77,3.12)
20,000–34,999	1.41	(0.92,2.16)	1.52	(0.86,2.71)	1.40	(0.72,2.73)
35,000–49,999	1.14	(0.71,1.83)	0.93	(0.49,1.79)	1.39	(0.68,2.86)
50,000+	1.00	Reference	1.00	Reference	1.00	Reference
Unknown	1.84 *	(1.17,2.91)	1.90 *	(1.00,3.59)	1.86	(0.93,3.74)
Employment status						
Employed	1.00	Reference	1.00	Reference	1.00	Reference
Unemployed	1.77 *	(1.02,3.08)	1.82	(0.77,4.30)	1.96	(0.94,4.11)
Homemaker/student	1.57 *	(1.08,2.27)	1.37	(0.42,4.53)	1.65 *	(1.09,2.49)
Retired	1.75 *	(1.26,2.44)	1.50	(0.89,2.51)	1.99 *	(1.27,3.10)
Unable to work	6.02 *	(3.77,9.60)	5.22 *	(2.40,11.39)	6.96 *	(3.84,12.62)
Health Insurance						
Yes	1.00	Reference	1.00	Reference	1.00	Reference
No	1.44 *	(1.03,2.02)	1.39	(0.84,2.30)	1.45	(0.92,2.31)
Sedentary lifestyle						
Yes	1.75 *	(1.41,2.17)	2.26 *	(1.58,3.23)	1.52 *	(1.16,2.01)
No	1.00	Reference	1.00	Reference	1.00	Reference
Obesity (based on BMI)						
Yes	1.45 *	(1.17,1.79)	1.47 *	(1.04,2.07)	1.47 *	(1.11,1.94)
No	1.00	Reference	1.00	Reference	1.00	Reference
Current cigarette use						
Yes	1.65 *	(1.30,2.09)	2.10 *	(1.45,3.03)	1.38 *	(1.01,1.91)
No	1.00	Reference	1.00	Reference	1.00	Reference
Chronic drinking						
Yes	2.13 *	(1.23,3.70)	2.71 *	(1.45,5.07)	1.14	(0.30,4.34)
No	1.00	Reference	1.00	Reference	1.00	Reference
Current activity limitation						
Yes	3.52 *	(2.83,4.40)	2.59 *	(1.78,3.76)	4.23 *	(3.19,5.60)
No	1.00	Reference	1.00	Reference	1.00	Reference
Diabetes						
Yes	3.22 *	(2.33,4.46)	4.13 *	(2.47,6.91)	2.83 *	(1.85,4.35)
No	1.00	Reference	1.00	Reference	1.00	Reference
Chi-Square	948.14 *		386.20 *		587.23 *	
df	32		31		31	

Source: Kansas Behavioral Risk Factor Surveillance Systems, 1993–1995; Notes: CI=confidence interval; * $p<0.05$.

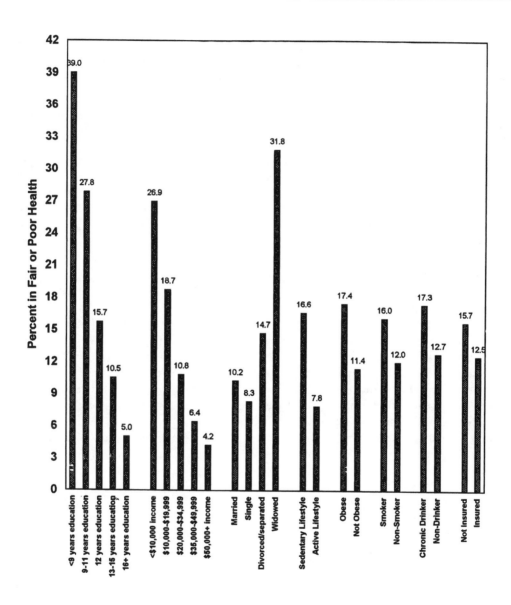

Figure 2
Self-Assessed Health Status by Social and Behavioral Characteristics: Kansas, 1993–1995

play a more significant role in women's than in men's subjective health. Employment status also plays a significant part in determining subjective health. After adjusting for age differences, the unemployed are almost 5 times as likely to rate their health as fair or poor as are employed people. Homemakers and students are about twice as likely as employed people to rate their health as fair or poor.

Table 8 also shows that the risk of assessing self health as fair or poor is substantially greater for Kansans who are obese, those lacking health care coverage, and those who smoke, drink heavily, or lead a sedentary lifestyle. After controlling for age differences, smokers, chronic drinkers, those lacking health insurance, and those leading a sedentary lifestyle are respectively over two times more likely than non-smokers, non-drinkers, the insured, and the physically active to describe their health as fair or poor.

Table 9 shows net variations in self-reported health among Kansans according to socioeconomic, behavioral, functional, and physical characteristics. The multivariate logistic regression models are presented for the total population as well as for men and women separately. As seen in Table 9, compared to their married counterparts, widowed men are more likely than widowed women to assess their health as fair or poor. Substantial education and income gradients in self-assessed health for the total population remain even after controlling for the other covariates. The higher the education and income levels, the lower the probability of assessing self health as fair or poor. However, *ceteris paribus*, education plays a very significant role in women's but not in men's subjective health, whereas income has a more powerful effect on men's than on women's subjective health. Furthermore, the risk of assessing self health as fair or poor is substantially greater for Kansans with diabetes, obesity, and activity limitation, and for those lacking health care coverage or those who report smoking, drinking heavily, or leading a sedentary lifestyle.

Recent Vitality

Tables 10 through 12 show substantial variations in recent vitality among adult Kansans according to a number of social and behavioral characteristics. The recent vitality measure obtained from the behavioral risk survey represents the average number of days during the past month the respondent felt very healthy and full of energy. An average Kansan aged 18 years or older reported feeling very healthy and full of energy approximately 19 out of the previous 30 days. People between the ages of 45–64 have, on average, 4 more days of vitality than those aged 18–24 years. Men reported feeling very healthy and full of energy 20 out of 30 days, while women reported feeling very healthy and full of energy 18 out of the past 30 days (see Table 10).

Ethnic differences in vitality are also substantial. Compared to whites, blacks and American Indians report on average 3 and 5 fewer good days respectively. The difference is very striking for American Indian men who on average report 10 fewer good days than white men (see Table 10). Those divorced or separated report almost 2 fewer good days than their currently married counterparts.

There are significant educational differences in reported vitality, which tend to be substantially larger for women than for men. Women with less than a high school education report 4 to 6 fewer good days than their college-educated counterparts. Furthermore, women who have some college education (but who did not complete their college degree) report 3 fewer days of feeling very good and energetic than women with a college degree. Household income shows a strong and consistent gradient, with those in upper income brackets reporting 6 to 7 more good days than their financially disadvantaged counterparts. Like education, income differences in vitality are substantially larger for women than for men.

Compared to the employed, homemakers and students, and unemployed individuals report 2 to

Table 10.

Recent Vitality (Mean Number of Days Feeling Very Healthy and Full of Energy During the Past Month) for Adults Aged 18 Years and Older, According to Selected Social and Behavioral Characteristics: Kansas, 1995

Characteristic	Both Sexes Combined (n=1,744)		Men (n=744)	Women (n=970)
	Mean Number of Days	Estimated Difference in Mean Number of Days (Age-Adjusted)	Estimated Difference (Age-Adjusted)	Estimated Difference (Age-Adjusted)
Total population	18.7	—	—	—
Age (years)				
18–24	16.0	Reference	Reference	Reference
25–34	17.9	1.8	2.7	1.1
35–44	18.6	2.6*	2.6*	2.3
45–64	20.3	4.2*	3.3*	4.9*
65+	19.0	3.0*	2.0*	3.9*
Sex				
Male	19.9	2.1*	—	—
Female	17.8	Reference	—	—
Race/ethnicity				
Non-Hispanic White	18.9	Reference	Reference	Reference
Non-Hispanic Black	16.0	−2.7*	−0.4	−3.8*
Hispanic	18.9	0.8	2.3	−1.6
Asian	20.1	1.6	1.6	0.4
American Indian	13.6	−5.3*	−9.6*	−1.7
Marital status				
Married	19.3	Reference	Reference	Reference
Single	17.6	0.0	−0.7	−1.7
Divorced/separated	17.7	−1.5*	−0.6	−1.7
Widowed	18.7	−1.1	−1.0	−0.9
Household size				
2 or more	19.0	1.0*	1.2	0.7
<2	18.1	Reference	Reference	Reference
Presence of children <18 years				
Yes	17.7	−1.6*	−0.9	−1.7*
No	19.4	Reference	Reference	Reference

Education (years)				
<9	18.3	−2.2	2.0	−6.1*
9–11	16.9	−3.1*	−2.0	−4.2*
12	18.5	−1.5*	−0.5	−2.7*
13–15	18.2	−1.6*	0.6	−3.2*
16+	20.0	Reference	Reference	Reference
Household income ($)				
<10,000	13.8	Reference	Reference	Reference*
10,000–19,999	18.1	4.5*	2.8	4.6
20,000–34,999	18.8	5.1*	3.2	5.4*
35,000–49,999	19.4	5.7*	2.9	6.7*
50,000+	20.4	6.5*	4.6*	6.7*
Unknown	18.6	4.5*	3.1	4.5*
Employment status				
Employed	19.3	Reference	Reference	Reference
Unemployed	14.8	−4.0*	−3.0	−3.8*
Homemaker/student	17.2	−1.5*	−1.1	−0.7
Retired	19.4	−0.8*	−2.6	0.5
Unable to work	9.3	−11.1*	−5.2	−13.8*
Sedentary lifestyle				
Yes	17.4	−3.2*	−2.2*	−4.0*
No	20.4	Reference	Reference	Reference
Obesity (based on BMI)				
Yes	17.3	−2.4*	−2.2*	−2.9*
No	19.3	Reference	Reference	Reference
Current cigarette use				
Yes	17.0	−2.2*	−1.8*	−2.9*
No	19.2	Reference	Reference	Reference
Chronic drinking				
Yes	15.8	−2.3*	−4.0*	−0.8*
No	18.8	Reference	Reference	Reference
Health insurance				
Yes	19.0	Reference	Reference	Reference
No	16.4	−2.0*	−2.1	−2.5*

Source: Kansas Behavioral Risk Factor Surveillance System Data File, 1995. * p<.05.

Table 11.

Multivariate Regressions Showing Adjusted Differentials in Recent Vitality (Mean Number of Days Feeling Very Healthy and Full of Energy) for Adults Aged 18 Years and Older, According to Selected Social and Behavioral Characteristics: Kansas, 1995 (n=1,744)

Covariate	Model 1			Model 2		
	Parameter Estimate (b)	SE(b)	p-value	Parameter Estimate (b)	SE(b)	p-value
Age (years)						
18–24						
25–34	1.994	1.043	0.056	1.821	1.031	0.078
35–44	2.652 *	1.073	0.014	2.730 *	1.081	0.012
45–64	3.541 **	1.087	0.001	4.252 **	1.094	0.000
65+	2.351	1.257	0.062	2.493	1.456	0.087
Sex						
Male	1.822	0.517	0.000	2.059 **	0.523	0.000
Female	Reference	Reference		Reference	Reference	
Race/ethnicity						
Non-Hispanic White	Reference	Reference		Reference	Reference	
Non-Hispanic Black	− 2.111	1.235	0.088	− 1.135	1.207	0.347
Hispanic	0.890	1.469	0.545	0.979	1.433	0.495
Asian	0.856	2.703	0.752	0.288	2.630	0.913
American Indian	− 4.989	2.704	0.065	− 3.212	2.644	0.225
Other	− 0.341	3.741	0.927	− 0.630	3.661	0.863
Marital status						
Married	Reference	Reference		Reference	Reference	
Single	− 0.857	0.886	0.334	− 0.343	0.877	0.696
Divorced/separated	− 1.113	0.825	0.177	− 0.193	0.832	0.817
Widowed	− 0.010	1.084	0.992	0.552	1.067	0.605
Unknown	− 1.580	2.998	0.598	− 0.656	2.925	0.823
Household size	0.209	0.453	0.644	− 0.075	0.450	0.867
Presence of children <18 years						
Yes	− 1.663 *	0.658	0.012	− 1.607 *	0.642	0.012
No	Reference	Reference		Reference	Reference	

Education (years)						
<9	−1.752	1.813	0.334	−0.106	1.788	0.953
9–11	−2.563 *	1.139	0.025	0.170	1.158	0.883
12	−1.228	0.651	0.059	0.252	0.670	0.707
13–15	−1.149	0.660	0.082	−0.217	0.660	0.742
16+	Reference	Reference			Reference	
Household income ($)						
<10,000					Reference	
10,000–19,999				3.184 **	1.114	0.004
20,000–34,999				3.183 **	1.077	0.003
35,000–49,999				3.239 **	1.204	0.007
50,000+				3.399 **	1.242	0.006
Unknown				2.765 *	1.208	0.022
Employment status						
Employed					Reference	
Unemployed				−1.968	1.663	0.237
Homemaker/student				−0.458	0.887	0.606
Retired				−0.480	1.067	0.653
Unable to work				−9.386 **	1.600	0.000
Sedentary lifestyle						
Yes				−2.782 **	0.504	0.000
No					Reference	
Obesity (based on BMI)						
Yes				−2.169 **	0.550	0.000
No					Reference	
Current cigarette use						
Yes				−1.436 *	0.618	0.020
No					Reference	
Chronic drinking						
Yes				−2.862	1.464	0.051
No					Reference	
Health insurance						
Yes					Reference	
No				−1.026	0.843	0.224
Intercept	17.104 **	1.589	0.000	16.132 **	1.838	0.000
R^2	0.038 **			0.102 **		
df	20			34		

Source: Kansas Behavioral Risk Factor Surveillance System Data File, 1995. * $p<0.05$. ** $p<0.01$.

Table 12.

Multivariate Regressions Showing Adjusted Differentials in Recent Vitality (Mean Number of Days Feeling Very Healthy and Full of Energy) for Men and Women Aged 18 Years and Older, According to Selected Social and Behavioral Characteristics: Kansas, 1995

Covariate	Men (n=744)			Women (n=970)		
	Parameter Estimate (b)	SE(b)	p-value	Parameter Estimate (b)	SE(b)	p-value
Age (years)						
18–24	Reference			Reference		
25–34	2.051	1.677	0.222	1.183	1.357	0.384
35–44	1.860	1.762	0.291	2.716 *	1.409	0.054
45–64	2.515	1.791	0.161	5.293 **	1.425	0.000
65+	1.797	2.383	0.451	2.912	1.881	0.122
Race/ethnicity						
Non-Hispanic White	Reference			Reference		
Non-Hispanic Black	0.021	2.012	0.992	− 1.667	1.507	0.269
Hispanic	3.279	2.005	0.102	− 1.978	2.086	0.343
Asian	1.144	3.317	0.730	0.914	4.468	0.838
American Indian	− 7.084	4.037	0.080	0.670	3.584	0.852
Other	− 1.557	5.505	0.777	0.091	5.156	0.986
Marital status						
Married	Reference			Reference		
Single	− 1.188	1.304	0.363	0.225	1.212	0.853
Divorced/separated	− 0.510	1.342	0.704	0.048	1.088	0.965
Widowed	− 0.550	2.244	0.806	0.130	1.304	0.921
Unknown	0.682	6.305	0.914	− 0.926	3.306	.0780
Household size	0.019	0.668	0.978	− 0.399	0.627	0.525
Presence of children <18 years						
Yes	− 1.633	0.963	0.090	− 1.388	0.907	0.126
No		Reference			Reference	
Education (years)						
<9	3.063	2.713	0.259	− 3.456	2.416	0.153
9–11	0.844	1.895	0.656	− 0.613	1.495	0.682
12	1.057	1.000	0.291	− 0.861	0.929	0.354
13–15	1.786	1.014	0.079	− 2.026 *	0.890	0.023
16+		Reference			Reference	

	Coef.			Coef.		
Household income ($)						
<10,000		Reference			Reference	
10,000–19,999	1.941	2.172	0.372	3.585 **	1.319	0.007
20,000–34,999	1.478	2.092	0.480	3.958 **	1.280	0.002
35,000–49,999	1.423	2.207	0.519	4.469 **	1.509	0.003
50,000+	2.492	2.245	0.267	3.722 *	1.581	0.019
Unknown	2.042	2.295	0.374	2.999 *	1.446	0.038
Employment status						
Employed		Reference			Reference	
Unemployed	– 2.752	2.979	0.356	– 1.033	2.056	0.615
Homemaker/student	– 1.688	2.156	0.434	0.324	0.995	0.745
Retired	– 2.708	1.705	0.113	1.309	1.381	0.344
Unable to work	– 4.176	2.781	0.134	– 11.844 **	1.967	0.000
Sedentary lifestyle						
Yes	– 2.153 **	0.787	0.006	– 3.415 **	0.665	0.000
No		Reference			Reference	
Obesity (based on BMI)						
Yes	– 2.298 **	0.819	0.005	– 2.043 **	0.750	0.007
No		Reference			Reference	
Current cigarette use						
Yes	– 1.463	0.932	0.117	– 1.400	0.844	0.098
No		Reference			Reference	
Chronic drinking						
Yes	– 3.421 *	1.638	0.037	– 1.330	4.171	0.750
No		Reference			Reference	
Health insurance						
Yes		Reference			Reference	
No	– 1.511	1.205	0.210	– 0.859	1.203	0.475
Intercept	19.431 **	3.101	0.000	16.775 **	2.351	0.000
R²	0.070 **			0.150 **		
df	33			33		

Source: Kansas Behavioral Risk Factor Surveillance System Data File, 1995. * p<0.05; ** p<0.01.

4 fewer good days. Not surprisingly, those engaged in unhealthy behaviors such as smoking, drinking, physical inactivity, and obesity have at least 2 fewer good days than their counterparts with a healthier lifestyle. Those lacking health insurance are expected to report 2 fewer good days than those with health care coverage.

Tables 11 and 12 show net variations in recent vitality according to socioeconomic and lifestyle characteristics. Model 1 in Table 11 shows significant educational differentials in vitality, after adjusting for age, sex, race/ethnicity, marital status, and household size and composition. Occupation and income were not controlled in this model, because education is antecedent to both. Model 2 in Table 11 shows the adjusted effect of household income, after controlling for education, occupation, and all other covariates in Model 1. Table 12 shows significantly lower levels of vitality among men who are obese, drink heavily, or those who lead a sedentary lifestyle; however, no significant differences in vitality among men remain according to age, race/ethnicity, marital status, education, occupation, and income. For women, on the other hand, age, education, occupation, income, obesity, and sedentary lifestyle differences in vitality remain significant and quite pronounced.

Prevalence of Diabetes

Prevalence of diagnosed diabetes in Kansas and associated socioeconomic and behavioral risk factors are shown in Tables 13 and 14. Five percent of Kansans report having been told by a doctor that they have diabetes, compared with 4.4 percent for the United States (the national median) and 2.5 percent for Montana. The risk of diabetes increases rapidly with increasing age, especially among men aged 45 years and older. After controlling for age differences, Hispanics and blacks report twice the risk of diabetes as whites (see Table 13). Similarly, after adjusting for age differences, those with less than 9 years of schooling have twice the risk of diabetes as those

with at least a college degree. Although there is not a consistent income gradient, those with household incomes less than $35,000 report almost 3 times higher risk of diabetes than those with incomes over $50,000. Not surprisingly, the risk of diabetes is increased two-fold among those who are obese.

Table 14 presents the results of the multivariate logistic regressions, showing net associations between socio-behavioral characteristics and the risk of diabetes among Kansans aged 18 years and older. Adjusting for socioeconomic factors reduced or eliminated significant racial, marital status, and education differentials in diabetes. Income and obesity, however, remained significant risk factors for diabetes even after controlling for the effects of other factors. *Ceteris paribus*, men with household incomes of less than $50,000 were 3 to 4 times more likely to report having diabetes than their counterparts with an income of $50,000 or more. The risk of diabetes was 74% higher for obese men and 146% higher for obese women compared to their non-obese counterparts.

SUMMARY AND CONCLUSIONS

THE evidence presented in this study indicates consistent and substantial improvements in the overall health of Kansans during the course of the twentieth century, particularly with respect to increases in life expectancy and reductions in overall mortality. However, the gains in these health measures have been relatively modest during the past several decades. Moreover, despite the overall improvement, racial and ethnic disparities in health and well-being do not appear to have diminished. Black Kansans continue to experience significantly poorer health than their white counterparts, as evidenced by their lower life expectancy, higher rates of infant mortality, and mortality from such major causes of death as heart disease, stroke, cancer, diabetes, liver cirrhosis, pneumonia and influenza, HIV/AIDS, homicide, and unintentional injuries.

Table 13.

Prevalence of Diabetes among Adults Aged 18 Years and Older, According to Selected Social and Behavioral Characteristics: Kansas, 1993–1995

Characteristic	Both Sexes Combined (n=4,882)				Men (n=2,135)	Women (n=2,747)
	Number	Rate (Percent)	Crude Rate Ratio	Age-Adjusted Relative Risk	Age-Adjusted Relative Risk	Age-Adjusted Relative Risk
Total population	243	5.0	—	—	—	—
Age (years)						
18–24	8	1.7	1.00	1.00	1.00	1.00
25–34	22	2.2	1.29	1.34	3.67	1.02
35–44	24	2.2	1.29	1.32	4.54	0.86
45–64	80	6.2	3.65	3.92*	11.49*	2.83*
65+	109	10.9	6.41	7.26*	33.53*	3.91*
Sex						
Male	96	5.4	1.20	0.97	—	—
Female	147	4.5	1.00	1.00	—	—
Race/ethnicity						
Non-Hispanic White	216	4.9	1.00	1.00	1.00	1.00
Non-Hispanic Black	15	7.3	1.49	1.88*	1.30	2.10*
Hispanic	10	6.1	1.25	1.88*	1.71	2.09
Asian	—	—	—	—	—	—
American Indian	2	5.4	1.10	1.23	1.44	1.02
Marital status						
Married	139	4.8	1.00	1.00	1.00	1.00
Single	15	1.9	0.53	0.70	0.58	0.88
Divorced/separated	39	6.1	1.27	1.50*	1.01	1.83*
Widowed	47	8.7	1.81	0.76	0.63	0.97
Education (years)						
<9	23	13.1	3.85	2.00*	1.80	2.23*
9–11	20	6.3	1.85	1.29	1.35	1.28
12	90	5.7	1.68	1.41	1.10	1.67*
13–15	65	4.4	1.29	1.30	1.04	1.52
16+	45	3.4	1.00	1.00	1.00	1.00

Household income ($)						
<10,000	22	6.0	3.16	2.62*	2.65	2.30*
10,000–19,999	57	6.9	3.63	2.98*	3.61*	2.49*
20,000–34,999	75	5.4	2.84	2.64*	3.54*	2.05*
35,000–49,999	24	2.8	1.47	1.48*	3.41*	0.52
50,000+	15	1.9	1.00	1.00	1.00	1.00
Unknown	50	7.6	4.00	2.65*	3.43*	2.15
Employment status						
Employed	101	3.1	1.00	1.00	1.00	1.00
Unemployed	6	5.2	1.67	1.86	1.84	1.77
Homemaker/student	16	3.4	1.10	1.08	—	1.07
Retired	103	10.7	3.45	1.47	1.86	1.21
Unable to work	17	15.3	4.94	4.24*	2.92	4.67*
Sedentary lifestyle						
Yes	146	5.2	1.11	0.95	0.80	1.09
No	97	4.7	1.00	1.00	1.00	1.00
Obesity (based on BMI)						
Yes	102	8.4	2.15	2.21*	1.75*	2.70*
No	141	3.9	1.00	1.00	1.00	1.00
Current cigarette use						
Yes	52	4.9	0.98	1.29	1.29	1.31
No	191	5.0	1.00	1.00	1.00	1.00

Source: Kansas Behavioral Risk Factor Surveillance Systems, 1993–1995. * $p < 0.05$.

Table 14.

Multivariate Logistic Regressions Showing Adjusted Differentials in the Risk of Diabetes among Adults Aged 18 Years and Older, According to Selected Social and Behavioral Characteristics: Kansas, 1993–1995

Covariate	Both Sexes Combined (n=4,882)			Men (n=2,135)			Women (n=2,747)		
	Odds Ratio	95% CI Lower	Upper	Odds Ratio	95% CI Lower	Upper	Odds Ratio	95% CI Lower	Upper
Age (years)	1.03*	1.02	1.05	1.04*	1.02	1.06	1.03*	1.01	1.04
Sex									
Male	0.97	0.72	1.29	—	—	—	—	—	—
Female	1.00	Reference		—	—	—	—	—	—
Race/ethnicity									
Non-Hispanic White	1.00	Reference		1.00	Reference		1.00	Reference	
Non-Hispanic Black	1.63	0.91	2.89	1.31	0.44	3.91	1.65	0.83	3.30
Hispanic	1.73	0.87	3.43	1.59	0.46	5.52	1.83	0.79	4.24
Asian	—	—	—	—	—	—	—	—	—
American Indian	0.90	0.21	3.95	1.30	0.15	11.03	0.72	0.09	5.68
Other	—	—	—	—	—	—	—	—	—
Marital status									
Married	1.00	Reference		1.00	Reference		1.00	Reference	
Single	0.57	0.32	1.04	0.55	0.20	1.49	0.70	0.33	1.50
Divorced/separated	1.28	0.81	2.03	0.93	0.42	2.08	1.53	0.85	2.75
Widowed	0.73	0.45	1.17	0.74	0.29	1.86	0.92	0.51	1.65
Unknown	2.85	0.78	10.39	3.99	0.43	36.90	2.65	0.53	13.15
Household size	1.20	0.92	1.55	1.20	0.79	1.83	1.23	0.87	1.74
Education (years)									
<9	1.41	0.78	2.52	1.39	0.57	3.39	1.50	0.68	3.33
9–11	0.74	0.41	1.34	0.83	0.34	2.02	0.70	0.31	1.56
12	0.98	0.66	1.46	0.76	0.42	1.39	1.13	0.66	1.93
13–15	0.98	0.65	1.48	0.79	0.42	1.50	1.10	0.64	1.90
16+	1.00	Reference		1.00	Reference		1.00	Reference	

Variable	Model 1 OR	95% CI	Model 2 OR	95% CI	Model 3 OR	95% CI
Household income ($)						
<10,000	2.12	0.99 – 4.56	2.47	0.59 – 10.39	1.54	0.60 – 3.97
10,000–19,999	2.77 *	1.47 – 5.25	3.94 *	1.42 – 10.95	1.99	0.87 – 4.53
20,000–34,999	2.58 *	1.43 – 4.66	3.65 *	1.44 – 9.25	1.85	0.86 – 3.98
35,000–49,999	1.41	0.73 – 2.75	3.60 *	1.38 – 9.40	0.48	0.17 – 1.38
50,000+	1.00	Reference	1.00	Reference	1.00	Reference
Unknown	2.64 *	1.39 – 5.00	3.59 *	1.30 – 9.92	1.99	0.87 – 4.53
Employment status						
Employed	1.00	Reference	1.00	Reference	1.00	Reference
Unemployed	1.63	0.68 – 3.91	1.52	0.33 – 6.86	1.53	0.51 – 4.57
Homemaker/student	1.02	0.58 – 1.80	—	—	0.98	0.54 – 1.78
Retired	1.40	0.89 – 2.18	1.75	0.88 – 3.51	1.16	0.64 – 2.09
Unable to work	3.42 *	1.87 – 6.25	2.69	0.85 – 8.49	3.33 *	1.60 – 6.93
Sedentary lifestyle						
Yes	0.87	0.66 – 1.15	0.76	0.49 – 1.18	0.96	0.67 – 1.37
No	1.00	Reference	1.00	Reference	1.00	Reference
Obesity (based on BMI)						
Yes	2.15 *	1.63 – 2.82	1.74 *	1.11 – 2.72	2.46 *	1.72 – 3.52
No	1.00	Reference	1.00	Reference	1.00	Reference
Current cigarette use						
Yes	1.24	0.88 – 1.75	1.39	0.81 – 2.39	1.17	0.75 – 1.84
No	1.00	Reference	1.00	Reference	1.00	Reference
Chi-Square	201.40 *		112.11 *		114.87 *	
df	26		25		25	

Source: Kansas Behavioral Risk Factor Surveillance Systems, 1993–1995. Notes: CI=confidence interval; * p<0.05.

Undoubtedly, significant improvements in Kansans' health would occur if racial and ethnic disparities in social capital as well as in access to social and economic resources were to be reduced.

Interstate and national comparisons on several health indicators (including life expectancy and mortality from several major causes of death) suggest that Kansans, on average, enjoy somewhat better health than their national counterparts. However, compared with some of its Midwestern neighbors (e.g., Iowa, North and South Dakota, Nebraska, and Minnesota) and New England states (e.g., Maine, New Hampshire, Vermont, Massachusetts, and Connecticut), Kansas does not fare as well. Health status also varies widely across the 105 Kansas counties. Nemaha, Washington, Mitchell, Chase and Sheridan counties generally have the highest levels of overall health in the state, while Wyandotte, Geary, Seward, Finney, and Sedgwick counties rank among the bottom in overall health (Singh, Wilkinson, Song et al. 1998).

The data presented here generally show substantial socioeconomic gradients in health, morbidity, and mortality among Kansans. Consistent with patterns observed nationally as well as in other industrialized countries, the empirical relationship between socioeconomic status and health is shown here to be not bipolar (i.e., the rich have better health than the poor). Rather, a graded relationship is found both at the individual and ecological levels. That is, as we move along the socioeconomic continuum, we see a corresponding improvement in health and mortality. For instance, people with a college degree enjoy significantly better health than those with some college education (but without a college diploma), who in turn enjoy better health than those who only have a high school education or less.

Although the present study uses a multivariate analytic strategy to measure the independent effects and complex interactions of various social and behavioral factors in determining health, morbidity, and mortality, a great deal of work remains to be done. Only a few measures of health are analyzed in this paper. Substantial gaps in data on health and morbidity measures remain, especially those on functional status and well-being, number of sick and work-loss days, loss of productivity, bed disability days, school absences or school-loss days, and so on. Community-level data on these health measures, especially at the county-level, are even more difficult to obtain. While national statistics on the prevalence of various diseases and morbidities can be derived from the U.S. National Health Interview Survey, there is no equivalent data system in Kansas. There is clearly a need to expand the scope of the existing annual sample surveys in the state (e.g., the Behavioral Risk Factor Surveillance System and the Kansas Poll) by adding additional questions on educational opportunity and aspirations, job security, social networks, social support, community solidarity, social integration and cohesion, sense of control over one's life, degree of autonomy and participation in the decision-making process in the home and the workplace, civic and political participation, and a number of other important social factors considered vital in understanding the mechanisms through which health inequalities are generated. Alternatively, new periodic statewide surveys, developed as a hybrid between the National Health Interview Survey and the National Opinion Research Center's General Social Survey (Davis and Smith 1996), may be carried out, which can provide data on a wide range of health and health care characteristics along with information on relevant social, cultural, psychological, economic, political, and environmental factors. Furthermore, a comprehensive social indicator program in Kansas can be established which can provide time-trend data on a wide array of social, economic, behavioral, health, and health care indicators at the state, county, and local levels. Record- and multi-level linkages of existing administrative health data sources (e.g., vital statistics, hospital discharge, and cancer registry) with census-based socioeconomic, demographic and environmental data may also be necessary in order to effectively measure the impact of macro-social structures and processes on individual health behaviors and health outcomes.

Substantial social differences in health and mortality documented here raise interesting research questions regarding the direct and indirect mechanisms through which social factors influence health. To what extent do changes in the social and economic environment of individuals and communities contribute to changes in individual and population health, independent of behavioral and medical care influences? How do macro societal factors such as educational and economic systems, income inequality, acculturation, and social segregation shape and constrain individual behaviors and use of medical services? How do we go about measuring the health impact of personal behaviors or medical care in the context of the larger social environment? Would the gains in health be any larger if we invested more in trying to improve people's social conditions, educational opportunities, and access to preventive health services than on high-technology medical care for a limited few? These are some of the key policy questions that we need to address as we continue to further advance our understanding of the determinants of health and mortality at the local and national levels.

REFERENCES

Adams, P. F., Marano, M. A. Current Estimates from the National Health Interview Survey, 1994. *Vital and Health Statistics* 10 (193): 1–520. (Hyattsville, MD: National Center for Health Statistics, 1995).

Amick, B. C., Levine, S., Tarlov, A. R., Walsh, D. C. (eds). *Society and Health.* (New York: Oxford University Press, 1995).

Anderson, R. N., Kochanek, K. D., Murphy, S. L. Report of Final Mortality Statistics, 1995. *Monthly Vital Statistics Report* 45 (11), supplement 2:1–80; 1997.

Blane, D., Brunner, E., and Wilkinson, R. G. (eds). *Health and Social Organization.* London and New York: Routledge Press; 1996.

Blane, D. Social Determinants of Health: Socioeconomic Status, Social Class, and Ethnicity. *American Journal of Public Health.* 85 (7): 903–905; 1995.

Bureau of Health Professions. *The Area Resource File (ARF), Public Use File Technical Documentation.* MD: Health Resources and Services Administration; 1997.

Centers for Disease Control and Prevention. *Kansas Health Profile, 1996*; 1996.

Cox, D. R. Regression models and life tables (with discussion). *J Royal Stat Soc.* 1972;40(B34):184–220.

Davis, J. A., Smith, T. W. *General Social Surveys, 1972–1996: Cumulative Databook.* Chicago: National Opinion Research Center; 1996.

Evans, R. G., Barer, M. L., Marmor, T. R. (eds). *Why Are Some People Healthy and Others Not? The Determinants of Health of Populations.* New York: Gruyter Press; 1994.

Hertzman, C., Kelly, S., Bobak, M. (eds). *East-West Life Expectancy Gap in Europe: Environmental and Non-Environmental Determinants.* Dordrecht, The Netherlands: Kluwer Academic Publishers; 1996.

Hoyert, D. L., Singh, G. K., Rosenberg, H. M. Sources of Data on Socioeconomic Differential Mortality in the United States. *Journal of Official Statistics, Statistics Sweden.* 1995; 11(3): 233–260.

Kposowa, A. J., Singh, G. K. The effects of marital status and social isolation on adult male homicides in the United States: evidence from the National Longitudinal Mortality Study. *J Quant Criminology.* 1994;10(3):277–289.

Jiobu, R. M. *Ethnicity and Inequality.* Albany, NY: State University of New York Press; 1990.

Kansas Department of Health and Environment. *Health Risk Behaviors of Kansans, 1992 to 1995.* Topeka, Kansas. 1997.

Kansas Department of Health and Environment. *Kansas Behavioral Risk Factor Surveillance System, 1992 to 1995 (Machine-Readable Data Files).* Topeka, Kansas; 1997.

Link, B. G., Phelan, J. C. Understanding the Sociodemographic Differences in Health: The Role of Fundamental Social Causes. *Am J Public Health.* 1996; 86 (4): 471–473.

Namboodiri, K. *Demographic Analysis: A Stochastic Approach.* San Diego and London: Academic Press; 1991.

Namboodiri, K., Suchindran, C. M. *Life Table Techniques and Their Applications.* Orlando, Fla: Academic Press; 1987.

National Longitudinal Mortality Study, 1979-89: Public Use File Documentation, Release 2. Bethesda, Md: National Heart, Lung and Blood Institute; 1995.

Pappas, G., Queen, S., Hadden, W., and Fisher, G. The Increasing Disparity in Mortality Between Socioeconomic Groups in the United States. *N Eng J Med.* 1993; 329: 103–109.

Powell-Griner, E., Anderson, J. E., Murphy, W. State- and Sex-Specific Prevalence of Selected Characteristics–Behavioral Risk Factor Surveillance System, 1994 and 1995. *MMWR.* 1997; 46 (SS-3):1–31.

Rogot, E., Sorlie, P. D., Johnson, N. J., and Schmitt, C. *A Mortality Study of 1.3 Million Persons by Demographic, Social, and Economic Factors, 1979-85 Follow-Up: U.S. National Longitudinal Mortality Study.* Washington, DC: Public Health Service; 1992. NIH publication 92–3297.

SAS Institute, Inc. *SAS/STAT Software: The PHREG Procedure, Version 6.* Cary, NC:SAS Institute; 1991.

SAS Institute, Inc. *SAS/STAT User's Guide: The LOGISTIC Procedure, Version 6.* 4th ed. Cary, NC:SAS Institute; 1989;2.

Singh, G. K., Wilkinson, A. V., Song, F. F., Rose, T. P., Adrian, M., Fonner, E., and Tarlov, A. R. *Health and Social Factors in Kansas: A Data and Chartbook, 1997-98.* Kansas Health Institute. Lawrence: KS: Allen Press; 1998.

Singh, G. K. Perinatal Health in Kansas: Social Differentials and Inequalities. *Kansas Health.* 1997; 1 (1):3.

Singh, G. K., Kposowa, A. J. Occupation-Specific Earnings Attainment of Asian Indians and Whites in the United States: Gender and Nativity Differentials Across Class Strata. *Appl Behav Sci Rev.* 1996; 4 (2):137–175.

Singh, G. K., Kochanek, K. D, and MacDorman, M. M. Advance Report of Final Mortality Statistics, 1994. *Monthly Vital Statistics Report.* 1996; 45 (3), supplement: 1–80.

Singh, G. K., Yu, S. M. US Childhood Mortality, 1950 through 1993: Trends and Socioeconomic Differentials. *Am J Public Health.* 1996; 86: 505–512.

Singh, G. K., Yu, S. M. Infant Mortality in the United States: Trends, Differentials, and Projections, 1950 through 2010. *Am J Public Health.* 1995; 85: 957–964.

Singh, G. K., Mathews, T. J., Clarke, S. C., Yannicos, T., and Smith, B. L. Annual Summary of Births, Marriages, Divorces, and Deaths: United States, 1994. *Monthly Vital Statistics Report.* 1995; 43 (13):1–44.

Singh, G. K., Kposowa, A. J. A comparative analysis of infant mortality in major Ohio cities: significance of sociobiological factors. *Appl Behav Sci Rev.* 1994;2(1):77–94.

Social Science and Medicine. Special Issue. Health Inequalities in Modern Societies and Beyond. Volume 44, Number 6. Great Britain: Pergamon; 1997.

Sommer, K. J. *Annual Summary of Vital Statistics of Kansas, 1996.* Kansas Department of Health and Environment. Topeka, Kansas; 1998.

Sorlie, P. D, Backlund, E., and Keller, J. B. US mortality by economic, demographic, and social characteristics: the National Longitudinal Mortality Study. *Am J Public Health.* 1995; 85:949–956.

Stambler, H. V. The Area Resource File–A Brief Look. *Public Health Rep.* 1988; 103:184–188.

Townsend, P., Davidson, N., and Whitehead, M. *Inequalities in Health.* London: Penguin; 1988.

Ventura, S. J., Martin, J. A., Curtin, S. C., and Mathews, T. J. Report of Final Natality Statistics, 1995. *Monthly Vital Statistics Report.* 1997; 45 (11), supplement:1–84.

Wilkinson, R. G. *Unhealthy Societies: The Afflictions of Inequality.* London and New York: Routledge Press; 1996.

Wilkinson, R. G. (ed). *Class and Health: Research and Longitudinal Data.* New York: Tavistock; 1986.

Williams, D. R., Collins, C. US Socioeconomic and Racial Differences in Health: Patterns and Explanations. *Ann Rev Sociol.* 1995; 21: 349–386.

Three

SOCIAL COHESION AND HEALTH

Ichiro Kawachi

Introduction

WHY are some communities healthier than others? For some time, social scientists have been aware of the enormous heterogeneity that exists in the well-being of communities within a single society. Thus some communities seem to prosper, possess effective political institutions, have law-abiding and healthy citizens, while other communities do not. Similarly, there is heterogeneity in well-being across states and regions within a single country, and even wider variations in cross-national comparisons. Until relatively recently, the standard epidemiological approach to explain such variations has tended to focus on individual differences. Instead of inquiring "Why are some societies healthier than others?", epidemiologists have asked "Why are some *individuals* healthy and others are not?" Implicit in such an approach is the view that communities are unhealthy because the individuals living within them have poor health habits, have genetic susceptibility to disease, or lack access to decent health care. But what if the determinants of variations between individuals are different from the determinants of variations between populations? In other words, can we identify characteristics of the social environment— i.e., *ecological* characteristics—that can promote or damage health, and yet are irreducible to the choices made by individuals?

Epidemiologists are trained to avoid the use of ecological variables, mainly because ecological analyses (the use of ecological variables to predict individual outcomes) is prone to the so-called ecological fallacy. But as Marmot[1] and others[2,3] have pointed out, "perhaps we should turn this fallacy on its head and argue that analyses of individual risks may be subject to the atomistic fallacy: analyses at the individual level may be inappropriate if we are seeking to determine social environmental causes of illness." Happily, a small but growing group of epidemiologists are beginning to apply this approach to practice. In response to the question "Why are some communities healthier than others?", epidemiologists are turning toward concepts developed in other disciplines, such as sociology and political science, where the influence of collective forces on individuals has always been taken seriously.

Emerging examples of ecological characteristics that hold promise in explaining population variations in health status include income

Paper prepared for the Proceedings of the Kansas Conference on Health and Its Determinants April 20–21, 1998, Wichita, Kansas.

inequality,[4-6] residential segregation,[7] [8] and social cohesion.[9] Each of these is an example of what Susser[2] referred to as obligate ecological variables, i.e., they are characteristics of groups, and cannot be reduced to properties of individuals. It makes no sense to talk about income inequality, residential segregation, or social cohesion measured at the individual level. Moreover, whether the community to which the individual belongs is segregated or socially cohesive depends to a large extent on the choices made by others. Identical individuals might therefore experience quite divergent health outcomes depending on the characteristics of the social environment in which they grow up and live. Proof of the existence of such "contextual effects" on health outcomes is one of the major tasks confronting those who investigate the social environment.

The purpose of the present chapter is to summarize research on one such area of active inquiry, viz., the relationship between social cohesion and health. To dispel any ambiguity that we are talking about a *societal* characteristic, the theoretical exposition will focus on a specific aspect of social cohesion: *civil society*, and its related concept, *social capital*.

CIVIL SOCIETY AND SOCIAL CAPITAL

THE concept of "civil society" (or "civic culture") has been talked about by political theorists for a long time. As described by Ralf Dahrendorf[10]:

"The term 'civil society' is more suggestive than precise. It suggests, for example, that people behave towards each other in a civilized manner; the suggestion is fully intended. It also suggests that its members enjoy the status of citizens, which again is intended. However, the core meaning of the concept is quite precise. Civil society describes the associations in which we conduct our lives, and that owe their existence to our needs and initiatives rather than to the state."

In other words, civil society is defined as that zone between the individual and the state, which is occupied by a crisscrossing network of voluntary associations. In turn, the web of social ties created by voluntary associations acts as the social glue that binds society together. Ever since Tocqueville,[11] a variety of advantages have been claimed for civil society, such as keeping individuals from becoming isolated, protecting them from the state, meeting needs that cannot be filled by government, and encouraging more active engagement in the life of the community whilst preserving a degree of choice. Theorists of civil society have further asserted that, by facilitating collective action, voluntary associations foster the economic development of communities, as well as the smooth functioning of representative democracy.[12-14]

More recently, the concept of *social capital* has been introduced to describe the kinds of resources that are potentially available to members who belong to a civil society. Social capital, as defined by its principal exponents,[15-17] consists of those features of social organization—such as networks of secondary associations, high levels of interpersonal trust, and norms of reciprocity—that facilitate collective action for mutual benefit. By definition, social capital is not a single entity, but can take a variety of forms. In principle, social capital describes any aspect of social relations that could serve as a resource for the achievement of desired ends. By definition, a civil society is one that is rich in stocks of social capital.

Although use of the term "social capital" can be traced back as early as 1961 (when Jane Jacobs[18] first used it in her classic treatise on urban planning), the more recent revival of interest in the concept was sparked by the publication of a book, *Making Democracy Work* (1993),[16] by political scientist Robert D. Putnam. The purpose of Putnam's 20-year study was to attempt to explain variations in the performance of local governments across twenty regions of Italy. The performance of civic institutions in each region of Italy was assessed by surveys, in-depth interviews, and a diverse set of policy indicators selected to gauge institutional responsiveness to constituents as well as their efficiency in conducting the public's business. The striking conclusion of Putnam's study was that the extent of civil society—as measured by stocks of social capital in each region—was the best predictor of the performance of regional government. In northern Italy, where citizens actively participate in civic associations—choral societies, soccer leagues, literary guilds and the like—regional governments were more "efficient in their internal operation, creative in their policy initiatives, and effective in implementing those initiatives."[16, p.81] By contrast, in southern Italy, where patterns of civic engagement were much weaker, local government tended to be corrupt and inefficient. Putnam explained his findings in terms of the way social capital enables citizens to cooperate with each other for mutual benefit, and hence overcome the dilemmas of collective action. Citizens living in areas characterized by high levels of social capital were more likely to trust their fellow citizens, and to value solidarity and equality. By contrast, social relations in regions with low social capital were characterized by proverbs such as "Damned is he who trusts another," "Don't make loans, don't give gifts, don't do good, for it will turn out bad for you," and "When you see the house of your neighbor on fire, carry water to your own."[16, p.144] In short, Putnam's research appeared to provide support for the view presented more than a half century earlier by Emile Durkheim:[19]

> "A nation can be maintained only if, between the State and the individual, there is interspersed a whole series of secondary groups near enough to the individuals to attract them strongly in their sphere of action and drag them, in this way, into the general torrent of social life."

What lessons, if any, can we in public health glean from Italy?

SOCIAL CAPITAL AND PUBLIC HEALTH

PUBLIC health researchers have been aware for some time that social cohesion and social integration are crucial for the maintenance of public health.[20] In what is perhaps the earliest example of ecological analysis, Durkheim[21] compared suicide statistics in European countries across time and space, and concluded that the lowest rates of suicide occurred in societies exhibiting the highest degrees of social integration, whether in domestic settings (low rates of divorce and widowhood), or as measured by the extent of religious affiliation or "collective sentiments" roused during political upheavals. Conversely, an excess of suicides occurred in societies undergoing various forms of dislocation and loosening of social bonds. Most importantly, whereas individuals at risk of committing suicide came and went, the *social suicide rate* in each society remained relatively stable—evidence of the power of social forces in shaping this phenomenon. In one of his most memorable passages, Durkheim concluded that:

> ". . . The social suicide-rate can be explained only sociologically. At any given moment the moral constitution of society establishes the contingent of voluntary deaths. There is, therefore, for each people a collective force of a definite amount of energy, impelling men to self-destruction. The victim's act which at first seem to express only his personal temperament are really the supplement and prolongation of a social condition which they express externally . . .

> "To explain his detachment from life the individual accuses his most immediately surrounding circumstances; life is sad to him because he is sad. Of course his sadness comes from him without in one sense, however not from one or another incident of his career *but rather from the group to which he belongs.*"[21, p. 299, emphasis added]

Studies using modern epidemiological methods have repeatedly corroborated Durkheim's original hypothesis that socially isolated *individuals* are at much higher risk of committing suicide (for example, see Kawachi et al.[22]; also chapter by

Lisa Berkman in this volume). Unfortunately, by focusing on individuals as the unit of analysis, modern epidemiology has tended to neglect Durkheim's more profound contribution, which was to approach society (as opposed to individuals) as the proper unit of analysis. In his treatise on the rules of sociological method, Durkheim contended: "The group thinks, feels and acts entirely differently from the way its members would if they were isolated. If therefore we begin by studying these members separately, we will understand nothing about what is taking place in the group." [23, p. 129] In other words, if we wish to understand what keeps some societies healthy yet others sick, then we had better search among social facts for explanations.

Empirical research linking social capital to health is still at a nascent stage. Nonetheless, three lines of evidence can be adduced: the case study approach; the ecological study; and the mixed-level study. Each of these is discussed in turn.

The Case Study Approach

The case study approach is the most qualitative, and the most susceptible to alternative explanations. Be that as it may, the most frequently cited case study of the effects of social cohesion on health is the example of the rural Pennsylvania community of Roseto.[24][25] Roseto (population 1,600) was first settled by immigrants from the same Italian village in 1882. In 1962, Stewart Wolf and colleagues launched a study in this town, intrigued by the observation that the mortality rate from heart attack in Roseto was 50% lower than in neighboring communities. The health advantage of Rosetans posed a medical paradox, since they smoked at the same rate as residents of neighboring towns, were just as overweight and sedentary, and their diet consisted of about the same amount of animal fat. The one feature that stood out about Roseto was that the townsfolk maintained close family ties and cohesive community relationships. Detailed comparisons of the extent of civic life in Roseto compared to the neighboring town of Bangor (population 5,000, with twice the age-adjusted mortality rate from heart disease) revealed that Roseto was endowed with 2.5 times the number of civic associations per capita.[26] Moreover, of those located in Roseto, 62.5% were locally-based, compared to Bangor organizations, of which 63.3% were branches of national groups.[27]

The "Roseto effect," as it came to be called, has been widely cited as evidence for the positive effects of social cohesion on longevity.[4][27][28] Even as this study was being carried out, however, the investigators observed the potential for major social change in Roseto. Interviews with the younger generation of Rosetans revealed that they were prepared to abandon their old community ways in favor of the more typically American behavior of neighboring towns. Having concluded that social cohesion served as a protection against cardiovascular mortality, the researchers predicted that anticipated changes in the community would result in the loss of this protection.[29] Beginning in the mid 1960s, as young people began to move away to seek jobs in neighboring towns and Roseto entered the mainstream of American life, the community's civic ties began to weaken. Informants complained about declining membership in their associations. Although Roseto continued to maintain a higher density of civic associations over Bangor throughout the three decades of the study, fully 40% of Roseto informants (compared to a third of those in Bangor) reported that their organizations had deteriorated or lost members over time. Whereas homes in Roseto used to be built with porches facing the neighbors across the street, beginning in the 1960s, new houses started to appear with porches attached at the back, overlooking private yards (Dr. Stewart Wolf: personal communication, 1996). The erosion of civic life in Roseto exactly coincided with the decade during which the heart attack rate in Roseto caught up with neighboring towns.[24 30]

The Ecological Study Approach

Examples of more quantitative approaches to studying social capital were demonstrated in two recently published studies.[9 31] Both studies attempted to assess the stock of social capital within geographic localities using a social survey approach. The strength of these studies is that they represent the first attempts to operationalize and quantify social capital as an ecologic characteristic. Their weakness consists of the fact that in doing so, the richness of social observation (such as gathered in the Roseto study) was lost. The study by Kawachi et al.[9] was conducted at a purely ecological level, while the one by Sampson et al.[31] represented a multi-level approach (to be discussed separately, below).

Kawachi et al.[9] carried out an ecological analysis of social capital in relation to state-level mortality rates in the USA. Indicators of social capital were obtained from the General Social Surveys conducted by the National Opinion Research Center between 1986 and 1990, and aggregated to the level of the state. Following Putnam's work,[17 32] items from the General Social Survey were chosen on the basis that they captured several of the core elements of social capital: density of associational membership, levels of interpersonal trust, and norms of reciprocity. Among other questions, the survey asked respondents about their membership in a wide variety of voluntary associations, including church groups, sports groups, hobby groups, fraternal organizations, labor unions and so on. Individual responses to these questions were aggregated up to the state level to create an indicator of per capita membership in voluntary groups. The General Social Surveys also asked residents in each state whether they thought "Most people would try to take advantage of you if they got the

chance" (an indicator of interpersonal mistrust), and whether "Most people can't be trusted"; and also, whether they agreed with "Most of the time people try to be helpful—or are they mostly looking out for themselves?" (perceived norms of reciprocity). In all, thirty-nine states were represented by the survey. After adjusting for potential sampling bias in the surveys, wide variations were observed between states in their stocks of social capital. For example, less than 25 percent of residents in North Dakota believed that "most people can't be trusted," compared to more than 60 percent in Alabama.

The indicators of social capital were strongly correlated with each other: civic mistrust to group membership ($r = -0.65$); mistrust to perceived lack of reciprocity ($r = 0.81$); and group membership to lack of reciprocity (-0.54) (all correlations, $P < 0.05$). In turn, each indicator of social capital was strikingly correlated with state mortality rates. Thus, per capita group membership in each state was strongly inversely correlated with age-adjusted all-cause mortality ($r = -0.49$, $p < 0.0001$). In regression analyses adjusted for household poverty rates, a one unit increment in the average per capita group membership was associated with a lower age-adjusted overall mortality rate of 66.8 deaths per 100,000 population (95% confidence interval: 26.0 to 107.5). Density of civic associational membership was similarly a predictor of deaths from coronary heart disease, malignant neoplasms, and infant mortality. Both the level of mistrust and perceived lack of reciprocity were also correlated with age-adjusted mortality rates ($r = 0.79$, and 0.71, respectively; $p < 0.0001$) (Figure 1).

In regression models, variations in the level of trust explained 58% of the variance in total mortality across states. Lower levels of trust were associated with higher rates of most major causes of death, including coronary heart disease, malignant neoplasms, cerebrovascular disease, un-

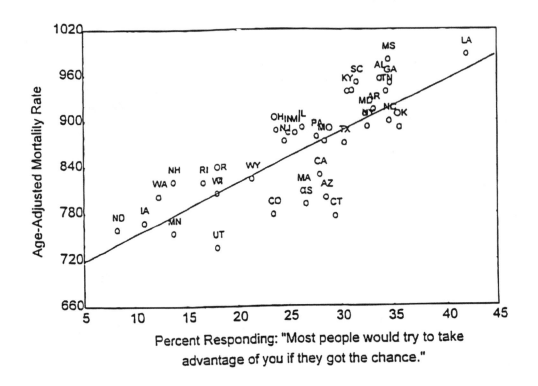

Figure 1
State-Level Correlation of Mistrust with Age-Adjusted Mortality Rates.
Reprinted from Kawachi et al. 1997

intentional injury, and infant mortality. If these associations are causal, then it was estimated that an increase in level of trust by one standard deviation, or 10%, would be associated with about a 9 percent lower level of overall mortality. One of the most striking associations observed was between stocks of social capital and rates of violent crime.[33] The lower the level of social capital, the higher the rate of violent crime, including homicide, aggravated assault, and burglary.

In fact, a long research tradition in criminology has postulated a link between social capital and crime, beginning with the early work of two criminologists from the Chicago School, Clif-

ford Shaw and Henry McKay (1942).[34] Shaw and McKay made the crucial discovery that the same socioeconomically disadvantaged areas in 21 US cities exhibited high delinquency rates over a span of several decades, despite changes in their racial and ethnic composition, thus indicating the persistent effects of the social environment within these communities on crime rates, regardless of what populations experienced them. This observation led Shaw and McKay to reject individualistic explanations of delinquency and focus instead on community processes that led to the apparent trans-generational transmission of criminal behavior. Social disorganization theory, which arose out of Shaw and McKay's work, has direct relevance for the theory of social capital.

Social disorganization has been defined as the "inability of a community structure to realize the common values of its residents and maintain effective social controls."[35] The social organizational approach views local communities and neighborhoods as complex systems of friendship, kinship, and acquaintanceship networks, as well as formal and informal associational ties rooted in family life and ongoing socialization processes.[36] From the perspective of crime control, it has been argued that residents of cohesive communities are better able to control violent behaviors and delinquency. Examples of such controls include: the supervision of leisure-time youth activities, intervention in street-corner congregation, and challenging youth "who seem to be up to no good."[36] Recently, social disorganization theory has been explicitly linked to the concept of social capital. The study, by Sampson et al.,[31] is an example of the third type of study, the multi-level analysis.

The Multi-Level Approach

Sampson and colleagues[31] examined the cross-sectional association between social capital measures and crime rates within Chicago neighborhoods. Measures of community characteristics were gathered from a community survey of 8,782 residents conducted in 1995 across 343 Chicago neighborhoods, where a neighborhood was defined as a geographic area equivalent to about 2–3 Census tracts. Residents were asked several questions related to social capital and social cohesion in their neighborhoods. On a five-point Likert scale, they were asked whether they agreed with statements, including: "people in this neighborhood can be trusted," "people around here are willing to help their neighbors," "this is a close-knit neighborhood," "people in this neighborhood generally don't get along with

each other," and "people in this neighborhood do not share the same values" (the last two items were reverse-coded). The resulting scale was then combined with responses to questions about the level of informal social control (whether neighbors would intervene in situations where children were engaging in delinquent behavior) to produce a summary index of "collective efficacy." Collective efficacy turned out to be significantly related to voluntary group participation (r = 0.45; p<0.01) as well as to neighborhood services (r = 0.21).

A major strength of this study was the authors' ability to control for a range of individual characteristics (such as age, socioeconomic status, gender, ethnicity, marital status, home ownership, and years in neighborhood) that may have confounded the cross-level relationship between the ecologic variable of interest (collective efficacy) and individual outcome (reports of violent victimization). In hierarchical statistical models adjusting for these potential individual-level confounds, the index of collective efficacy was significantly inversely associated with perceived neighborhood violence as well as violent victimization. As an independent check, the authors also examined the relationship of collective efficacy to 1995 homicide rates in the neighborhoods. A 2 standard deviation elevation in neighborhood collective efficacy was associated with a 39.7% reduction in the expected homicide rate.

As a further example of multi-level analysis, Kawachi et al.[37] carried out a study of the relationship between state-level social capital and individual self-rated health. Self-rated health ("Would you say your overall health is excellent, very good, good, fair, or poor?") was assessed among 167,259 individuals residing in 39 U.S. states, sampled by the Centers for Disease Control's Behavioral Risk Factor Surveillance System (BRFSS). Social capital indicators, aggregated to the state level, were obtained from the National

Opinion Research Center's General Surveys, described above.[9] Indicators of social capital included levels of interpersonal trust (% citizens responding "Most people can be trusted"), norms of reciprocity (% citizens responding "Most people are helpful"), and per capita membership in voluntary associations. Logistic regression was carried out with the SUDAAN procedure to estimate the odds ratios of fair/poor health (vs. excellent/good health). Similar to the study by Sampson et al.,[31] a strength of this study was the availability of information on individual-level confounds, including health insurance coverage, smoking status, overweight, as well as sociodemographic characteristics such as household income level, educational attainment, and whether the individual lived alone.

As expected, strong associations were found between individual risk factors (e.g., low income, low education, smoking, obesity, lack of access to health care) and poor self-rated health. However, even after adjusting for these proximal variables, individuals living in areas with low social capital were at increased risk of poor self-rated health. For example, the adjusted odds ratio for fair/poor health associated with living in areas with the lowest levels of social trust was 1.41 (95% confidence interval: 1.33 to 1.50) compared to living in high-trust states (Table 1). In other words, these findings were consistent with an apparent contextual effect of state-level social capital on individual well-being, independent of the more proximal predictors of self-rated health.

MECHANISMS LINKING SOCIAL CAPITAL TO HEALTH

THE mechanisms linking social capital to health outcomes have not been fully elucidated. There are several plausible paths by which socially isolated *individuals* experience increased risk of poor health outcomes, due to their limited access to resources ranging from instrumental aid, information flows, to emotional support (see

chapter by Lisa Berkman in this book). However, the mechanisms linking social capital to health outcomes might be different from those linking social networks to individual health. Here it is important to distinguish the *contextual* effects of living in an area depleted of social capital, from its *compositional* effects. On the one hand, an ecologic-level correlation between low social capital and poor health could be entirely accounted for by the fact that more socially isolated individuals reside in areas lacking in social capital (a compositional effect). Socially isolated individuals are more likely to be concentrated in communities that are depleted in social capital, because such places provide fewer opportunities for individuals to form local ties.[38] However, the persistent effect of social capital on self-rated health after adjusting for a marker of individual isolation (i.e., living alone)[37] suggests that social capital is also likely to exert a *contextual* effect on health as well.

Some of the contextual effects of social capital may involve psychosocial effects of living in hostile social environments.[4] States with low levels of interpersonal trust are less likely to invest in human security, and to be less generous with their provisions for social safety nets. For example, mistrust was highly inversely correlated ($r = -0.7$) with the maximum welfare grant as a percentage of per capita income in each state (Figure 2).[37]

Needless to say, less generous states are likely to provide less hospitable environments for vulnerable segments of the population, e.g., women and children who depend on welfare. Much work remains to be carried out in documenting the psychosocial pathways linking social cohesion, social capital, and health.

SOCIAL CAPITAL IN DIFFERENT POPULATION SUB-GROUPS

CONCERN has been raised recently about the decline of social capital in American society over the past three decades.[32]

Table 1.

Multi-level logistic regression results. Odds ratios and 95% confidence intervals (CI) of individuals reporting fair/poor health according to levels of social trust, adjusted for individual-level characteristics (Reprinted from Kawachi et al. 1999)

Independent Variables	Odds ratio for fair/poor health	
	Model 1[1]	Model 2[2]
Low trust[3]	1.68 (1.58 - 1.79)	1.41 (1.33 - 1.50)
Medium trust	1.19 (1.13 - 1.26)	1.14 (1.08 - 1.21)
High trust	1.00	1.00
Age (yrs)	1.04 (1.04 - 1.04)	
Age:		
< 25 yrs		0.74 (0.67 - 0.81)
25-39		1.00
40-64		2.38 (2.26 - 2.50)
65+		4.80 (4.52 - 5.10)
Male	0.92 (0.88 - 0.95)	1.05 (1.01 - 1.09)
Race:		
Black	2.01 (1.91 - 2.11)	1.33 (1.27 - 1.40)
White	1.00	1.00
Other	1.84 (1.71 - 1.98)	1.43 (1.33 - 1.55)
Living alone		1.93 (1.34 - 2.80)
Income:		
< $10,000		5.95 (5.58 - 6.34)
$10,000-14,999		4.39 (4.00 - 4.60)
$15,000-19,999		3.01 (2.80 - 3.23)
$20,000-24,999		2.42 (2.25 - 2.60)
$25,000-34,999		1.88 (1.75 - 2.01)
$35,000+		1.00
Missing		2.97 (2.79 - 3.17)
Current smoker		1.51 (1.45 - 1.57)
Obese		1.70 (1.64 - 1.77)
Health insurance coverage		0.73 (0.70 - 0.78)
Recent checkup		1.39 (1.32 - 1.46)

[1]Adjusted for age (as continuous variable), gender, and race.

[2]Adjusted for age (as categorical variable), gender, race, household income, living alone, current smoking status, obesity, health insurance coverage, and health checkup in last 2 years.

[3]Percent responding on the General Social Surveys that "most people can't be trusted."

Low trust states were: AL, AR, LA, MS, TN, WV (mean % mistrust = 59.4%; range: 56.0-61.6%).

Medium trust states were: AK, CA, CO, CT, FL, GA, IL, IN, IA, KY, MD, MA, MI, MO, NH, NJ, NY, NC, OH, OK, OR, PA, RI, SC, TX, UT, VA, WA (mean % mistrust = 42.9%; range: 33.4 - 51.7%).

High trust states were: KS, NE, ND, WI, WY (mean % mistrust = 26.7; range: 21.2 - 32.6%).

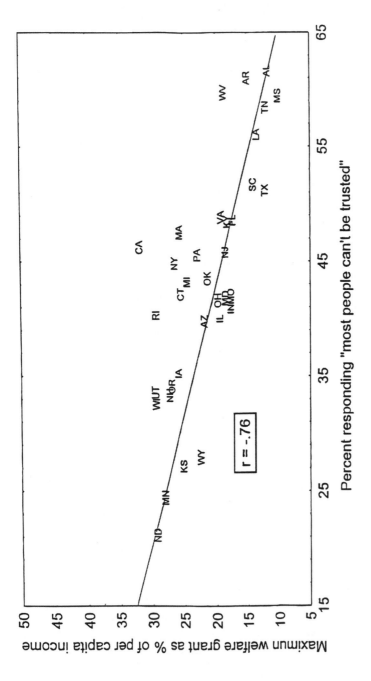

Figure 2
Scatterplot of Levels of Interpersonal Trust and the Maximum Welfare Grant
as a Percentage of Per Capita Income in Each State

Between 1960 and 1993, the proportion of Americans saying that most people can be trusted fell by more than a third, from 58% to 37%.[32] Membership in all sorts of voluntary associations has also dropped. While the causes of the decline in civil society are still debated,[39] the consequences of these trends are likely to be disproportionately borne by poor and working-class Americans, because, as one observer remarked:

> "When the social fabric thins, more affluent people can buy their way out with private schools, guarded or gated communities, private social clubs, and individual psychotherapy (about which one scholarly critic subtitled a book *The Purchase of Friendship*). People with less purchasing power obtain these needs socially, or go without." [40, p. 355]

Consistent with this view, Kawachi et al.[37] found that the self-rated health of individuals belonging to the lowest income stratum (household income less than $10,000) appeared to be most adversely affected by residing in states with low stocks of social capital. (At the same time, it is impossible to ignore the feedback loop running in the direction from poverty → disinvestment in social capital. As Banfield[41] observed about impoverished villagers in Southern Italy, trusting others is to gamble on the expectation that they will reciprocate, rather than abuse your trust. Under conditions of extreme poverty, one has no margin for error, i.e., one cannot afford to gamble because if one's trust is abused—if a loan is not repaid, for example—one's entire family must starve. Unfortunately, the presence of such feedback loops implies the presence of vicious cycles of poverty → mistrust → further economic backwardness).

In addition to inequalities in the vertical dimension, access to social capital may also be patterned along horizontal (or ascriptive) dimensions, i.e., by gender and race. Although social capital has many characteristics of a public good whose benefits are potentially available to all members within a social structure, in reality, some types of social capital may not be readily accessible to all strata of society. For example, many voluntary groups have historically excluded women and ethnic minorities. Kawachi et al.[37] found that voluntary group membership had a weaker effect on the health of women compared to interpersonal trust and norms of reciprocity. The case study of Roseto (discussed above) sheds some light on this observation. More than one-third of the clubs and associations in Roseto admitted men only, compared with one-quarter in neighboring Bangor. Interestingly, though the cardio-protective effect of living in Roseto was apparent in both sexes, lower overall mortality was found only among Roseto men.[26]

African-Americans may be similarly disadvantaged in their access to social capital, whether because of residential segregation, labor market exclusion, or other forms of discrimination both overt and covert.[20] For instance, Kennedy and Kawachi et al.[42] recently examined the relationship between collective racial prejudice and mortality rates among African-Americans. Collective prejudice can be conceptualized as a lack of respect that one group displays toward another. In the words of Miller and Ferroggiaro,[43] "respect and self-respect are central components of an enlarged concept of citizenship . . . Respect affects how we are treated, what help from others is likely, what economic arrangements others are willing to engage in with us, when reciprocity can be expected." In other words, respect acts as a resource for individuals, and should be considered a component of the stock of *social capital* of a society[43]—i.e., a component of interpersonal trust and social obligation that are essential for minimizing the risks of poor physical, psychological, or social health.[44] Collective prejudice is usually accompanied by a breakdown of social trust between members or groups within society, and the consequent disinvestment in social capital. Poor health status arises in such societies because the community fails to invest in, and assume responsibility for, the collective well-being of its members.[44][45]

In the analysis by Kennedy and Kawachi et al.[42] collective prejudice was operationalized at the state level by aggregating responses to a question on the General Social Survey that asked: "On the average blacks have worse jobs, income, and housing than white people. Do you think the differences are: (a) Mainly due to discrimination? (yes/no); (b) Because most blacks have less in-born ability to learn? (yes/no); (c) Because most blacks don't have the chance for education that it takes to rise out of poverty? (yes/no); and (d) Because most blacks just don't have the motivation or will power to pull themselves up out of poverty? (yes/no)." The two indicators of collective prejudice—i.e., the proportion of residents in each state who responded that blacks had less innate ability, or less willpower—were highly correlated with each other ($r = 0.81$). In turn, each indicator was strikingly correlated with black mortality rates. A one percent increase in the prevalence of those who believed that blacks lacked innate ability was associated with an increase in age-adjusted black mortality rate of 359.8 per 100,000 (95% confidence interval: 187.5 to 532.1 deaths per 100,000). The effect of collective prejudice on black mortality remained undiminished after adjusting for median income and poverty levels. Together with median income and poverty, the indicators of prejudice could account for between 22 to 28 percent of the between-state variance in black mortality.[42]

There are numerous mechanisms by which prejudice might lead to worse health outcomes for African-Americans. For instance, racial prejudice may affect African-Americans' chances of employment. Kirschenman and Neckerman[46] conducted interviews of 185 Chicago-area employers to determine the extent of racial stereotypes. Employers' characteriza-

tions of black workers mirrored pervasive racial stereotypes, i.e., that black workers were "unskilled, uneducated, illiterate, dishonest, lacking initiative, unmotivated, involved with drugs and gangs, did not understand work, had no personal charm, were unstable, lacked a work ethic, and had no family life or role models." Unfortunately, the low trust expressed in such views tends to become self-fulfilling prophecy. For example, employers' views may bias evaluation of job performance, and influence job placement: workers perceived to have lower productivity may be given less on-site job training. In turn, antagonism between workers and employers, supervisors, or customers may end up genuinely reducing productivity. Thus every party ends up paying for the costs of low social capital.

REFINING THE MEASUREMENT OF SOCIAL CAPITAL

MUCH work is needed to refine the approach to the measurement of social capital. We need to integrate knowledge from other disciplines. In the field of community psychology, several survey instruments have been developed which overlap considerably with elements of social capital.[47] Examples of these constructs include: psychological sense of community[48][49]; neighborhood cohesion[50]; and community competence.[51][52]

"Psychological sense of community" is a construct that has been theoretically defined along four dimensions: *membership* (the sense of feeling part of a group); *influence* (a bi-directional concept that refers to the sense that the individual matters to the group, and that the group can influence its members, thereby creating cohesiveness through community norms); *integration* (the sense that members' needs will be met by the resources received through their membership in the group); and *shared emotional connection* (the sense of shared history in the community).[49] At least 30 studies have been published which directly attempted to measure this construct, although as Hill[53] concluded in a recent review: "The development of a standardized, operational definition of the construct has eluded researchers. At least five measures of the construct have been developed, and there is still a lack of agreement as to what specific dimensions make up psychological sense of community."

On the other hand, despite differences in the approach to measurement across studies, community psychologists do appear to agree on two points: that "psychological sense of community" refers to a collective characteristic, not to individual relationships and behaviors; and that, being an aggregate variable, it is most usefully measured and studied at the community level.[53] Furthermore, the actual instruments that have been developed to measure "psychological sense of community" tap several individual items that have direct relevance to a community's stock of social capital, e.g., participation of members in churches or local neighborhood associations (PTA, youth groups, business/civic groups); whether community leaders can be trusted; whether people in the neighborhood are sociable; and whether people can depend on each other for help.[54-58]

Other measures of community—including community competence and neighborhood cohesion—similarly appear to tap into aspects of social capital, e.g., the feeling that one can rely on neighbors, and the belief that potential help is available[50]; the existence of norms of reciprocity and mutual aid; and citizens' participation in local associations.[52 59] Given the considerable headway that community psychologists have made in this area, further refinement in the operationalization and measurement of social capital is likely to come about as a result of collaboration with researchers in this field.

Ideally, social capital should be measured via the community survey approach. But what if survey data are not available? Is it possible to impute social capital from routinely collected data, such as the Census? Use of Census data to construct indices of social capital admittedly involves imprecision. Nevertheless, in the absence of community survey data, there are theoretically defensible reasons for resorting to the use of such proxies as the percent of single parent-headed households, the unemployment rate, residential stability, voting turnout, and crime rates. Although these variables tap several other aspects of communities (e.g., neighborhood deprivation), each of these variables can be theoretically linked to dimensions of social capital, such as the extent of civic engagement and the formation of interpersonal trust between citizens. An example of this proxy type of approach was illustrated by the analysis of Singh and Song in the *Data and Chartbook of Health and Social Factors in Kansas*.[60]

SOCIAL COHESION AND HEALTH: IMPLICATIONS FOR KANSAS

USING routinely available social indicator data, Singh and Song[60] constructed a Kansas county-level index of "social stability and integration," consisting of 9 indicators of family instability (proportion of single-parent households, female divorce rate), social integration and solidarity (% home ownership, % population living on farms), as well as measures of urbanization, household crowding, and unemployment rate. The internal reliability for the index was 0.91. Indices of child health and overall health status across the 105 counties in Kansas were then regressed on this index of social stability/integration. The regressions indicated that the index of social integration was strongly associated with child health as well as with overall health (which included cause-specific mortality rates, crime rates, and teen pregnancy). The magnitude of the association between community health and the index of social integration

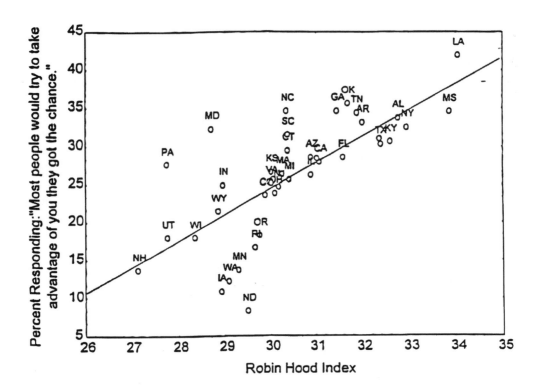

Figure 3
State-Level Correlation Between Income Inequality and Mistrust
(Reprinted from Kawachi et al. 1997).

was found to be twice as strong as that found with an index of socioeconomic status (which included measures of income, education, and income inequality). The indices of social integration and socioeconomic status together accounted for 89 percent of the variance in child health and 93 percent of the variance in overall health across counties.

In cross-state comparisons, according to the General Social Surveys, Kansas tends to rank in the top decile of states in terms of levels of social capital. For instance, Kansas was 4th out of 39 states in terms of per capita voluntary group membership; only Wyoming, Washington, and Utah ranked higher.[9] Similarly, Kansas ranked among the three least distrustful states in terms of public opinion (Figure 2). In life expectancy terms, Kansas ranked in the top quartile of the United States in 1990.

SOCIAL CAPITAL AND PUBLIC POLICY

A considerable gulf still remains between theory and practice: if social capital turns out in fact to be important for public health, we still have a limited understanding of what interventions are appropriate to remedy the situation. Interventions to rebuild civil society depend on a fuller understanding of the causal antecedents of social capital.

Recently, Kawachi et al.[9] have speculated that the surge in economic inequality in American society during the past 20 years may have contributed to the decline in social cohesion (see also the chapter by Richard Wilkinson in this volume). In 1975, the wealthiest 1 percent of American families owned 22 percent of total wealth, whereas currently they are estimated to own 42 percent.[61] Similarly dramatic trends have been documented in the distribution of income across American households.[62] These trends in inequality may have caused the social fabric to unravel, as Americans from all social strata (but especially the affluent) have withdrawn from civic life and retreated into enclaves defined by patterns of increasing residential segregation.[63] At the level of states, there is certainly a striking correlation between the Robin Hood Index—a measure of income inequality closely correlated with the Gini coefficient—and levels of mistrust (r = 0.76) (Figure 3).[9]

Whether policies to ameliorate such trends in economic and residential polarization could reverse the decline in civil society remains to be seen.

Some analysts have argued that government action (for example, through the provision of social services) is more likely to crowd out volunteerism and civic engagement, than to encourage the building of a civil society.[64] Yet others[39][65] have pointed out that throughout history, civic society has depended on the support of the state. Thus:

> "Philanthropy and mutual aid, churches and private universities, depend upon tax exemptions. Labor unions need legal recognition and guarantees against 'unfair labor practices.' Professional associations need state support for their licensing procedures. And across the entire range of association,

individual men and women need to be protected against the power of officials, employers, experts, party bosses, factory foremen, directors, priests, parents, patrons; and small and weak groups need to be protected against large and powerful ones. For civil society, left to itself, generates radically unequal power relationships, which only state power can challenge."[65, p. 302]

CONCLUSIONS

THE present chapter began by posing the question: Why are some communities healthy while others are not? The research on civil society and social capital marks the beginning of an endeavor to identify and characterize the health-enhancing features of the social environment. The theory and concepts are borrowed from political theory and sociology. But as the research increasingly demonstrates, the health of the public is inextricably entwined with the political, economic, and social arrangements of society at large.

At a defining moment during the recent rise of economic rationalism, Margaret Thatcher made her famous pronouncement: "There is no such thing as Society. There are individual men and women and there are families." To which Durkheim would have responded: Society matters. For if we truly believe that societal characteristics cannot be reduced to the sum of choices made by individuals, then we had better take seriously the notion that improvement in population health requires improvement in the social environment.[1] The formidable intellectual task confronting students of civil society is to restore the role of Society in the preservation and maintenance of well-being of its members.

NOTES

1. Marmot, M. Improvement of social environment to improve health. *Lancet* 1998; 351: 57–60.

2. Susser, M. The logic in ecological: I. The logic of analysis. *Am J Public Health* 1994; 84: 825–829.

3. Schwartz, S. The fallacy of the ecologic fallacy: the potential misuse of a concept and the consequences. *Am J Public Health* 1994; 84: 819–824.

4. Wilkinson, R. G. *Unhealthy Societies. The Afflictions of Inequality*. London: Routledge, 1996.

5. Kennedy, B. P., Kawachi, I., and Prothrow-Stith, D. Income distribution and mortality: Test of the Robin Hood Index in the United States. *Br Med J* 1996; 312: 1004–1007.

6. Kaplan, G. A., Pamuk E., Lynch, J. W., Cohen, R. D., and Balfour, J. L. Income inequality and mortality in the United States. *Br Med J* 1996; 312: 999–1003.

7. LaVeist, T. A. Segregation, poverty, and empowerment: Health consequences for African Americans. *The Milbank Quarterly* 1993; 71: 41–64.

8. Polednak, A. P. *Segregation, poverty, and mortality in urban African Americans*. New York: Oxford University Press, 1997.

9. Kawachi, I., Kennedy, B. P., Lochner, K., and Prothrow-Stith, D. Social capital, income inequality, and mortality. *American Journal of Public Health* 1997; 87: 1491–1498.

10. Dahrendorf, R. A precarious balance: economic opportunity, civil society, and political liberty. *The Responsive Community* 1995; Summer (5): 13–39.

11. de Tocqueville, A. (1835). *Democracy in America*. New York: Vintage Books, 1945.

12. Smith, C. and Freedman, A. *Voluntary Associations. Perspectives on the Literature*. Cambridge, MA: Harvard University Press, 1972.

13. Inglehart, R. *Culture Shift in Advanced Industrial Society*. Princeton, NJ: Princeton University Press, 1990.

14. Fukuyama, F. *Trust. The social virtues and the creation of prosperity*. New York: The Free Press, 1995.

15. Coleman, J. S. *Foundations of Social Theory*. Cambridge, MA: Harvard University Press, 1990.

16. Putnam, R. D. *Making Democracy Work. Civic Traditions in Modern Italy*. Princeton, NJ: Princeton University Press, 1993.

17. Putnam, R. D. The prosperous community. Social capital and public life. *The American Prospect* 1993; 13: 35–42.

18. Jacobs, J. (1961). *The Death and Life of Great American Cities*. New York: Vintage Books, 1992.

19. Durkheim, E. (1933). *The Division of Labor in Society*. New York: Macmillan, 1933.

20. Kawachi, I., Kennedy, B. P. Health and social cohesion: why care about income inequality? *Br Med J* 1997; 314: 1037–1040.

21. Durkheim, E. *Suicide* (1897). Ed. George Simpson, transl. J.A. Spaulding and G. Simpson. New York: The Free Press, 1951.

22. Kawachi, I., Colditz, G. A., Ascherio, A., Rimm, E. B., Giovannucci, E., Stampfer, M. J., and Willett, W. C. A prospective study of social networks in relation to total mortality and cardiovascular disease incidence in men. *J Epidemiol Comm Health* 1996; 50: 245–251.

23. Durkheim, E. (1938). *The Rules of Sociological Method*. Ed. Steven Lukes, transl. W.D. Halls. New York: The Free Press, 1982.

24. Bruhn, J. and Wolf, S. *The Roseto Story: An Anatomy of Health*. Norman, OK: Oklahoma University Press, 1979.

25. Wolf, S., Bruhn, J. *The Power of Clan: a 25 year prospective study of Roseto, PA*. New Brunswick, NJ: Transaction Publishers, 1992.

26. Lasker, J. N., Egolf, B. P., and Wolf, S. Community social change and mortality. *Soc Sci Med* 1994; 39: 53–62.

27. Amick, B. C. III, Levine, S. Introduction. In: B.C. Amick III, Levine, S., Tarlov, A. R., and Walsh, D. (eds). *Society and Health*. New York: Oxford University Press, 1995.

28. Kawachi, I., Kennedy, B. P., Lochner, K. Long live community. Social capital as public health. *The American Prospect* 1997, November/December, 56–59.

29. Bruhn, J., Phillips, B., and Wolf, S. Social readjustment and illness patterns: comparison between first, second, and third generation Italian-Americans living in the same community. *J Psychosom Med* 1972: 16; 387–394.

30. Egolf, B., Lasker, J., Wolf, S., and Potvin, L. The Roseto effect: A 50-year comparison of mortality rates. *Am J Public Health* 1992; 82: 1089–92.

31. Sampson, R. J., Raudenbush, S. W., and Earls, F. Neighborhoods and violent crime: a multilevel study of collective efficacy. *Science* 1977; 277: 918–924.

32. Putnam, R. D. Bowling alone: America's declining social capital. *J of Democracy* 1995; 6: 65–78.

33. Wilkinson, R. G., Kawachi, I., and Kennedy, B. P. Mortality, the social environment, crime and violence. *Sociology of Health and Illness* 1998; 20 (5): 578–597.

34. Shaw, C., McKay, H. *Juvenile Delinquency and Urban Areas*. Chicago: University of Chicago Press, 1942.

35. Sampson, R. J., Groves, W. B. Community structure and crime: Testing social-disorganization theory. *American Journal of Sociology* 1989; 94, 774–802.

36. Sampson, R. J. The Community. In: James Q. Wilson and Petersilia, J. (eds). *Crime*. San Francisco: Institute for Contemporary Studies, 1996: pp. 193–216.

37. Kawachi, I., Kennedy, B. P., and Glass, R. Social capital and self-rated health: A mixed-level analysis. *American Journal of Public Health* 1999; 89: 1187–1193.

38. Sampson, R. J. Local friendship ties and community attachment in mass society: a multilevel systemic model. *Am Sociol Rev* 1988; 53: 766–79.

39. Skocpol, T. Unraveling from above. *The American Prospect* 1996; 25 (March-April): 20–25.

40. Kuttner, R. *Everything for Sale. The virtues and limits of markets*. New York: Alfred Knopf, 1997.

41. Banfield, E. *The moral basis of a backward society*. Chicago: Free Press, 1958.

42. Kennedy, B. P., Kawachi, I., Lochner, K., Jones, C. P., and Prothrow-Stith, D. (Dis)respect and black mortality. *Ethnicity and Disease* 1997; 7: 207–214.

43. Miller, S. M., Ferroggiaro, K. M. *Poverty and Race* 1996; 5(1): 1–14.

44. Aday, L. A. Health status of vulnerable populations. *Annu Rev Public Health* 1994; 15: 487–509.

45. Kawachi, I., Levine, S., Miller, S. M., Lasch, K., and Amick, B. Income inequality and life expectancy: theory, research and policy. Joint Program on Society and Health Working Paper series. Boston, MA: New England Medical Center, Working Paper No. 94-2, 1994.

46. Kirschenman, J., Neckerman, K. M. "We'd love to hire them but . . ." The Meaning of Race for Employers. In: Jencks, C., Peterson, P. E. (eds). *The Urban Underclass*. Washington, DC: The Brookings Institute, 1991.

47. Lochner, K., Kawachi, I., and Kennedy, B. P. Social capital: a guide to its measurement. *Health and Place* 1999 (in press).

48. Chavis, D. M., Hogge, J. H., and McMillan, D. W. Sense of community through Brunswick's Lens: a first look. *Journal of Community Psychology* 1986; 14: 24–40.

49. McMillan, D. W., Chavis, D. M. Sense of community: a definition and theory. *Journal of Community Psychology* 1986; 14: 6–23.

50. Buckner, J. C. The development of an instrument to measure neighborhood cohesion. *American Journal of Community Psychology* 1988; 16: 771–91.

51. Cottrell, L. S. The competent community. In: Kaplan, B. H., Wilson, R. N., Leighton, A. H. (eds). *Further Explorations in Social Psychiatry*. New York: Basic Books, 1976.

52. Eng, E., Parker, E. Measuring community competence in the Mississippi Delta: The interface between program evaluation and empowerment. *Health Education Quarterly* 1994; 21: 199–220.

53. Hill, J. L. Psychological sense of community: Suggestions for future research. *Journal of Community Psychology* 1996; 24: 431–8.

54. Doolittle, R., MacDonald, D. Communication and a sense of community in a metropolitan neighborhood: A factor analytic examination. *Communication Quarterly* 1978; 26: 2–7.

55. Glynn, T. Psychological sense of community: Measurement and application. *Human Relations* 1981; 34: 789–818.

56. Davidson, W. and Cotter, P. Measurement of sense of community within the sphere of city. *Journal of Applied Social Psychology* 1986; 16: 608–19.

57. Davidson, W. and Cotter, P. Psychological sense of community and support for public school taxes. *American Journal of Community Psychology* 1993; 21: 59–66.

58. Davidson, W., Cotter, P., and Stovall, J. Social predisposition for the development of sense of community. *Psychological Reports* 1991; 68: 817–18.

59. Goeppinger, J., Baglioni, A. J. Community competence: a positive approach to needs assessment. *American Journal of Community Psychology* 1985; 13: 507–23.

60. Singh, G. K., and Song, F. F. Social Indicators. In: *Health and Social Factors in Kansas. A Data and Chartbook,*

1997–98. Singh, G. K., Wilkinson, A. V., Song, F. F., Rose, T. P., Adrian, M., Fonner, E. Jr, and Tarlov, A. R. (eds). Topeka, KS: Kansas Health Institute, 1998.

61. Fischer, C. S., Hout, M., Sanchez, M., et al. *Inequality by Design: Cracking the Bell Curve Myth*. Princeton: Princeton University Press, 1996.

62. Krugman, P. *Peddling prosperity*. New York: W. W. Norton & Co, 1994.

63. Jargowsky, P. Take the money and run: Economic segregation in U.S. metropolitan areas. *American Sociological Review* 1996; 61: 984–99.

64. McKnight, J. *The careless society: community and its counterfeits*. New York: Basic Books, 1995.

65. Walzer, M. The idea of civil society. *Dissent* 1991 (Spring): 293–304.

Four

BUILDING HEALTHY COMMUNITIES

*Stephen B. Fawcett, Vincent T. Francisco, Derek Hyra,
Adrienne Paine-Andrews, Jerry A. Schultz, Stergios Russos,
Jacqueline L. Fisher, and Paul Evensen*

HEALTHY COMMUNITIES:
A PARABLE OF TWO PATHS

IN the early 1920's, the people of Prairie Center and Sunflower enjoyed a rich community life. There were strong ties among neighbors. People supported each other in many informal ways; through churches, in conversations at the local cafe, and on front porches. Adults cared for children not their own. When Billy or Maria did something wrong, their parents were sure to hear about it. People trusted others to look out for them.

Gradually life changed in each community. Growth from nearby urban areas added people with limited ties to the community. Local zoning laws—and regional planning—separated the places where people worked from those where they lived. Roads now cut through established neighborhoods, making it necessary to take the car to places people used to walk.

Individuals and families made new choices about how to use their time. Rather than visit neighbors, people stayed at home and watched television. Increasingly, both adults worked outside the home; often at several low-paying jobs to meet family needs. As a result, there were fewer

adults to mind what kids were doing. All these individual choices and constraints added up: community folks had less contact with their neighbors, with their children, and with others' children.

In Prairie Center, things changed gradually, and so did the way local people addressed their problems. As drug use and violence increased in the 1980's and 1990's, the local media put the blame on youth and their parents. Following advice from outside experts, the county jail was expanded at considerable cost. This left less public money for education and health. Those who could afford it sent their children to private schools. Those who could went out of town for health care. Poor people suffered the most; sharp cuts in public assistance could not be made up by local churches and charities.

People still cared deeply about their OWN children and family members. But the sense was that each person and family should take care of themselves. Many people were increasingly distrustful of THEM. "Them" was all those outside the family.

The people of Sunflower took a different approach. A tragedy in the late-1980's, deaths of two children in a drug-related incident, got people's attention. They began a process of community renewal. They started a dialogue about what really mattered to local people, and what values they shared. They identified a common purpose: creating a caring place for all children.

The people of Sunflower began to work together in new ways. They formed action teams that cut across the usual boundaries, including both the powerful and those "labeled" people, such as youth and low-income families, who were seen by some as the problem. Now a diverse group of citizens, public officials, clergy, service providers, and business people joined hands. They worked to transform schools, businesses, health and human service organizations, the faith community, and other valued assets. They established benchmarks for success—all kids succeeding in school, less drug and alcohol use, fewer teen pregnancies, fewer children living in poverty, and adults employed in decent jobs. They coordinated efforts in what they called the "Sunflower Partnership."

Gradually, people started to notice a difference with the unfolding of community changes, both large and small, in Sunflower. Several major businesses allowed flextime for their employees so they could help children. The school district expanded the hours of neighborhood schools, creating safe places for children after school. The faith community collected "pledges" to care for others. City government officials approved new guidelines for tax abatements that rewarded businesses for creating better paying jobs for the unemployed and working poor.

Taken together, these hundreds of changes improved community life. The differences could be seen: slowly, gradually. They also produced results: kids did better in school, fewer kids got in trouble, the neighborhoods were safer, and children and adults were more successful. There was more to be done, of course, but people saw signs of progress.

People from diverse backgrounds connected with each other in neighborhoods, workplaces, and around issues that mattered to them. They minded each other's children. They looked out for one another. They worked together in common purpose. In short, local people were more fully involved in the ongoing work of building a healthy community.

BUILDING HEALTHY COMMUNITIES: SOME ORIENTING IDEAS

BUILDING healthy communities is the process of people working together to address health and development concerns that matter to them. As a process of community development[1], it is ongoing and gradual; not a one-time response to a political issue, such as crime, or an isolated campaign to address a crisis such as a drug-related tragedy. As a continuum of outcomes, it unfolds over time as incremental community (and systems) change, and related improvement in more distant indicators. Social ties and trust may contribute to, and result from, people working together in common purpose. Several orienting ideas help us understand this process of "building healthy communities."

Community refers to people who share a common place, experience, or interest. People may come together around issues that affect their place: the local block, neighborhood, city, town, or workplace. They may also connect because of shared experience, such as discrimination, due to race, ethnicity, disability, income, or gender. Finally, people may find common purpose based on shared interests, such as concern with addressing child hunger, neighborhood safety, or drug use. In dialogue, we discover the commonality and diversity of experiences and interests that can unite people in place-based work.

Health (of individuals) can be defined as a state of complete physical, mental, and social well-being.[2] It refers to "a state of well-being and the capability to function in the face of challenging circumstances".[3] Health is not merely the absence of disease or infirmity.[4] Health is seen as a resource for everyday life, not the objective of living.[5]

Community health, also known as population health, refers to the state of collective well-being of people who share a common place or experience. What's the level of well-being for all of us who share this place? For our children and adolescents? For adults and older adults in our community? For the poor?

Community health and development issues that matter to local communities include those affecting: a) Physical well-being; for example, decent jobs, adequate housing, violence and public safety, child hunger and nutrition, teen pregnancy, cardiovascular diseases, and injury; b) Mental well-being; for instance, substance abuse, academic failure, depression, and having meaningful work; and c) Social well-being; for example, caring relationships between children and adults, independent living of older adults, and support among family members, peers, and neighbors. Efforts to improve population health focus on changing the conditions in which health occurs.[6]

Determinants of health refer to conditions that affect health and well-being.[7] These include the: a) social environment and prosperity (e.g., family structure; educational system; health services; social networks; social class; household income; disparity of income); b) physical environment (e.g., barriers in the physical design of the environment; exposure to hazards and toxic substances; poor housing conditions and overcrowding); and c) genetic endowment (i.e., hereditary factors that increase or decrease risk for health outcomes; e.g., the biological basis for alcoholism, mental disorders, and heart disease).[8] *Social determinants* refer to those environmental features, such as trust and social ties, that affect health and well-being through relationships and exchanges among people.

SOCIAL DETERMINANTS, SOCIAL CAPITAL, AND COMMUNITY CAPACITY

POPULATION-LEVEL research— with whole communities, states, and nations—suggests the strong effects of economic circumstances and social features on a community's health status. For example, Wilkinson's[9] cross-national, comparative research showed a strong correlation between income inequality, the gap between those with most and least income, and death from a variety of causes. Kaplan and colleagues,[10] using data from all 50 states of the United States, demonstrated a similar relationship between income distribution and mortality. Also, research with British civil servants by Marmot and colleagues[11] suggests a strong inverse relationship between social class (i.e., job classification) and mortality. In a rare experimental study, a marked increase in income (due to a negative income tax) resulted in improved health outcomes (i.e., fewer low-birthweight babies).[12] In a comprehensive review of the literature on social determinants of health, Feinstein[13] concluded that there is a strong and consistent link between wealth, education, and health outcomes. Yet income disparity has grown in the United States since 1973, with the rich getting richer and the poor getting poorer.[14 15]

The idea of *social capital*—civic engagement and trusting relationships among people—is thought to help explain how income is associated with outcomes in health and development.[16 17] Kawachi and colleagues[18] examined the relationships among income inequality, social capital (civic engagement and level of trusting relationships) and health outcome (all-cause mortality) at the state level. Their research suggests that the more social capital (civic engagement and trust), the better the health outcome. Further, researchers speculate that a decline in social capital—people watching more television, and accordingly, less engaged with their neighbors—

may help explain a rise in a variety of adverse societal outcomes.[19] [20]

Less clear are the mechanisms by which social determinants (including poverty and social capital) might influence health and development outcomes. For example, does social capital increase the likelihood that people will be able to transform the environment in ways that improve health? Perhaps when people trust each other, they are more likely to be engaged in community building efforts. Or, is social capital a by-product of successful efforts to transform communities, and related health improvement? Perhaps as communities improve, more people get involved and trusting relationships are developed. Or, does increased social capital affect health directly? For instance, a sense of belonging may reduce stress and improve physical and mental health. Do other factors—perhaps poverty and income disparity, and related stressors and barriers—affect the conditions under which both health and social ties occur? Perhaps the stressors of trying to meet basic needs in the face of poverty reduce access to health resources and the basic conditions that affect health. Also, social comparisons that focus on disparities in wealth between community members may limit their willingness to connect with others, or to get involved on their behalf. Further research may help clarify how income inequality and social capital—and related variables—interact to affect community health and development.

Although social scientists[21] [22] have asserted the importance of social capital and cited possible reasons for its apparent decline, few have brought forth tangible ways of how communities can propagate it.[23] [24] One promising strategy for enhancing social capital—and less directly, income inequality and community health—is to support collaborative partnerships. Collaborative partnerships are ecological systems[25] that encourage community engagement around local concerns.[26] They create niches of opportunity for, and reduce barriers to, successful community engagement; and, thereby, may increase trust.

They can encourage community engagement that transforms the local environment, and the broader policy and systems changes that produce a more equitable distribution of resources.[27] By increasing civic engagement and equality of opportunity and result, collaborative partnerships focus on two variables associated with health and development outcomes: social capital and income inequality.

Finally, success in addressing the determinants of health may be related to community capacity. *Community capacity* refers to the ability of local people to work together to affect conditions and outcomes that matter to them; and to do so over time, and across concerns.[28] [29] Markers of community capacity include community action and resulting change in conditions and outcomes (e.g., community and systems change; improvement in community-level indicators). To reflect capacity, community (systems) changes should occur *over time* (i.e., be sustained) and *across concerns* (i.e., when a new issue or goal is identified, changes are brought about related to these new goal areas).

UNDERSTANDING THE CONTEXT
OF PUBLIC PROBLEM SOLVING

BUILDING healthy communities requires public problem solving: people engaged in addressing issues of health and development that matter to them. Community-wide engagement in public problem solving is affected by our assumptions about the nature of public life, problems, and solutions.[30] Some assumptions, such as that solving problems together builds trust, may advance common work; others, such as "nothing works," may impede it.

First, assumptions about the nature of public life—and who is responsible for public problems—can enhance or impede the work.[31] Two myths may be central to disengagement of citizens from public life: first, the notion that public life is a battleground for selfish interests; and second, that public life is only for experts, officials, and celebrities.[32] Business and special interests do have disproportionate influence; and public life does bring together people with different values, and disagreement, even conflict, may result. But self-interest and conflict are not the core of public life. Indeed, public life is also a vehicle for individual and community growth. We all have a public life. Through ties in our family and workplace, and with friends and neighbors, we help each other deal with what matters: serving and being served, protecting and being protected.

Second, beliefs about the nature of public problems—for example, whether problems originate in people[33] or in their environments[34]—may limit or advance community engagement in problem solving. Too often, we frame public problems as being in *those* people abusing substances or in *that* group with the high crime rate.[35] This prevents others from seeing how the problem affects their lives, and from participating in the solution. More truthfully, public problems are shared by all of us. For example, the health and development outcomes for a child born addicted to drugs are not only related to conditions in the past and current environment; they are also tied to future economic security and well-being for that child, his or her family, and the community. Crime and violence associated with poverty not only affect the businesses, playgrounds, and streets of low-income neighborhoods; they extend into, and originate from, the surrounding community.

Similarly, societal issues—such as child health, academic success, or substance abuse—do not fit into neat categories. The factors, such as social support or access to resources, that put people at risk for (or protect them against) one outcome affect other outcomes as well.[36] Defining problems more inclusively, as interconnected with other issues, allows us to see their, and our, interdependence.

Finally, how we define a problem also affects how we attempt to solve it. Limiting myths about solutions are tied to false assumptions of independence: that my problems are separate from yours; and, therefore, my solutions should be too. This valuing of individual effort is evident in beliefs like "Government causes problems, it doesn't solve them," or that "Only I can solve my problems." Although these assertions might be rooted in some partial truths—for example, that personal responsibility is important—they can also discourage people from working together to solve public problems. To build healthy communities, we must discover the assets of individuals and organizations—including those thought to be part of the problem—that can be brought together in common purpose.[37]

ADVANCING THE WORK TOGETHER: SOME PRINCIPLES, ASSUMPTIONS, AND VALUES

DETERMINATION of community health—what causes collective well-being—is complex and multidimensional.[38] Health and development outcomes are affected by an array of interrelated personal and group factors (including competence and biological capacity) and environmental factors (including support and resources, barriers and hazards, preventive and treatment services, poverty, policies, and culture). For example, a mother and father with several low-paying jobs have limited time for their children and may smoke cigarettes to cope with the financial stress. Their young children may spend less time in adequate childcare and have higher exposure to second-hand smoke and other environmental hazards (e.g., cockroaches and lead paint) from poor housing. Limited engagement with adults may diminish early childhood development; exposure to environmental hazards may increase their risks for chronic disease; and these may interact to reduce prospects for academic achievement and adequate employment, for the children and for their children.

The work of building healthy communities requires the ongoing contribution of—and trust among—individuals and organizations from all sectors or parts of the community. The related determinants of community health demand solutions from multiple sectors (e.g., business, health organizations, media, and government).[39][40] Singular and fragmented approaches that target one issue (e.g., a campaign to reduce tobacco use) or sector (e.g., health organizations or schools) are unlikely to effect community-level outcomes. Rather, promoting community health is a developmental process: an unfolding of integrated, comprehensive, community and systems changes toward common goals.

Some Guiding Principles, Assumptions, and Values

When made explicit, assumptions and values help others to critically evaluate the work and to understand what success would look like for practitioners.[41] Table 1 outlines 10 principles, assumptions, and values for guiding the work of building healthy communities. For example, Principle #3 highlights the value of community self-determination: a healthy community is a local product with priority issues and strategies best determined by those most affected by the concern. Similarly, Principle #9 underscores the importance of building capacity to address what matters to local people over time and across concerns. Taken together, these 10 principles, assumptions, and values may help guide the interconnected work of a diverse group of people and organizations in transforming the conditions that affect community health. Such development efforts involve interdependent relationships

---

Table 1

Some Principles, Assumptions, and Values that Guide the Work of Building Healthy Communities

1. Community health improvement involves the *population* as a whole, not merely individuals at risk for specific physical, mental, or social conditions.
2. Community health requires changes in both the *behaviors* of large numbers of individuals *and* the *conditions* or social determinants that affect health and development.
3. A healthy community is a *local product* with priority issues and strategies best determined by those most affected by the concern.
4. Freedom and justice require reducing income disparities to promote optimal *health and development for all.*
5. Since health and development outcomes are caused by *multiple factors,* single interventions are likely to be insufficient.
6. The conditions that affect a particular health or development concern are often *interconnected* with those affecting other *concerns.*
7. Since the behaviors that affect health and development occur among a variety of people in an *array of contexts,* community improvement requires engagement of diverse groups through *multiple sectors* of the community.
8. Statewide and community partnerships, support organizations, and grantmakers are *catalysts for change*: they attempt to convene important parties, broker relationships, and leverage needed resources.
9. The aim of support organizations is to *build capacity* to address what matters to people over time and across concerns.
10. Community health and development involves *interdependent relationships* among multiple parties in which none can function fully without the cooperation of others.

among multiple parties that share risks, resources, and responsibilities for the work.[42]

Toward Broad Collaborative Partnerships

Efforts to build healthy communities require broad collaborative partnerships in common purpose. This demands horizontal integration—organizations linked across sectors (e.g., school, business, government)—and vertical integration, connections across multiple levels (e.g., neighborhood, community, county, state, region). Multilevel collaboration should include several key partners, including state and community partnerships, support organizations, and grantmakers and governmental agencies.

STATE AND COMMUNITY PARTNERSHIPS
Collaborative partnerships link organizations drawn from all relevant community sectors. For example, a community partnership to promote child health might engage citizens and agency representatives in transforming the media, businesses, schools, civic and community organizations, youth organizations, local government, health organizations, the faith community, and financial institutions. Each sector can contribute to the initiative's efforts by intervening with specific risk (and protective) factors, such as social support or access to services, or broader social determinants of health, such as income inequality and educational opportunity.

SUPPORT AND INTERMEDIARY ORGANIZATIONS
Some local, regional, and statewide organizations, such as university research centers, provide technical assistance and evaluation in support of statewide and community partnerships. These intermediary organizations can enhance the capacity of community partners by building on core competencies for doing the work (e.g., community assessment, strategic planning, advocacy). Intermediary organizations help assess the needs of collaborative partnerships and provide support that is timely, appropriate, and responsive. For example, state and county health departments and research organizations can assist community partners by developing health data systems that provide county-level data and other information useful for making decisions. Similarly, university research and public service centers can support collaborative planning, community intervention, and community evaluation to enhance both understanding and improvement of community efforts.

GRANTMAKERS AND GOVERNMENTAL AGENCIES
Foundations and governmental agencies can help create the conditions for community partnerships to be successful. First, grantmakers often use requests for proposals to convene groups around common purpose. Second, they provide the multi-year resources needed by both statewide and community partners and intermediary organizations to conduct the agreed-upon work. Third, they broker connections among those working in the same community or on common issues. Fourth, funders also help leverage funding and other resources for comprehensive efforts. Finally, grantmakers and governmental agencies can also help make outcome matter in multi-year grants by awarding bonus grants and outcome dividends contingent on evidence of attaining objectives and outcomes.

BUILDING CAPACITY FOR
COMMUNITY AND SYSTEMS CHANGE:
A THEORY OF CHANGE

A THEORY of change describes how the initiative should work.[43] Figure 1 outlines the framework used by our University of Kansas Work Group to help understand, support, and document the process by which collaborative partnerships do their work. How-to information to support implementation of the theory of change is available on the Internet-based Community Tool Box, *http://ctb.lsi.ukans.edu/*. Based on related models,[44][45] this framework for building capacity for community and systems change

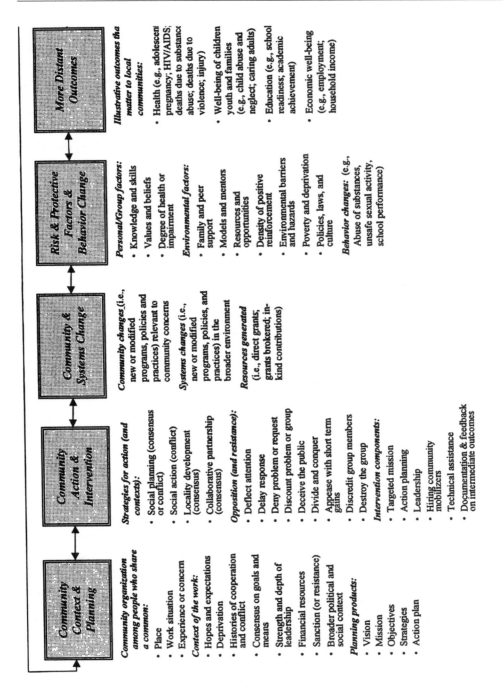

Figure 1

Building Capacity for Community and Systems Change

includes five components: 1) community context and planning, 2) community action and intervention, 3) community and systems change, 4) risk and protective factors and behavior change, and 5) improving more distant outcomes.

The model is *interactive*. For example, an understanding of the community context, and the ongoing process of collaborative planning, should guide community action and intervention. Similarly, feedback on the effects of the locally determined intervention on community and systems change should influence the context and ongoing planning. The model is also iterative or repeating. For example, achieved levels of improvement in more distant outcomes, such as reduced rates of violence or improved academic success, should lead to a renewed cycle of collaborative planning and intervention for these or other issues that matter to local communities.

Community Context and Planning

The *context*—people's past and current experiences, their dreams for a better life, and the conditions under which people act—frames the practice of promoting community health and development. People's hopes and expectations, such as about whether things can change, influence their willingness to engage in community problem solving. Job and family demands, past histories of responsiveness from those in power, and intensive problems or deprivation may limit people's participation in collaborative planning and other future-oriented community efforts. Individual and group histories of cooperation and conflict, such as gains or losses from prior collaborative or competitive efforts, also affect willingness to work together. Consensus (or lack of agreement) on current goals and means also influences community participation in collective problem solving.

Strong and deep leadership—having a diverse and dispersed team with vision, competence, and persistence—can help inspire and sustain community efforts to address health and develop-

ment issues. Financial resources, such as for hiring community organizers to follow through on action plans, also affect the rate of change. Sanction (or resistance) from the community, or those in authority, influences the likelihood and effectiveness of change. Finally, the broader political and social context, such as political instability or mass protest, may affect the nature of community action and the chances that those in power will respond favorably to the group's efforts to bring about systems change.

Collaborative planning is a critical and ongoing aspect of the process of community organization and change for health improvement. People come together to identify issues that matter to them such as drug use, job opportunities, the quality of schools, decent housing, or crime. Community-level indicators, such as archival records of the levels of school failure or violence, help substantiate community concerns and provide benchmarks for detecting improvements on these more distal outcomes.

Inventories of community assets, such as people and materials, help detect resources that can be mobilized in change efforts.[46] Strategic planning can be used to help clarify the community's vision, mission, objectives, and strategies of change. In action planning, local people identify "community changes"—new or modified programs, policies, and practices—to be sought in each relevant sector of the community (e.g., schools, business, government). Similarly, organized community groups may seek "systems changes," new or modified policies and practices at a broader level, such as revised regional planning guidelines to minimize the concentration of poverty in low-income neighborhoods. Community and support teams, such as found in community-based organizations or university-based research organizations, may assist community members in the process of promoting community health and development. In their ongoing planning, community organization efforts bring together people and organizations with diverse experiences and resources—

including poor people, ethnic minorities, youth, elders, and those already with power—to cooperatively plan and implement changes in the community.

Community Action and Intervention

Local planning and analysis of the context help guide *how* community people take action on what matters to them: the strategies for change.[47] [48] For example, where the goal is building community capacity and there is consensus on the issues, locality or community development may be a particularly appropriate strategy for bringing people together to pursue a common purpose. Each strategy for promoting community health invokes its own set of intervention components and elements.

Community action often begets a variety of forms of opposition or resistance.[49] Even a relatively benign self-help effort to fix up low-income housing may run into resistance from local officials, evidenced by their deflecting responsibility to others or delaying needed construction permits. Similarly, efforts by a community partnership to redistribute resources from law enforcement to substance abuse prevention will likely be opposed by agencies with interests at stake (and their allies), such as by discounting the value of prevention approaches, denying requests for information, or challenging the legitimacy of the partnership.

Opposition should also be expected when people agree on ends but not means. Consider the case of a public health initiative to reduce teen pregnancy that promotes abstinence and safe sex for those who choose to be sexually active. Opponents may attempt to divide the group on religious grounds (e.g., those for, or against, contraception), or deceive others about the group's purposes (e.g., they are encouraging teens to have sex). When the aim is to redistribute significant power or resources—perhaps by using lawsuits, sit-ins, boycotts, or other disruptive tactics—strong opposition is inevitable. In-

tensive opposition may include attempts to divide members and conquer the weaker organization, appease the group with buyouts that provide short-term gain, discredit leaders with personal attacks, or destroy the organization through a smear campaign in the local media. Community organizations may respond to the opposition, in turn, with appropriate counteractions, such as by reframing the issues, or by going public with opponents' tactics.[50]

Community and Systems Change

Community and systems changes are important intermediate outcomes of community health and development efforts.[51] Community change consists of new or modified programs (e.g., an intergenerational mentoring program), policies (e.g., a business policy to hire local residents for construction jobs in the neighborhood), or practices (e.g., opening public parks to late-night supervised recreation for youth) related to the mission.[52] Similarly, broader systems changes might include a new program of a nearby community college to support computer information networks in community-based organizations, or a change in grantmaking policy to award outcome dividends for improvement in community-level indicators, such as levels of academic performance or affordable housing. Community and systems change may both accompany, and be facilitated by, social ties and trust among affected parties.

Generating resources for community health and development efforts is another desired intermediate outcome. These may include direct grants given and received, funding brokered through relationships with other grantmakers, and in-kind contributions such as professional services and materials. Community leadership, grantmakers and governmental institutions, and intermediary and support organizations collaborate on documenting and communicating information about accomplishments and outcomes. They also assist in generating (or brokering) resources that can be used to reduce income inequalities and promote community improvement.

Risk and Protective Factors and Behavior Change

A primary purpose of community and systems change is to alter the context in which people relate to each other. Some features of the person or environment, such as social isolation, may increase the likelihood of adverse outcomes; these are known as risk factors. By contrast, protective factors, such as strong social ties, may decrease the chances of risk behaviors and related adverse outcomes.[53] For example, youth violence may be related to a variety of personal and group factors such as knowledge about the consequences of violence, skill in conflict resolution, and existing health and cognitive abilities of youth and their peers, parents, and guardians. Environmental factors that may affect youth violence include supervision and support from family and friends, models for caring relationships, basic resources, and opportunities for supervised alternative activities after school. Similarly, the amount of social approval and disapproval available for caring (or punitive) relationships with others, poverty and deprivation, and opportunity also add to risk (or protection). Changes in the community (and broader system), and related positive changes in risk and protective factors for the concern, may effect changes in behavior of large numbers of people and associated improvement in more delayed outcomes.

More Distant Outcomes

Improvements in more distant outcomes, such as reducing violence or increasing employment rates and family incomes, are the ultimate goals of efforts to build capacity for community health and development. Data on community-level indicators sensitive to local concerns (e.g., the percentage of new housing units affordable by those currently without adequate housing) help assess the extent of progress on community-identified

issues associated with development efforts. An annual community report card might communicate information about the state of well-being in the community, trends on community-referenced indicators, and important community changes and success stories related to shared community goals.

Linking Intermediate and More Distant Outcomes: A Working Hypothesis

A central question for this theory of change is under what conditions are community and systems changes—an intermediate outcome—associated with more distant outcomes. When are changes in programs, policies and practices sufficient to effect community-level outcomes related to group goals (e.g., reduced rates of violence or academic failure)?

Our working hypothesis is that, to effect more distant outcomes, community and systems change must be of sufficient: a) amount (i.e., by goal; e.g., reduce teen pregnancy, increase childhood immunizations), b) intensity of behavior change strategy (i.e., providing information and enhancing skills, facilitating support, modifying access and barriers, changing incentives and disincentives, modifying policies), c) duration (i.e., one-time event, more than once, ongoing), and d) penetration (i.e., to targets of change, such as children or elected officials, through sectors or channels of influence, such as schools or faith organizations, and place-based efforts, such as in specific cities or neighborhoods).

To examine this question, we review multiple case studies for which we have longitudinal data on both community and systems change (an intermediate outcome) and community-level indicators (a more distant marker). For example, to test this working hypothesis with a multi-site initiative to prevent adolescent pregnancy, we might examine whether variations in more distant outcomes (i.e., estimated pregnancy rates) are associated with community and systems changes of varying: a) amount, b) intensity of behavior change strategy (i.e., improving access to contraceptives, not merely providing information), c) duration (i.e., some ongoing policy and curricular changes, not just one-time social activities), and d) penetration to targets of change (i.e., business leaders, as well as youth) through sectors or channels of influence (i.e., faith organizations and businesses, as well as schools), and place-based efforts (i.e., concentrated in specific neighborhoods where youth might be at particular risk).

SOME FACTORS AFFECTING COLLABORATIVE PARTNERSHIPS FOR COMMUNITY HEALTH

OVER nearly a decade, our University of Kansas Work Group has used iterations of this theory of change to help understand—and improve—the functioning of collaborative partnerships for community health and development. We have learned from, and with, over 30 state and local partnerships. The varied contexts included cities, urban neighborhoods, tribes, and rural communities. The partnerships addressed an array of issues including prevention of adolescent substance abuse,[54] adolescent pregnancy,[55] cardiovascular diseases,[56] and promotion of youth development, health and human services, rural health, and urban community development.

In a multiple case study design,[57] our Work Group used a common measurement system to document the unfolding of community and systems changes over time.[58] [59] We also used qualitative research methods to identify critical events, such as a change in leadership, in the life history of the partnerships. Using graphs of trends over time, we looked for discontinuities in the pattern of community and systems change, and correlated events that might have effected observed increases (or decreases) in the rate of changes in the environment. By examining whether effects were replicated across different case studies, we were able to examine the generality of a finding that a particular factor, such as

action planning, is associated with increases in the rate of change.

This analysis yielded seven factors or events often associated with marked variations in the rate of community and systems change. Although further research may help determine whether the relationships are causal, their consistency across collaborative partnerships, communities, goal areas, and time is quite remarkable. The following seven factors suggest promising practices for enhancing the functioning of collaborative partnerships.

Targeted Mission

Having a clear focus—a targeted mission—is one of the most significant contributors to the rate of community and systems change. For initiatives with a targeted mission (e.g., preventing substance abuse or promoting child health), we have seen substantially higher rates of community change than for broad, unfocused "healthy communities" initiatives with no clearly articulated purpose.

Action Planning

Action planning refers to identifying specific objectives for community and systems change in all relevant sectors of the environment. In the process of action planning, community partnerships identify the actions that will bring about the community changes rated as more important and feasible, and identify who will take those actions, by when they will be done, and what resources (and communication) are needed to get the job done.[60] The completion of action planning, in the context of a targeted mission, has consistently resulted in marked increases in the rates of community and systems change.

Change in (loss of) Leadership

Involving leaders with a clear vision of how the environment can be transformed to improve community health and development can accelerate the number and intensity of community and system changes. When such leaders leave the initiative, however, the rate of change often diminishes markedly. A change to such a leader—from one with a less clear vision—can have a facilitating effect. Such leaders see community change goals as niches of opportunity for civic engagement, identify a broader array of change agents (including people affected by the problem), and help create mechanisms by which local people's accomplishments are celebrated.

Resources for Community Mobilizers

One thing that is very clear is that there needs to be a catalyst—let's call them community mobilizers—to facilitate the efforts of the partnership. They provide follow-up on agreed upon actions. Hiring community mobilizers or organizers has consistently led to increases in rates of community and systems change.

Documentation and Feedback on Intermediate Outcomes

In the business of community health and development, the product is the capacity of community members to effect change leading to improvement in community-determined outcomes. Such efforts track intermediate markers, such as community and systems change, and benchmarks for more distant community-level outcomes. Tracking the unfolding of community and systems changes over time, and the events that affect them, can help community leadership understand, celebrate, and improve the functioning of collaborative partnerships.

Technical Assistance

Good leaders work to attract persons with complementary skills, and to enhance the capacity of team members to do the work. Core competencies for doing the work of community health and development—for instance, in action planning or advocacy—often transcend the variety of specific (targeted) missions of the initiatives and specialized training of people doing the

work. The goal of technical assistance is to build community capacity: the ability of local people to effect valued community and systems change—and related more distant outcomes—over time, and across concerns or goal areas.

Making Outcome Matter

Finally, grantmakers and governmental agencies can greatly facilitate the progress of an initiative by making explicit the contingencies on goal attainment and outcomes achieved. For example, following an announcement from a foundation program officer that continued funding for a multi-year grant to a community partnership was contingent on evidence of progress, the rate of community change increased dramatically.[61] Although untested, promising methods of rewarding results include providing bonus grants for those initiatives that implement important changes and intervention components, and awarding outcome dividends by which communities receive funds saved from improvements in community-level indicators (e.g., rates of teen pregnancy or unemployment).

TEN RECOMMENDATIONS FOR BUILDING HEALTHY COMMUNITIES

BUILDING healthy communities is a local process and product. But the work of local communities can be enhanced by a broader support system, including statewide partnerships, intermediary and support organizations, and grantmakers and governmental agencies. While the former must do the local work, the latter can help create conditions under which it is easier and more likely to be successful. Based on the preceding analysis, ten specific recommendations for building capacity for community change and improvement follow:

1. In collaboration with statewide and community partnerships, grantmakers and governmental agencies should develop and implement a social marketing plan to promote civic engagement in building healthy communities.

- If the marketing plan is successful, larger numbers of people will say (and act accordingly): a) "Things need to change," b) "Working together, we can change things," c) "We should change things," and d) "We must embed programs and policies consistent with these values and goals in our public and private institutions."
- Messages should refute the myths that reduce civic engagement (e.g., those experiencing public problems are to blame; nothing works).
- Messages should focus on empowering insights that encourage community involvement (e.g., to reduce and prevent problems, we must change the environments in which people make choices).
- Messages should promote widespread adoption of specific ideas (e.g., "we are in this together") and practices (e.g., become a mentor or friend to a child not your own). The communications plan should tailor its strategies to reach relevant audiences (e.g., parents and guardians, youth, religious leaders, business leaders).
- A communications plan should be developed and implemented in collaboration with community partnerships to promote awareness of their local goals and accomplishments (e.g., community and systems changes; improvements in the lives of individuals; success stories; community champions).
- Use traditional (e.g., print media, storytelling) and modern methods of communication (e.g., broadcast media, the Internet) to disseminate success stories about effective community efforts to promote health and development, and lessons learned in doing the work.

2. Convene statewide and local collaborative partnerships to create comprehensive opportunity structures for civic engagement and promotion of community health and development.
   - Grant funds should help establish and maintain broad multi-issue community partnerships. This would help focus on targeted issues (e.g., task forces for teen pregnancy; employment) within a structure (e.g., action committees for each sector such as schools) that permits coordinated efforts on interrelated issues.
   - Partnerships should involve both influential people (those with access to power) and those most affected by the issue (including youth, the poor, and others experiencing the "problem").
   - Coordinated action committees (and related action plans) should provide multiple niches for community engagement in transforming all relevant sectors of the community (e.g., schools, business, health organizations, media, human service organizations, government, civic organizations, faith community).
   - Funding partnerships—among grantmakers in the public, private, and foundation sectors—should help coordinate investments in the same place (e.g., neighborhood, county). They should also permit integrated work across bureaucratic boundaries (e.g., integrated grants for health, education, and economic development).

3. Provide information to help focus collaborative efforts on issues and options that most affect health and development, and that matter to local communities.
   - Support organizations should provide information about the social determinants of health and development—highlighting the contributions of poverty and education—to help focus community objectives on reducing the number of children and families in poverty and on increasing early child development, school readiness, and academic achievement.
   - Support organizations should provide information about the incidence (new cases) and prevalence (existing cases) of more specific health and development outcomes (e.g., the rate of adolescent pregnancy) to suggest candidate objectives for statewide and community partnerships.
   - Collaborative partnerships should convene community listening sessions—and assess and analyze community needs and assets—to influence selection of locally-determined objectives and strategies.
   - Support organizations should develop and communicate a theory of change (e.g., building capacity for community and systems change) that helps guide the work.

4. Support action planning and community intervention that focuses attention on changes in the environment that advance the locally-determined mission and objectives.
   - Planning should begin early and be ongoing. Annual action planning can renew efforts; regular updates on progress (and adjustments) can enhance communication and coordination.
   - Promote widespread adoption of promising interventions—what works—while permitting adaptation to fit local conditions.
   - Focus on transforming the environment in

which behavior related to health and development occurs: personal and group factors (e.g., experience and competence) and environmental influences (e.g., social support, resources and opportunities, policies).

- Information about factors that increase risk for (or protect against) adverse health and development outcomes can help focus attention on strategic intervention components and changes in the environment.
- Seek balance in interventions: universal efforts to reach a broad audience and targeted programs of sufficient intensity to affect outcomes with those at higher risk.

5. Provide coordinated investments in collaborative partnerships for community health—including support for community leadership and change agents—which are large enough and long enough to make a difference.

- Fund community partnerships long enough to make a difference (e.g., 5 to 10 years).
- Provide resources to hire community mobilizers or organizers to follow up and support the work of action committees.
- Continue to generate "small wins" that reward collaborative efforts more immediately while also tackling larger systems changes that demand longer-term engagement.
- Promote sustainability of successful community partnerships by gradual reduction in long-term funding. Promote institutionalization of their more effective interventions by incorporating them into existing budgets.

6. Use a variety of methods to build capacity for doing the work.

- Enhance personal contact among those doing (and supporting) the work. Seek to build the trusting relationships necessary for people to learn from each other.
- Use distance education methods (e.g., teleconferencing, the Internet) to create and connect distributed learning communities of people doing the work. (This should be accompanied by investment in hardware, materials, training, and support to promote access to, and use of, new technologies.)
- Use the Internet (e.g., the Community Tool Box, *http://ctb.lsi.ukans.edu/*) to disseminate "how-to" information for core competencies of building healthy communities (e.g., community assessment, strategic planning, advocacy, community evaluation).
- Link newer community partnerships with those

more experienced; and more established leaders with newer generations of leadership.

7. Document the process of community and systems change—new or modified programs, policies, and practices—to enhance mutual learning, accountability, and community improvement.

- Collaborate with leaders of initiatives to develop meaningful ways to present and use data on community and systems change to promote mid-course adjustments and to attract resources.
- Acknowledge, honor, and celebrate those organizations and community champions that bring about significant community and systems changes.
- Use data on community and systems change to promote mid-course adjustments.
- Provide feedback on key variables in the theory of change: a) the amount of community or systems change by goal (e.g., unemployment, youth development), b) intensity of strategy (e.g., providing information, modifying access), c) duration of the change (e.g., one-time event, ongoing), and d) penetration of the change to reach those at risk (including settings and places experienced by high-risk sub-groups).
- Examine trends and patterns in community and systems change over time to identify factors (e.g., action planning) that may affect the rates of change.
- Use an annual state-of-the-partnership report to encourage accountability of statewide and community partnerships to the community and to funders.

8. Make outcome matter.

- Establish and report on agreed-upon intermediate outcomes—such as high rates of important community and systems changes—for community-determined goals.
- Establish and report on agreed-upon more distant outcomes—and related community-level indicators or benchmarks (e.g., estimated pregnancy rate)—for community-determined goals.
- Establish and report on benchmarks for broader social determinants of health and development (i.e., disparity of income; educational attainment).
- Make annual renewal of community investments contingent on evidence of progress (e.g., high rates of community and systems change; improvements in behavior and other benchmarks).

- Award bonus grants (e.g., cash awards) to encourage progress in implementation and outstanding accomplishments of community and systems change.
- Award outcome dividends to reward improvements in longer-term community-level outcomes (e.g., permit communities to reinvest the money saved by reductions in rates of adolescent pregnancy to address other community-determined goals).

9. Develop broad collaborative partnerships—including among statewide and community partnerships, intermediary and support organizations, and grantmakers and governmental agencies—to create a comprehensive and integrated support system for promoting community health and development.
   - Create broad collaborative partnerships among diverse organizations and institutions that share risks, resources, and responsibilities for community improvement.
   - Modify reward and opportunity structures within private and public institutions to support civic engagement in public problem solving (e.g., hiring, promotion, and flextime policies of organizations that encourage civic engagement).
   - Statewide and community partnerships, intermediary and support organizations, and grantmakers and governmental agencies should act as catalysts for change by convening people around important health and development concerns, brokering access to people who can help address community issues, and leveraging resources that few communities could access themselves.

10. Future research and dissemination should help understand and enhance the mechanisms that affect community health and development.
    - Examine whether (and how) reductions in poverty (and income inequality) and improvements in education effect improvements in community-level indicators of health and development.
    - Examine the conditions under which community and systems change (i.e., amount of change by goal, intensity of behavior change strategy, duration, and penetration of target groups) are associated with improvements in more distant community-level indicators (e.g., rates of adolescent pregnancy, child abuse and neglect, employment, high school completion).

- Disseminate information about "what works" and promising practices for building healthy communities, through a variety of appropriate channels of influence (e.g., print and broadcast media, professional associations, the Internet).

CONCLUSION

A HEALTHY community is a form of living democracy: people working together—across the usual boundaries—to address what matters to them. As citizens, we have a duty to shape the basic conditions that affect our lives, and the lives of those with whom we share a common place or experience.[62][63] Insofar as building healthy communities is a democratic process, it can create cohesion and reduce mistrust among a diverse group of people. In transforming local communities, we are guided by shared values and principles—including equality of opportunity and social justice—that bind us in common purpose.[64] As citizens, we share a responsibility to work together to solve our common problems.

Community health and well-being are affected by the conditions, modifiable features of the environment, in which people lead their lives. Some social determinants, such as inequality of wealth and poor education, exert strong negative influences on community health; and social capital, including trust and social ties, may enhance it. Future research, perhaps using more ecological assessments,[65] should help us better understand these complex and reciprocal influences. Practice should focus on community and systems changes that transform the context in which health and development are determined. Critical reflection—among collaborative partnerships, support organizations, and grantmakers—should examine how well we are transforming the conditions under which health and development occur.

Building healthy communities blends the particular and the universal, the local and broader contexts.[66] Such efforts are grounded in the local: the family, the neighborhood, and other familiar communities of interest and place. As such, they build on the shared values and social relationships that inspire trust and build social capital.[67] But to be effective, we must also engage diverse groups—people and organizations "not like us"—and transform the broader conditions—the policies and practices—that affect local work. This requires courage, doubt, and faith: to trust those outside our immediate experience, to question what is, and to believe that together we can make a difference.

Building healthy communities requires an ecological view: seeing the web of interconnectedness that binds people, problems, solutions, and contexts. Systems changes create niches of opportunity for civic engagement, make the work easier, and enhance its value for more people in more places. In a healthy community, individuals pursue common purpose—not for the sake of community alone, but because addressing issues larger than us gives meaning to our lives.

The work of building healthy communities takes time: of us, of our children, and of our children's children. A Jewish proverb counsels: "You are not bound to finish the work, but neither are you free to give it up".[68] In our emerging ties across place and time, we join others in creating environments worthy of all our children, and in providing models for future generations to engage in this good work.

ACKNOWLEDGMENTS

W E gratefully acknowledge the contributions of our colleagues and teachers in community-based organizations and foundations who deeply influenced our thinking about building healthy communities. Past and current colleagues at our Work Group who shaped these ideas include Jannette Berkley-Patton, Kari Harris, Rhonda Lewis, Christine Lopez, Michael McAfee, Jenette Nagy, Kim Richter, Ella Williams, and Thurman Williams. This was presented as an invited address to the 1998 Kansas Conference on Health and Its Determinants, sponsored by the Kansas Health Institute and the Kansas Health Foundation. Work, on which this summary report is based, was supported by grants from the Kansas Health Foundation, the John D. and Catherine T. MacArthur Foundation, the Ewing Marion Kauffman Foundation, the Kansas Alcohol and Drug Abuse Services Commission, the Greater Kansas City Community Foundation, and the Robert Wood Johnson Foundation. Reprints may be obtained from the first author, Work Group on Health Promotion and Community Development, 4082 Dole Center, University of Kansas, Lawrence, KS 66045. (U.S.A.)

NOTES

1. Fawcett, S. B., Paine, A. L., Francisco, V. T., and Vliet, M. (1993). Promoting health through community development. In D. Glenwick and L. A. Jason (Eds.), *Promoting health and mental health in children, youth, and families*, pp. 233–255. New York: Haworth Press.

2. World Health Organization. (1987). Ottawa charter for health promotion. *Health Promotion*, 1–4, iii–v.

3. Institute of Medicine. (1997). Committee on Using Performance Monitoring to Improve Community Health: Durch, J.S., Bailey, L.A., and Stoto, M.A. (Eds). *Improving health in the community: A role for performance monitoring*. Washington, D.C.: National Academy Press.

4. World Health Organization. (1987).

5. World Health Organization. (1987).

6. Institute of Medicine. (1988). *The future of public health*. Washington, D.C.: National Academy Press.

7. Institute of Medicine. (1997).

8. Institute of Medicine. (1997).

9. Wilkinson, R. G. (1996). *Unhealthy societies: The afflictions of inequality*. London, England: Routledge.

10. Kaplan, G. A., Pamuk, E., Lynch, J. W., Cohen, R. D., and Balfour, J. L. (1996). Income inequality and mortality in the United States. *British Medical Journal, 312*, 999–1003.

11. Marmot, M. G. Smith, G. D., Stansfeld, S., Patel, C., North, F., Head, J. White, I., Brunner, E. and Feeney, A. (1991). Health inequality among British civil servants: The Whitehall II study. *The Lancet, 337* (8), 1387–1393.

12. Kehrer, B. H., and Wolin, C. M. (1979). Impact of income maintenance on low birthweight: Evidence from the Gary experiment. *Journal of Human Resources, 14,* 435–462.

13. Feinstein, J. (1993). The relationship between socioeconomic status and health: A review of the literature. *Milbank Quarterly, 71,* 279–322.

14. Brofenbrenner, U., McClelland, P., Wethington, E., Moen, P., and Ceci, S. J. (1996). *The state of Americans: This generation and the next.* New York: The Free Press.

15. Bernstein, J., and Mishel, L. (1997). Has income inequality stopped growing? *Monthly Labor Review, 120* (12), 3–16.

16. Putnam, R. D. (1993). *Making democracy work.* Princeton, NJ: Princeton University Press.

17. Wilkinson, R. G. (1996).

18. Kawachi, I., Kennedy, B. P., Lochner, K., and Prothrow-Stith, D. (1997). Social capital, income inequality, and mortality. *American Journal of Public Health, 87*(9), 1484–1490.

19. Putnam, R. D. (1993).

20. Putnam, R. D. (1995). Bowling alone: America's declining social capital. *Journal of Democracy, 6*(1), 64–78.

21. Putnam, R. D. (1993).

22. Putnam, R. D. (1995).

23. Feinstein, J. (1993).

24. Kawachi, I. et al. (1997).

25. Barker, R. G. (1968). *Ecological psychology.* Stanford, CA: Stanford University Press.

26. Fawcett, S. B., Paine-Andrews, A., Francisco, V. T., Schultz, J. A., Richter, K. P., Lewis, R. K., Williams, E. L., Harris, K. J., Berkley, J. Y., Fisher, J. L., and Lopez, C. M. (1995). Using empowerment theory to support community initiatives for health and development. *American Journal of Community Psychology, 23*(5), 667–697.

27. Orfield, M. (1997). *Metropolitics: A regional agenda for community and stability.* Washington, D.C.: Brookings Institution Press.

28. Fawcett, S. B., Paine-Andrews, A., Francisco, V. T., Schultz, J., Richter, K. P., Berkley-Patton, J., Fisher, J. L.,

Lewis, R. K., Lopez, C. M., Russos, S., Williams, E., Harris, K. J., and Evenson, P. (in press). Evaluating community initiatives for health and development. In I. Rootman, D. McQueen et al. (Eds.) *Evaluating health promotion approaches.* Copenhagen, Denmark: Work Health Organization—Europe.

29. Goodman, R. M., Speers, M. A., McLeroy, K., Fawcett, S., Kegler, M., Parker, E., Smith, S., Sterling, T., and Wallerstein, N. (1998). Identifying and defining the dimensions of community capacity to provide a basis for measurement. *Health Education and Behavior, 25*(3), 258–278.

30. Lappe, F. M. and DuBois, P. M. (1994). *The quickening of America: Rebuilding our nation, remaking our lives.* San Francisco, CA: Jossey-Bass.

31. Schorr, L. B. (1997). *Common purpose: Strengthening families and neighborhoods to rebuild America.* New York: Anchor Books, Doubleday.

32. Lappe, F. M. and DuBois, P. M. (1994).

33. Herrnstein, R. J. and Murray, C. (1994). *The bell curve: Intelligence and class in American life.* New York: Free Press.

34. Wilson, W. J. (1996). *When work disappears: The world of the new urban poor.* New York: Knopf.

35. Ryan, W. (1971). *Blaming the victim.* New York: Vintage Books.

36. Institute of Medicine. (1997).

37. Kretzman, J. P., and McKnight, J. L. (1993). *Building communities from the inside out: A path toward finding and mobilizing a community's assets.* Chicago: ACTA Publications.

38. Institute of Medicine. (1997).

39. Aguirre-Molina, M. (1996). Community-based approaches for the prevention of alcohol, tobacco, and other drug use. *Annual Review of Public Health, 17,* 337–358.

40. Institute of Medicine. (1988).

41. Fawcett, S. B. (1991). Some values guiding community research and action. *Journal of Applied Behavioral Analysis, 24,* 621–636.

42. Himmelman, A. T. (1992). Communities working collaboratively for a change. (Monograph available from the author, 1406 West Lake, Suite 209, Minneapolis, MN 55408).

43. Schorr, L. B. (1997).

44. Fawcett, S. B. et al. (1993).

45. Green, L. W. and Kreuter, M. W. (1991). *Health promotion planning: An educational and environmental approach,* 2nd ed. Mountain View, CA: Mayfield.

46. Kretzman, J. P. and McKnight, J. L. (1993).

47. Fawcett, S. B. (1999). Some lessons on community organization and change. In Rothman, J. (Ed.), *Reflections on community organization: Enduring themes and critical issues.* Itasca, IL: F.E. Peacock Publishers.

48. Rothman, J. (Ed.) (1999). *Reflections on community organization: Enduring themes and critical issues.* Itasca, IL: F.E. Peacock Publishers.

49. Altman, D. G., Balcazar, F. E., Fawcett, S. B., Seekins, T., and Young, J. Q. (1994). *Public health advocacy: Creating community change to improve health.* Palo Alto, CA: Stanford Center for Research in Disease Prevention.

50. Altman et al. (1994).

51. Schorr, L. B. (1997).

52. Francisco, V.T., Paine, A.L., and Fawcett, S. B. (1993). A methodology for monitoring and evaluating community coalitions. *Health Education Research: Theory and Practice, 8*(3), 403–416.

53. Hawkins, D. and Catalano, R. (1992). *Communities that care.* San Francisco, CA: Jossey-Bass.

54. Fawcett, S. B., Lewis, R. K., Paine-Andrews, A., Francisco, V. T., Richter, K. P., Williams, E. L., and Copple, B. (1997). Evaluating community coalitions for the prevention of substance abuse: The case of Project Freedom. *Health Education and Behavior, 24*(6), 812–828.

55. Paine-Andrews, A., Vincent, M. L., Fawcett, S. B., Campuzano, M. K., Harris, K., Lewis, R., Williams, E., and Fisher, J. (1996). Replicating a community-based initiative for the prevention of adolescent pregnancy: From South Carolina to Kansas. *Family and Community Health, 19*(1), 14–30.

56. Paine-Andrews, A., Harris, K. J., Fawcett, S. B., Richter, K. P., Lewis, R. K., Francisco, V. T., Johnston, J., and Coen, S. (1997). Evaluating a statewide partnership for reducing risks for chronic diseases. *Journal of Community Health, 22*(5), 343–359.

57. Yin, R. K. (1988). *Case study research: Design and methods.* Newbury Park, CA: Sage.

58. Fawcett, S. B. et al. (in press).

59. Francisco, V. T. et al. (1993).

60. Work Group on Health Promotion and Community Development. (March, 1998). *Community Tool Box,* Chapter 6, Strategic Planning [Online]. Internet address: *http://ctb.lsi.ukans.edu/.*

61. Fawcett, S. B. et al. (1997).

62. Lappe, F. M. and DuBois, P. M. (1994).

63. Sclove, R. E. (1995). *Democracy and technology.* New York: Guilford Press.

64. Citrin, T. (1998). Topics for our times: Public health—community or commodity? Reflections on Healthy Communities. *American Journal of Public Health, 88*(3), 351–352.

65. Raudenbusch, S. W. (1997). *Toward a science of ecological assessment: A model for the systematic social observation of neighborhoods.* Unpublished paper presented at the annual meeting of the American Society of Criminology, San Diego, November, 1997.

66. Carroll, J. (1997). *Neighborhoods and citizenship.* Lecture at the Boston Public Library, Boston, Massachusetts. Broadcast by C-SPAN television network. November 15, 1997.

67. Fukuyama, F. (1995). *Trust: The social virtues and the creation of prosperity.* New York: The Free Press.

68. Walzer, M. (1998). Pluralism and social democracy. *Dissent,* Winter issue, 47–53.

Part Two

CHILD DEVELOPMENT AND HEALTH

Five

SOCIAL AND EDUCATIONAL INDICATORS OF CHILDHOOD WELL-BEING IN KANSAS

Thanne Rose and Frank Song

EARLY chilhood experiences have a great impact on success in adult life, including influence on cognitive and social skills, imagination and creativity, mental health, and self-esteem.[1] One of the key indicators of a nation's overall development is the development and well-being of its children. Yet, how children are doing is a function of external influences well beyond their control, such as social policy and environment. Does a common philosophy exist in local communities regarding childhood well-being? Policies, "those laws, regulations, formal and informal rules and understandings that are adopted on a collective basis to guide individual and collective behavior . . .", may have a direct, immediate influence on structural characteristics or services considered routine parts of a child's social environment: increasing health-insurance coverage, expanding early Head Start and "parents as teachers" programs, requiring an adult-to-child ratio in the child care and school settings, privatizing adoption and foster care for children, to name a few.[2, 3, 4]

In this chapter we explore indicators of the social environment of childhood to enhance our understanding of the characteristics influencing favorable outcomes for children, such as gradu-ating from high school. High school graduation is an outcome associated with lowered risks of violence, substance abuse, teen pregnancy, and crime in adulthood.[5, 6] The term "indicators" is used here in the broadest sense, to accommodate the various kinds of information about children currently available on the county level for most of the population of Kansas. Sometimes the types of data are related to services or interventions, sometimes a process or a direct outcome measure. Social environment in the early years of childhood includes primarily the home, child-care environment (in-home and center-based), school, church, and library. Each of these environments has certain structural and process characteristics that may influence favorable outcomes in later years.

The prism shown in Figure 1 is a metaphor for understanding the interplay between the learning opportunities for children (services or interventions), the child (and the individual differences of genes and environment) and outcomes of well-being. Natural light reaches the prism, moves through the medium of the prism, changing directions slightly and emerging from the prism as perceptible and distinct colors (outcomes). Each child encounters opportunities

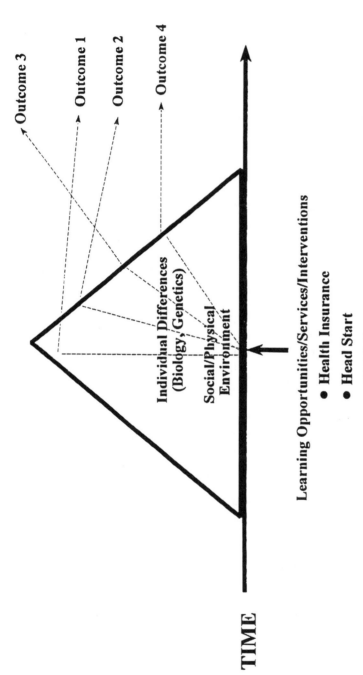

Figure 1
Early Childhood and Social and Educational Outcomes of Well-being:
A Prism as a Metaphor

to learn within the context of a social environment, resulting in a variety of outcomes, some of them discernible and measurable. Each favorable outcome has some probability of occurring that is a function of the individual differences averaged across all children.

Figure 2 shows conceptually how data are combined at the county level using information from partners within Kansas. Indicators about childhood well-being and social environment are obtained from a combination of community-based sources and the organizations within the Kansas State Government responsible for delivering, licensing, regulating, or enforcing various services. Like most states, Kansas has a variety of communities (and counties) reflecting more rural or more urban oriented social environments for children. Household characteristics, age composition, and regional population density are included to determine whether the relationships of interest are modified in some way by general characteristics in the population.

An example of a social environment providing opportunities for children is the public library. Public librarians develop and offer various programs targeting children in specific age-groups. The children's programs help in the development of literacy as well as in the use of language skills, both of which are important to school success.[7] These programs also reinforce and improve existing skills, learned either in the home through parent-child interactions or at the place of schooling through teacher-child interactions.[8] In more rural areas of Kansas, it is not atypical for a child to attend five library programs and check out over 25 books per year from the local public library.[9]

Table 1 provides an overview of the variables considered for analysis. We used some basic guidelines to reduce the size of the original pool of variables about childhood well-being. First, we consulted the research literature for variable inclusion and located that information from the partner-organization within Kansas.[10–13] Next, if new data were summarized on an aggregate

level other than on the county level, we restructured it so that it could be analyzed on the county level. If two variables were strongly correlated (for example, divorce rate and single-parent household) but one variable captured more realistically the social environment (single-parent household), then we included the more valid indicator even though a slightly larger variance may have been explained by using the other variable.

We used a standard correlation and multiple regression approach, with the unit of observation at the county level.[14, 15] The correlation matrix provided an initial impression of the interrelationships among the pool of independent variables and between the dependent variable (high school graduate rate) and each independent variable. Absolute values of correlation equal to or greater than 0.3 were included in the models.

Bivariate analysis showed that a high student-teacher ratio, free or reduced school meals, child-abuse rate, urban setting, single-parent household, divorce rate, child poverty, unemployment rate, out-of-home placement, were highly significant and negatively related to high school graduation rate. Income, parent education level, ratio of adults over 60 to children under 15 years of age (an approximation of the younger and older part of the population not working full-time in the community) and child-care availability were positively correlated with high school graduation rate. Public-library variables such as library program attendance per child, library-book transactions per child, inter-library loans per child given size of library (based on bound books and volumes) were marginally correlated with high school graduation. In more agricultural counties, lower out-of-home placement, lower levels of (reported) child abuse, higher student-teacher ratio, higher oldest-to-youngest dependency ratios, and greater public-library utilization were associated with graduation from high school. In the final models, at least 75 percent of the variance was explained by including the terms student-to-teacher ratio,

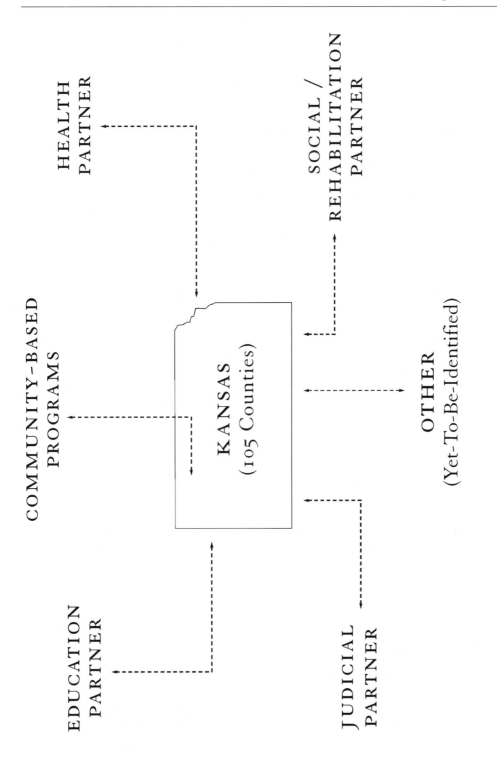

Figure 2
County-Level Linkage of Data About Children Among Partners Within the Organizational Structure of Kansas State Government

Table 1.

Overview of Variables Considered for analysis by Indicator Type and Aggregate-Level

Indicator	County Level	County-Group Level	State Level
Care Environment	◆ child-care slots ◆ out-of-home placement ◆ head start participation ◆ teen pregnancy ◆ juvenile arrest ◆ single-parent household	◆ type of licensed, regulated child care	◆ parent requests about time, type, age of child in child-care setting
Public Schools	◆ free/reduced-price meals at school ◆ student-teacher ratio ◆ average daily attendance pre-K, K ◆ average daily attendance 1–12 ◆ high school graduation rate	◆ enrollment ◆ violent acts, suspensions, expulsions, dropouts ◆ academic-skills assessments (school district size) ◆ future plans of high school graduates	
Public Libraries	◆ attendance at children's programs ◆ library transactions of children's materials ◆ interlibrary loan per child		
General Population Characteristics	◆ G1 (retired)-to-G3 (dependents) ratio ◆ percent of population in agriculture ◆ per-capita income ◆ persons per square mile		

single-parent household, teen pregnancy rate, and free/reduced meals. Student attendance in public schools and variables about public library utilization did not improve significantly the fit in the series of final multi-variate models.

Ideally we would like to use a multidimensional measure of early child development, an index similar to the child health and development index.[16] We foresee better and more complete data, leading to the identification of a more "upstream" outcome reflecting favorable outcomes in the early years of childhood. Currently, assessment of such skills as reading and math among primary-school-age children exist only on the state level.

Immediate social environment does influence a child's ability to reach educational goals. In most cases, single-parent households, divorce, or a broken family will be associated with lower income, a sense of insecurity, incompleteness of care and love, distraction of attention from studies, and emotional stress. Children in these situations may also have to work part-time to help the family, distracting them from giving their full attention to study. Teen pregnancy increases the demands on the time and energy of young people, resulting in their dropping out of school. The more students a teacher has responsibility for, the less personal attention he or she can offer to a given student during school time. Streamlining the opportunities for young children to acquire and reinforce learning skills in the home, child-care setting, library, and school is optimal.

If we can combine our knowledge of the organizational structure of Kansas government and what part of the structure collects the data that is reflected in the indices of childhood (population) well-being, then we know what information should be given to partners on the county and community levels to improve these measures of well-being. Partners in Kansas now have tangible measures of their county's well-being and can begin to invest in their community's health. There are opportunities to share ideas across communities within a county and to track the progress over time. Perhaps a common philosophy about childhood well-being can emerge through this process.

With this data are some reliability and validity issues worth mentioning, such as under-reporting and differences in degree of reporting by subgroups of the populations. In Kansas, community-based programs serve a vital function in helping interpret numbers in ways we often have not thought of, because these programs may be getting more complete information on the community level than is reflected on the county or state level. Actively incorporating new and more complete information will bring greater clarity to the interpretation of findings in the future.

NOTES

1. Carnegie Corporation of New York. *Starting Points: Meeting the Needs of Our Youngest Children: The Report of the Carnegie Task Force on Meeting the Needs of Young Children.* New York: Carnegie Corporation of New York, 1994.

2. Governor Graves, "State of State '98", www.ink.org/public/governor/stotst98.html. (1998): pp. 1–5.

3. Feild, T. (1996). *Managed Care and Child Welfare: Are They Compatible? Conceptual Issues in Managed Care for Child Welfare.* Institute for Human Services Management.

4. Wallack, L. (1990) *Media Advocacy: Promoting Health through Mass Communication.* In: Glanz, F., Lewis, F. M. Health Behavior and Health Education: Theory, Research and Practice. 370–386.

5. Maynard, R. A. and Garry, E. M. (January 1997). *Adolescent Motherhood: Implications for the Juvenile Justice System.* (Fact Sheet #50). *Office of Juvenile Justice and Delinquency Prevention.* U.S. Department of Justice, Office of Justice Programs.

6. Greenwood, P., Model, K. E., Rydell, C. P., Chisea, J. (May 1996). *"Diverting Children From a Life of Crime: What Are the Costs and Benefits?"* *RAND Research Brief.* The RAND Corporation, Santa Monica, California.

7. Snow, Catherine E. (May 1983). "Literacy and Language: Relationships during the Preschool Years." *Harvard Educational Review.* Vol. 53 (2):165–189.

8. Hart, B. and Risley, T. R. (1995). Meaningful Differences in the Everyday Experience of Young American Children. Maryland: Paul H. Brookes Publishing Co.

9. Bird, R. (1997). Kansas Public Library Services. 1996 Directory and Statistics. Topeka, Kansas: Library Development Division, Kansas State Library.

10. Kansas Action for Children, Inc. *Kansas Kids Count Data Book*. Topeka, Kansas, 1996.

11. University of Kansas. *Kansas Statistical Abstract 1997*. Lawrence, Kansas: Institute for Public Policy and Business Research.

12. Kansas State Board of Education website (1997): www.ksbe.state.ks.us./cgi-bin/list.state.

13. Kansas Association of Child Care Resource and Referral Agency (July 1996–December 1997). *Data Details*.

14. Green, S. B., Salkind, N. J., Akey, T. M. *Using SPSS for Windows: Analyzing and Understanding Data*. New Jersey: Prentice Hall, 1997.

15. Afifi, A. A., Clark, V. Computer-aided Multivariate Analysis, Third Edition. [city]: Chapman and Hall, 1996. pp. 83–221.

16. Singh, G. K., Wilkinson, A. V., Song, F. F. et al. (1998). *Health and Social Factors in Kansas: A Data and Chartbook, 1997–1998*. Topeka, Kansas: Kansas Health Institute.

Six

EARLY INFLUENCES ON DEVELOPMENT AND SOCIAL INEQUALITIES: AN ATTACHMENT THEORY PERSPECTIVE

Peter Fonagy and Anna Higgitt

T HE discipline of developmental psychopathology has become a dominant and unifying framework in modern child psychiatry and psychopathology (Cicchetti and Cohen 1995; Miller and Lewis 1990). The central concern is predicting maladaptive patterns of development and identifying the mechanisms by which psychosocial and biological factors influence this. Models which emerge from research into risk and protective factors have tended to be quite complex, neither specific nor linear (e.g., Seifer, Sameroff, Anagnostopolou, and Elias 1992). Crucially, the work of Rutter (1987) has demonstrated that risk conditions occur simultaneously and the number rather than the type of risk factors is predictive of outcome.

It is beyond the scope of this chapter to summarize the extensive literature on risk and protective factors. Instead, emphasis will be given to those risk factors likely to have a bearing on social inequalities in health, and particularly those which are amenable to preventative intervention. Five sets of factors will be considered in the first part of this chapter: biological factors, family and social factors, parenting factors, attachment, and the influence of nonmaternal care. The chapter concludes with a review of recent preventative

interventions, and some recommendations for action.

DEVELOPMENTAL FACTORS IN THE CREATION OF SOCIAL INEQUALITIES

Biological Factors

Biological compromise (e.g. premature birth, low birthweight, serious medical illness) significantly influences infant outcome, although the aggregation of risk factors means that outcomes for most etiologies exist along a continuum. Rates of biological compromise are not equally distributed across social groups. For example, low birthweight (LBW < 2,500 g) has a prevalence of 6% in white, middle class U.S. women and 15% in low socioeconomic status (SES), ethnic minority teenagers who tend to be single (unmarried) mothers (Paneth 1995). The multi-site *Infant Health and Development Project* (Korner et al. 1993) found in a large cohort of premature infants that compromised outcome (IQ < 85 at 3 years) was unevenly distributed. In a signal detection analysis, race had greatest sensitivity and specificity in predicting outcome, followed by maternal education, and then medical complications; birthweight was a insignificant predictor.

The differences were quite dramatic. Whereas 90% of infants of poorly educated black mothers with medical complications had compromised outcome, only 9% of white infants with well-educated parents fell into this category regardless of birth complications. A multi-faceted psychosocial intervention was successful in reducing the former figure to 50%, while the same intervention for the middle class group only yielded a 2% change. These figures underscore the overwhelming importance of psychosocial factors in determining the outcome of apparently biological risks. Other biological variables, such as maternal smoking during pregnancy (Wakschlag et al. 1997), appear to be independent of psychosocial factors, however.

Genetic influences are increasingly seen as relevant to the outcomes associated with social inequalities (Plomin 1994). The *MacArthur Longitudinal Twin Study* has provided important information concerning genetic factors in behavioral inhibition. The biological predisposition for wariness in response to unfamiliar events is evident from infancy (Kagan, Reznick, and Snidman 1988; 1991). While behavioral inhibition is quite unstable between 14 and 24 months (Robinson et al. 1992), the change is due to genetic rather than environmental factors (Plomin et al. 1993), suggesting that genes may turn off and on at different ages (Cherny et al. 1994). Genes are also "context dependent." For example, in the *MacArthur Longitudinal Twin Study*, the comparison of identical and fraternal twins revealed continued genetic influence on empathic responses (e.g., showing cognitive, emotional, and behavioral arousal in response to the distress of another) at 24 and 36 months. Testing conditions, however, had a dramatic influence. Genetic factors predominated children's empathic responses when an unfamiliar tester was the source of distress. But when the mother was the potential object of empathy, the predominant influences were specific to the mother; they were of a shared environmental type (Robinson, Zahn-Waxler, and Emde 1998). It seems that socialization influences shared by the twins in their interactions with the parents and others were a major influence with mothers but not with the tester, and in the latter context, genetic influences could more readily manifest. Thus genetic influences, even where present, should not be considered environmentally immutable. It is conceivable that the social context of low SES status may serve to inhibit or trigger genetic propensities.

Social and Family Factors

Social class, and particularly poverty, has been found repeatedly to predict developmental outcomes of childhood. The relationships are generally indirect, acting through variables influencing (a) the availability of resources (such as nutrition, housing and medical care); (b) lifestyles and attitudes (neighborhood quality, accidents, exposure to toxic substances); and (c) the social and emotional context in which the child develops (parenting skills, maltreatment, marital disharmony, quality of care).

Infants and young children growing up in poverty are more likely than affluent children to have health problems (such as lead poisoning, failure to thrive, otitis media, iron deficiency anemia), cognitive delays, and behavioral problems (Klerman 1991; McLoyd 1990; Parker, Greer, and Zuckerman 1988; Pollitt 1994; Ramey and Campbell 1991; Wise and Meyers 1988). In Kansas, Sudden Infant Death Syndrome, which accounts for 16% of infant deaths, is on average 4–5 times higher in infants with mothers with less than a high school diploma than it is amongst those with a college education (Singh 1998).

The effect of low socioeconomic status (SES) on social development and delinquency is particularly strong when experienced in early childhood (Elder and Rockwell 1979). Young children with low SES are not only exposed more frequently to risk factors, but also experience more serious consequences from these risks (Bradley et al. 1994b). They are more vulnerable to negative life events such as single parenthood, social isolation, and loss of employment. Moreover, severe levels of early environmental and social deprivation have been shown to be associated with significant neurodevelopmental deficits. Recent work exploring the sequelae of extreme deprivation experienced by Romanian infants (Perry 1997) has shown that in late-adopted (after 8 months) orphans functional MRI scans revealed significant fronto-temporal deficits at 4 years of age despite high levels of post-adoption care. It is important to note in this context that studies of attachment security in this sample revealed an unexpectedly high prevalence of insecure (particularly disorganized) attachment patterns specifically in the late-adopted group. The early-adopted group, while more likely to be insecure than normal controls, was no more likely to manifest disorganized attachment patterns. Perry's formulation of these data suggests that chronic arousal and the long-term presence of high cortisol levels in the brain is the cause of the abnormalities.

Family instability is more prevalent in underprivileged groups, and conflict associated with instability has a powerful negative influence on child development. Marital conflict predicts abnormal infant behavior and conduct problems in toddlers (Easterbrooks and Emde 1986; Jouriles et al., 1991), and has a greater negative influence than parental loss through death or divorce (Hetherington, Cox, and Cox 1982; Loeber and Stouthamer-Loeber 1986). Evidence suggests overt expressions of inter-parental anger, the expression of physical hostility, child-rearing disagreements, and a lack of resolution of conflicts account for the higher risks associated with family instability (Cummings, Ianotti, and Zahn-Waxler 1985; Cummings, Zahn-Waxler, and Radke-Yarrow 1981; Easterbrooks, Cummings, and Emde 1994; Grych and Fincham 1990). Intra-parental intimacy, on the other hand, has a benign influence on infant development (Cox et al. 1989; Howes and Markman 1989).

Single, socially isolated young mothers constitute a particularly high risk group. A significant minority of Kansas mothers is single mothers (25% of births between 1989 and 1994 were to single mothers), and their children have injury rates that are twice those of children in two-parent families (Roberts and Pless 1995). Moreover, in Kansas, as in the rest of the U.S., 13% of infants are born to teen mothers, the majority unmarried (Singh 1998). Adolescent parenthood is a well-established risk factor in infant development with a markedly skewed social distribution (Hechtman 1989). Deficiencies in the parenting behavior of adolescent mothers may account for this. They are more passive, less stimulating, smile and talk less, give more commands, are more restrictive, physically intrusive and punitive, and are less satisfied with mothering (Coll et al. 1986; Culp et al. 1988; Passino et al. 1993; Whitman et al. 1987). These parental behaviors are associated with relatively poor cognitive and linguistic outcomes, as well as impulsivity, aggression, and social withdrawal in the child (Hart et al. 1992; Osofsky, Hann, and Peebles 1993; Spieker and Bensley 1994; Weiss et al. 1992).

Maltreatment of the young child is another well-demonstrated risk factor with significant associations with social class (Cicchetti and Toth 1995). In fact, after controlling for the impact of low SES, physical and emotional maltreatment remain significant but less powerful influences (Herrenkohl et al. 1995). The causal paths involve biological aspects, as early maltreatment has profound neurodevelopmental as well as behavioral sequelae (Cicchetti and Toth 1995; Hart, Gunnar, and Cicchetti 1995).

Maltreated youngsters show many social and emotional problems, including indiscriminate sociability, poor affect regulation, heightened levels of aggression, social withdrawal, inconsistent and unpredictable signals, and disorganized attachment (Carlson et al. 1989; Cicchetti and Barnett 1991; Crittenden, Partridge, and Clausen 1991). Perhaps most critically, there appear to be major dysfunctions of self-development. Schneider-Rosen and Cicchetti (1991) demonstrated that these children show less positive affect in response to their image in the mirror. Beeghly and Cicchetti (1994) demonstrated a specific deficit in the use of internal state words. This and other evidence reviewed by Fonagy and Target (Fonagy and Target 1997) suggests that early maltreatment may undermine crucial aspects of the infant-caregiver interpersonal interchange, an interchange which underpins the child's acquisition of an adequate understanding of how the mind works. Their limited understanding of the nature of mental states—how beliefs and desires determine human behavior—undermines their capacity to interact adequately with their caregivers and their peers, forcing them to use action rather than words both to influence the behavior of others and to regulate their own internal states.

The Quality of Parenting

Child-rearing practices powerfully impact on child development. The strength of the relationship between quality of parenting and socioeconomic status is moderate (Belsky 1984; Bradley and Caldwell 1984). Mothers from low socioeconomic groups tend to provide less warmth and affection, less variety in social and cultural experiences, and more punitive caregiving (Fox, Platz, and Bentley 1995; Koblinsky, Morgan, and Anderson 1997; Smith and Brooks-Gunn 1997; Socolar, in press). In combination, such practices are associated with poor outcomes, including lower IQ, emotional and behavioral problems. For example, the multi-site Infant Health and Development Program showed that harsh parental discipline, in the context of low maternal warmth, was associated with a 12-point deficit in the IQ scores of girls (Smith and Brooks-Gunn 1997).

Power assertion rather than supportive guidance in parenting is linked with the development of externalizing behavioral disorders (Belsky, Woodworth, and Crnic 1996; Crockenberg and Litman 1991; Power and Chapieski 1986). In a study of over 1,000 young children, using videotape observations of mother-child interaction at 6–15 months, ratings of mothers' sensitivity (e.g., positive regard, non-intrusiveness, sensitivity to non-distress expression) predicted non-compliant behavior in the child at two and three years (NICHD Early Child Care Research Network 1998). By contrast, a good relationship with one parent (marked by warmth and the absence of criticism) has been shown to have a substantial protective effect against the development of conduct disorder (Farrington and West 1981; McCord 1986; Pulkkinen 1983; Rutter 1979; Werner and Smith 1982). These patterns are established early. When parents make predominantly "do demands" ("come and eat," "put your shirt on") to two- and three-year olds, rather than "don't demands" ("don't wander off," "don't go around in you pajamas all day"), as well as expressing positive affect, the child's level of compliance is enhanced (Kochanska and Aksan 1995; Kuczynski and Kochanska 1995).

Current evidence suggests that a number of pathways are simultaneously involved in mediating the influence of low socioeconomic status on parenting. Restricted access to resources such as a safe environment, play materials, outings, and other social learning experiences may have a direct effect on caregiving (Watson et al. 1996). Factors associated with poverty (e.g., low maternal IQ, lack of knowledge of child development) may limit parenting skills. Additionally, poverty may create stresses that limit the quality of parenting and/or create marital conflict (McAdoo 1988; Patterson 1986). Psychological distress resulting from an excess of negative life events and difficulties and the absence or disruption of marital bonds can also precipitate parenting behaviors such as punitiveness, inconsistency and unresponsiveness (Lempers, Clarke-Lempers, and Simons 1989). Low SES adults have often experienced adversity during their own childhood, which prepares them poorly for the needs of their own children (Egeland, Jacobovitz, and Sroufe 1988). However, the extent and quality of social support available to low SES mothers may moderate the impact of poverty on parenting (Burchinal, Follmer, and Bryant 1996).

Genetic evidence suggests that the most important aspects of family environmental influences on development are those unique to each sibling in the same family. One study of parenting style (Reiss et al. 1995) measured three domains of parenting (warmth/support, conflict/negativity, and monitoring/control) in 708 families. These families had at least two same-sex adolescent siblings: monozygotic or dizygotic twins, ordinary siblings, full siblings in step-families, half siblings in step-families, or genetically unrelated siblings in step-families. Harsh, aggressive, explosive and inconsistent parenting showed strong associations with antisocial behavior. Overall, 60% of the variance in adolescent antisocial behavior could be accounted for by conflictual and negative parental behavior directed specifically at the adolescent. Interestingly, the same attitudes toward the siblings signaled a less pathological outcome in the adolescent.

Parental psychopathology represents a major risk factor for child development and the more severe and chronic the parent's disorder, the more likely there is to be a deleterious impact upon the child (Bassuk et al. 1997; Seifer and Dickstein 1993). There is no evidence, however, to suggest that specific disorders are associated with specific early developmental outcomes. The impact of parental disturbance may well be indirect, identifying parents likely to exhibit problematic parenting (Lyons-Ruth, Connell, and Grunebaum 1990).

Maternal depression is particularly relevant in lower socioeconomic status, high-risk samples, and has been intensively studied (Campbell, Cohn, and Meyers 1995; Field et al. 1990; Lyons-Ruth et al. 1990). Disturbances in mother-infant engagement characteristic of depressed mothers are less evident in middle class samples (Murray et al. 1996). The pathogenic aspects of disadvan-

taged, depressed mothers' interactions with their children may be either "withdrawn-unavailable" or "hostile-intrusive." Both have been shown to interfere with cognitive and emotional development (Murray and Cooper 1997). For example, in one study of 353 couples, maternal disorder and infant behavior at three months predicted disturbance of the mother-infant interaction, which in turn predicted infant behavior problems at two years, independent of early infant behavioral problems (Laucht, Esser, and Schmidt 1994). It has also been shown that infants whose mothers are still depressed when the infants are six months old begin to show growth retardation, neurophysiological abnormalities, and developmental delay (e.g., Field 1995). Infants manifest right frontal EEG asymmetry (which may be a marker for a bias toward the expression of negative emotion) as well as lowered vagal tone and elevated levels of adrenaline and noradrenaline (Dawson et al. 1992, 1995; Field et al. 1995).

Substance abuse is also strongly associated with social inequalities. It compromises early childhood development, but there is little evidence that this is due to prenatal drug exposure (Halpern 1993). Rather, the combination of biological and psychosocial risk factors associated with drug abuse (such as inadequate nutrition and poor prenatal care, which compromise fetal growth) has been shown to have deleterious effects upon development (Lester and Tronick 1994). Drug exposure is likely to affect CNS development as a function of timing, dose, and duration (Tronick et al. in press), but their impact is likely to be moderated by factors unrelated to the nature of the exposure. Such families are also characterized by parental psychopathology, a disorganized caregiving environment with multiple caregivers, exposure to violence, and a lack of resources for essentials (Haller et al. 1993).

Security of Attachment as a Mediator of Psychosocial Risk

Theoretical and empirical considerations both point to the security of infant attachment as a mediating factor for other forms of psychosocial risk. John Bowlby (1988), the originator of attachment theory, asserted that resilience in the face of stressful life events in later life is determined by the pattern of attachment developed during the early years. Laboratory procedures are available for the reliable assessment of attachment patterns in early and middle childhood. In adolescence and adulthood, measures of narrative coherence in accounts of early childhood are used. Of particular relevance here are insecure attachment patterns that either suppress attachment behaviors (avoidant infant, dismissing adult), or that intensify the signaling of distress yet reject attempts at soothing (resistant infant, preoccupied adult). A further category of individuals exhibit anomalous, even bizarre behaviors toward the caregiver or manifest disoriented, confused, emotionally unintegrated descriptions in narratives of loss or trauma as adults. Such disorganized or unresolved patterns are held to be indicative of an absence of coherent affect-regulation strategies (Crittenden 1995; Main and Hesse 1990; Main and Solomon 1990; Solomon, George, and Dejong 1995).

Attachment classifications have substantial stability from infancy to later development. Recent studies have shown a 70–80% continuity between infancy and adult assessments of attachment (Hamilton 1994; Main 1997; Waters et al. 1995). Securely attached infants tend to grow up to be healthier in terms of social relationships and emotional adjustment; to be more competent in terms of language skill and achievement; and to have a more positive self-image than insecurely attached ones. Infants who are disorganized in their attachment are most likely to develop substantial social problems at school and to exhibit aggression and a variety of psychiatric difficulties (Lyons-Ruth 1996; Moss et al. 1996; Solomon et al. 1995).

Social inequalities predict security of attachment, with social advantage usually associated with secure attachment (Belsky 1996; Murray et al. 1996; NICHD Early Child Care Research Network 1997; Shaw and Vondraa 1993; Spieker and Booth 1988). In an inner-city study, for example, only 24% of infants were found to be securely attached, and 32% were considered to be insecure/disorganized (Broussard 1995). In middle class samples, 65% are normally securely attached and 10% disorganized (van IJzendoorn et al. 1992). To some extent, a mother's attachment security may protect the child from some common aspects of social deprivation, such as marital disharmony (Das Eiden, Teti, and Corns 1995).

Attachment status has biological as well as psychosocial aspects. The physiological correlates of insecure attachment suggest a long-term vulnerability to stress-related illnesses. Insecure infants (especially those with disorganized patterns of attachment) have increased reactivity of the hypothalamic-pituitary-adrenal axis (Nachmias et al. 1996; Spangler and Grossman 1993). Work with rats and monkeys demonstrated that the mother-infant relationship acts as a regulator of the developing neural system in infants (Hofer 1996) and maternal deprivation results in the withdrawal of a number of different hidden regulatory processes. Thus, increased HPA activity may be an indication of the absence of the regulatory effect of prior mother-infant interaction. Animal studies that selectively deprive the infant of different elements of the normal mother-infant interaction demonstrate that HPA responses to such deprivation are quite specific. Withdrawal of nutrient supply specifically affects the adreno-cortical response, whereas withdrawal of ano-genital licking impacts the pituitary level (Sucheki et al. 1995). The separation-induced premature release from regulation has long-term effects on subsequent neuro-regulatory development. It manifests, for example, in susceptibility to immobilization-induced gastric ulceration (Ackerman 1980; Weiner 1996). These findings have complex implications for humans. Inadequate early care may lead to dysfunction because of the failure of the normal smooth modulation and coordination of physiological function, affect and behavior into a coherent and stable diurnal pattern (Hofer 1996). In infant animals the source of the regulation is behavioral. In human mother-infant interaction regulation is at the level of rapid interchanges of subjective expectations (mental representations of relationships). The beneficial effect of social support on health may operate through the regaining of interactional regulators (Hofer 1996).

Perhaps most relevant to social inequalities are the findings concerning the intergenerational consistencies of attachment classifications. A number of laboratories have reported that the infant's attachment classification to the parent appears to be predicted accurately by the attachment classification of that parent, obtained before the birth of the child (Benoit and Parker 1994; Fonagy, Steele, and Steele 1991; Steele, Steele, and Fonagy 1996; van IJzendoorn 1995). The parents' quality of attachment predicts the infant's attachment to its parents which may, in its turn, influence that young person's ability to parent his or her own child. Determinants of parenting ability are rarely used as goals in preventative interventions, yet mental health promotion initiatives should be ensuring long-term wellness.

Studies of Child-Care

Twenty percent of children are in child-care of some type, the rate higher in urban than in rural areas (Singh 1998). There is a long-standing debate concerning the impact of non-maternal care on infant-mother attachment (Fox and Fein 1990; Karen 1994; Rutter 1981). Daily separations from the mother could, according to attachment theory, undermine the child's expectations about the parent's availability (Sroufe 1988) or the mother's sensitivity with the child (Brazelton 1985). Studies in the 1980s reported that insecurity (anxious-avoidance) seemed to be associated with over 20 hours a week of child-care during the first year of life (Belsky and Rovine 1988; Clarke-Stewart 1989; Lamb and Sternberg

1990). Other studies reported that non-maternal care in the first year predicted increased behavioral problems at three and four years (Baydar and Brooks-Gunn 1991; Volling and Feagans 1995) and in school-age children (Barton and Schwarz 1981; Haskins 1985). Early and extensive care has been shown to predict later maladjustment in Bermuda (McCartney et al. 1982), Italy (Varin et al. 1994), Sweden (Sternberg et al. 1991), and Norway (Borge and Mehuish 1995).

More recent studies no longer report this association, however. A definitive study of 1,153 mother-infant dyads (NICHD Early Child Care Research Network 1997) found no significant differences in attachment security related to child-care participation, other than a temporary increase in caregiver-perceived problems at age two. A combination of maternal and child-care factors were, however, shown to be powerful predictors of attachment outcome. For example, children who received less sensitive caregiving both in child-care and from their mothers were almost twice as likely to be insecure as children with less risk from these sources. However, high quality child-care appeared, in some measure, to compensate for maternal insensitivity. The child's gender also complicated the picture, with time in day-care increasing insecurity for boys, but decreasing it somewhat for girls. Boys are generally more vulnerable to psychosocial stressors. The NICHD investigation offers good evidence to support the benign nature of the social and economic pressure upon women to return to work rapidly after the birth of a child, but underscores the importance of the relationship with the primary caregiver as a determinant of infant outcome.

Social inequalities are most evident in terms of the quality of non-maternal child-care that may be available to a working mother. On the whole studies demonstrate that when quality of care is high, any adverse effects associated with early, extensive, and continuous care are mitigated, eliminated entirely, or even reversed (e.g., Andersson 1989; Field 1991; Howes and Olenick 1986;

Howes, Phillips, and Whitebook 1992; Phillips, McCartney, and Scarr 1987). For example, in one study children in high quality center-based care between six and twelve months were rated as less anxious, more prosocial, and less troubled by transitions to school at age eight (Andersson 1992). In the NICHD study (NICHD Early Child Care Research Network 1998), quality of care was the most consistent child-care variable predicting compliance and problem behavior. The amount of variance accounted for was modest, but these analyses controlled for income levels, thus attenuating the association. Additionally, the amount of experience a child had with groups of other children predicted less problematic and more cooperative functioning in the NICHD study and other reports (Clarke-Stewart, Gruber, and Fitzgerald 1994; Vandell 1979). However, group experience appears to be helpful only when introduced in the second year of life; in the first year it is associated with more mother-reported problems (NICHD Early Child Care Research Network 1996).

The NICHD studies showed that child behavior was best predicted by quality of mothering, irrespective of non-maternal care. However, the experience of non-maternal care strongly influences maternal behavior toward the child (NICHD Early Child Care Network 1997). For example, the time spent in non-maternal care negatively correlates with observed ratings of maternal sensitivity at six months and positively correlates with maternal negativity at 15 months. If maternal sensitivity is controlled for, most of the significant associations between child behavior and non-maternal care disappear. Similar results were reported in a more detailed study of a smaller sample (Belsky 1998), where fathering was also found to be more negative when families relied extensively on non-maternal child-care arrangements.

Hence, the risk associated with non-maternal care may be mediated by the impairment of parental sensitivity associated with early, extensive, and continuous non-maternal child care. Time away from the child may undermine the parent's ability to get to know the child well which may, in turn, compromise the parent's capacity to manage the child's behavior effectively. Alternatively, parents managing the demands of work and child-care might simply lack the energy and patience to offer adequate parenting. It appears, then, that time in care may not directly cause the development of problem behaviors, but it might do so by influencing family processes. This suggests that attempts to reduce the negative effects of child-care arrangements should focus upon the parenting processes in the home rather than trying to improve the quality of non-maternal care. Furthermore, time in care in the baby's first six months predicts poorer patterns of mother-child interaction when the children are two or three years of age. These findings have clear implications for parental leave policies and practices.

Summary: A Relationship Focus

The child's relationship with a caregiver appears to be critical to understanding and addressing social inequalities in child development. Many of the stresses associated with low SES impact on the child by diminishing the quality of the relationship to his/her caregiver. These limitations may manifest as inadequate child care, insensitive caregiving, harsh or negative discipline, maltreatment, psychiatric illness, or in some other manner. Thus, strengthening the relationship is likely to be effective in a wide range of domains of child development.

This perspective is strongly endorsed in the U.S. Department of Health and Human Services' guidelines for launching the *Early Head Start* program, a program for 0–3 year olds and their families (Department of Health and Human Services 1994).

"Child caregiver relationships . . . are critical for providing infants and toddlers support, encouragement, continuity and emotional nourishment necessary for healthy development and the development of healthy attachments. . . . Within the context of caregiving relationships, the infant builds a sense of what is expected, what feels right . . . as well as skills and incentives for social turn-taking, reciprocity, and cooperation. The infant's activities are nourished and channeled in appropriate ways so as to encourage a sense of initiative and self-directedness. During the toddler period, the child, through repeated interactions with emotionally available caregivers, also begins to learn basic skills and self-control, emotional regulation and negotiation. Empathy for others and prosocial tendencies for caring and helping also develop during toddlerhood as well as the emotions of pride and shame; experiencing and learning about these capacities require responsive caregiving relationships in the midst of life's inevitable stresses and challenges . . . A sense of pleasure, interest and exploration, early imaginative capacities, and the sharing of positive emotions also begin in infancy—all of which require repeated and consistent caregiver relationship experiences and form a basis for social competence that carries through toddlerhood and the preschool period. . . ." (U.S. Department of Health and Human Services 1994, p.7).

STUDIES ON THE PREVENTION OF INEQUALITIES IN HEALTH

Overview of the Evidence on Primary Prevention
Initially, prevention research was impeded by inconsistent terminology and inadequate research design. Research has rapidly accelerated over the past two decades, to a point where relatively confident statements may now be made about the efficacy of a variety of preventative and health promoting strategies in children and adolescents (Cowen 1997). A critical debate concerning the value of prevention (Marlowe and Weinberg 1983) triggered three important milestones in the field (Koretz and Moscicki 1997):

1. In 1993 the National Institute of Mental Health Steering Committee of the National Prevention Research Conferences (National Institute of Mental Health 1993) provided an integrated summary of NIMH scientific activities in prevention research. It defined the relevant concepts of prevention, delineated appropriate methodologies and recommended future developments.
2. The Institute of Medicine report by the Committee on the Prevention of Mental Disorder (Mrazek and Haggerty 1994) described the Prevention Intervention Research Cycle for the development and testing of interventions. It also proposed a model of prevention interventions (Gordon 1983) which classified these on the basis of risk status into universal (low risk), selective (medium risk), and indicated (high risk) strategies.
3. The NIMH Prevention Research Plan (National Institute of Mental Health 1995) consolidated the recommendations from the 1993 Steering Committee report and the 1994 Institute of Medicine report into practical research objectives.

A further critical contribution was Durlak and Wells' (1997) meta-analytic review of 177 controlled primary prevention programs for children. The studies reviewed had a primary mental health thrust. They excluded studies designed to effect academic achievement or to prevent drug use and offered strong evidence for the efficacy of mental health promotion in strengthening behavioral and social adaptation. The mean effect size (ES) was 0.34, comparable in size to those reported for other types of psychological, health, educational, and behavioral interventions; for example, programs to prevent smoking and alcohol use in children tend to obtain effect sizes between 0.29 and 0.36 (Bruvold 1993; Tobler 1992). Positive effect sizes were found for both competence enhancement and problem reduction outcomes; in the 25% of studies with follow-up data, initial success was maintained.

Primary prevention studies may be distinguished along two dimensions (Cowen 1986; Price 1986). In the first dimension, programs are either person- or environment-centered interventions. The former target a risk population directly, while the latter attempt to change individuals indirectly by modifying the environment (e.g., through modification of child-rearing techniques, or teachers' management of the classroom). In designing intervention techniques, the former draw on the clinical literature while the latter attempt more widespread social change using developmental, social psychology, or sociological principles. The risk status of the target population defines the second dimension: (a) a universal strategy is applied to all members in an available population (e.g., all children in a particular nursery); (b) the selective approach targets an at-risk group who are not yet dysfunctional (e.g., children of alcoholic parents); (c) the transition approach targets individuals about to experience potentially stressful life events (e.g., divorcing parents). The large majority of interventions are person- rather than environment-centered and use the universal or transition approach.

Prevention Programs
Targeting First-Time Mothers

Programs that target first-time mothers tend to be very effective (ES=0.87). This effect size compares favorably with those for treatments such as bypass surgery or chemotherapy for certain cancers, which all fall below 0.5 (Lipsey 1990). Transition programs (offering reassurance and support around the birth of the first child and both social support and child-rearing assistance) yield substantial benefits in the reduction of problems (ES=0.93) and in the enhancement of competencies (ES=0.81).

The *Infant Health and Development Program* (Brooks-Gunn et al. 1994) was a large study aimed at reducing the educational, health, and behavioral risks associated with low birthweight. One third of the 985 infants across eight sites were randomly selected for a program involving home visits (weekly in the first year and biweekly for two further years), educational programs in specially designed preschools (four hours per day), and parent group meetings. There was a

significant impact on IQ, health status, and behavior (CBCL) during the period of intervention (in the first three years p<0.001). The observed group differences were related to improvements in learning materials and the range of stimulation, modeling of social maturity, and warm acceptance of the child (Bradley et al. 1994a). High father involvement, particularly for the black ethnic group, was associated with better outcome in terms of IQ (Yogman, Kindlon, and Earls 1995). On five-year follow-up, however, only the heavier babies (2,001 to 2,500 g) continued to show IQ benefits (p<0.008) and neither group manifested significant health or behavior benefits. The limited long-term affects underscore the fact that the mere physical presence and educational and supportive input of a home visitor is unlikely to benefit disadvantaged mothers in the long-term. Two other large (n=2,235 and 1,654) randomized controlled trials with high-risk families demonstrated in fact that home visits offering social support and education only had no discernible advantage for disadvantaged mothers or their infants (Oda, Heilbron, and Taylor 1995; Villar et al. 1992).

The *Pre-natal Infancy Project* (or *Elmeira Project*), conducted by David Olds and his colleagues, was based on the 'ecological' developmental model of Bronfenbrenner (1979), and was more comprehensive than the program described above. This model assumed an interdependence amongst social systems operating simultaneously; high risk was seen as a combination of unhealthy maternal behavior, dysfunctional infant caregiving, and a stressful social environment. The sample (low SES, single young mothers) was recruited before the 25th week of pregnancy. Home nurse visits throughout the first two years of life (weekly for the first six weeks, then decreasing to once every six weeks during the second year) included an educational component (risk behaviors), parenting techniques, enhancement of social support, and advice. Benefits were evident from childbirth, and during the first two years there was a 32% reduction in emergency room visits, particularly for injuries and ingestions (56%) (Olds et al. 1986b). There was also a reduction in verified child abuse, from 19% to 4%, amongst unmarried teenage parents (Olds et al. 1986a). It was found that fewer restrictions and punishments were used and more intellectually stimulating material was available. Once the nurse home visits ceased (in the 3rd and 4th year) the differences in the rates of child abuse and neglect between the two groups were reduced and so was the difference in the children's intelligence scores (Olds, Henderson, and Kitzman 1994a). However, significant differences in the number of injuries and ingestions were maintained, as well as a clear reduction in behavioral problems, and there were lasting IQ gains in the children of mothers who smoked during pregnancy (Olds, Henderson, and Tatelbaum 1994b). The financial investment in the scheme was recovered in terms of government savings by the time the child was 4 years old (Olds et al. 1993). Follow-up after 15 years revealed that nurse-visited mothers in the highest risk group (low SES, unmarried) continued to have fewer births, to claim less aid, to show lower impairments due to alcohol and other drugs, and to have fewer arrests or convictions (Olds et al. 1997). The 50% reduction of verified reports of child neglect or abuse was particularly notable.

Kitzman and colleagues (1997) have replicated the findings of the Elmeira Project in Memphis, Tennessee, with a somewhat larger sample of primarily African-American women. There was a reduction in pregnancy-induced hypertension (from 20% to 13%), in presentations of children with injuries or ingestions, and in the number of second pregnancies over the two-year period (from 47% to 36%). More of the mothers in the nurse-visited group breastfed their infants (26% vs. 16%). Additionally, these mothers provided more facilitative home environments, reported higher levels of perceived mastery (which is also a likely protective factor against child maltreatment), and held fewer beliefs that are consistent with neglect and child abuse (e.g., lack of empa-

thy, unrealistic expectations of infants, and beliefs in corporal punishment).

The strongest effects in both these studies may have originated from the long-term impact of structural changes in the mothers' lives associated with the home visits. For example, delaying their next pregnancy and entering productive employment improved their child's chances (Olds et al. 1988). Similarly, the long-term success of the *Mother-Child Home Program of Verbal Interaction Project* (Levenstein 1992) may well have been due to parents in the experimental group deciding, as a consequence of these interactions, to send their children to preschool (95% vs. 74%). Thus, the engagement of parents is an essential precondition for the success of a program, even when this is focused principally upon children.

We believe that successful preventive interventions require a relationship-based approach. Two successful programs where long-term follow-up data are available had principal goals of improving parent-child communication, and strengthening parent-child relationships (Johnson and Walker 1987a; Lally, Mangione, and Honig 1988). The fostering of an affectionate relationship between mother and infant brought about a reduction in problem behaviors in mid-childhood (7–12 years) (Johnson and Walker 1987a) and early adolescence (15 years) (Lally et al. 1988). Significant gains in infant development were demonstrated in association with improved mother-infant relationship in about half of the 12 studies that included long-term follow-up (see review by Lojkasek, Cohen, and Muir 1994). Furthermore, observational studies indicate that many aspects of risk (socioeconomic status, maternal psychopathology) are, to some degree, mediated by the low quality of mother-child interaction (e.g., Dodge, Pettit, and Bates 1994; Harnish et al. 1995). Thus, the fostering of a positive affectionate relationship between the mother and the infant and the strengthening of the mother's self-perceived efficacy in relation to her parenting role are the likely effective aspects of these programs.

Many different home visitation programs for first-time mothers have been promoted, but only a relatively small minority are effective (Olds and Kitzman 1993). When they are effective, benefits are surprisingly large and widespread, even extending to younger siblings of mothers who had been visited (Seitz and Apfel 1994). Several major home visitation programs are currently under way in the United States, including the *San Diego Healthy Families America Clinical Trial* and *Hawaii's Healthy Start Home Visitation Program*. Additionally, a major multi-site initiative (*Early Head Start*) is underway. A Rand Corporation report (Karoly et al. 1998) has confirmed the fiscal benefits of home visitation in the United States. These preventative approaches are most beneficial for young, low SES mothers. The programs target the mothers' health behaviors, child-care practices, family planning, educational achievements, participation in the workforce, and their self-confidence for meeting life challenges. Evidence now shows that the social welfare of teenage mothers could not be greatly affected by policies that simply delayed their childbearing but changed little else (Maynard 1997).

Important questions remain concerning the characteristics of a successful home visiting program (Moffitt 1997). These include: (a) the content and structure of effective programs; (b) the most appropriate target population (low SES, young, primaparous); (c) the minimum effective home visiting package; (d) methods of delivering the service (training, staffing, organization); and (e) conditions of delivery (mandatory or voluntary, local, regional or statewide).

Transition Programs for Children of Divorce

Durlak and Wells' (1997) work included seven, mainly brief, group programs, which all aimed to help children understand and cope with changes resulting from parental disharmony. The *Children of Divorce Intervention Program* from San Francisco is a good example (Alpert-Gillis, Pedro-Carroll, and Cowen 1989). Overall, 64% of children in such programs were better off than those in the control group (ES = 0.36). The benefits were felt both in terms of a reduction of problems (ES = 0.38) and an enhancement of competency (ES = 0.33). Whilst significant, these effect sizes are not particularly encouraging and probably reflect the brevity of the interventions offered. In another study, Wolchik and colleagues (1993) identified five potential mediators of children's adjustment to divorce. They designed an intervention to influence each of these potential mediators, but found that only one, the quality of the mother-child relationship, was strongly related to outcomes. This highlights the centrality of the relationship (attachment) perspective in prevention, as well as the importance of a theoretically coherent model in designing preventative interventions.

An alternative perspective is to assist the parents through their divorce in order to reduce the risk for the child. In the U.S., state legislatures and court administrative districts have implemented educational programs with the aim of instructing parents on reducing marital conflicts and creating non-adversarial post-divorce environments (Biondi 1996). A survey of 102 parent education programs established for this purpose throughout the U.S. has been reported by Braver and colleagues (1996). Most programs covered topics on the impact of divorce on children and the benefits of parental cooperation and more than half were mandatory. Unfortunately, most programs do not aim to enhance parental competence (e.g., conflict management, positive parenting) and it is unlikely that they achieve much for the children involved. Yet the potential of such programs is great. Indeed, one report of a child-focused class demonstrated dramatic lowering of child exposure to parental conflict and greater willingness for shared parenting at six-month follow-up (Arbuthnot and Gordon 1996).

The Prevention of Maltreatment

Perhaps of most significance are findings that physical maltreatment and neglect can, it seems, be prevented by home visits (Gray et al. 1979a, 1979b; Hardy and Streett 1989; Larson 1980; Olds et al. 1986a), although not all studies demonstrate significant benefit (e.g., Barth 1991; Whipple and Wilson 1996). MacMillan and colleagues (1994a, 1994b), in a review of this literature, concluded that "extended home visitation can prevent child physical abuse and neglect among families with one or more of the risk-markers of single parenthood, teenage parent status and poverty" (MacMillan et al. 1994a, p.854). Evidence on the prevention of sexual abuse is less compelling (MacMillan et al. 1994b). Nevertheless, in view of the well-documented and serious sequelae of childhood maltreatment (Cicchetti and Toth 1995), these findings are of the utmost importance to preventative health care.

It is emerging that parents at risk of physical abuse can be relatively readily identified. In one study, a representative sample of first-time mothers was asked to disclose their abuse history by questionnaire and then asked if they would accept services designed for expectant parents who were mistreated as children. Overall, 15% of these women acknowledged such experience, and 70% of these, along with 26% of those who denied abuse, expressed interest in these services. Further targeting of an intervention could be based on demographic information concerning single parenting, socioeconomic status, young maternal age, and social isolation (Christmas, Wodarski, and Smokowski 1996). Parent education programs for such groups demonstrate cost-effective benefits, not only in terms of a reduced risk of maltreatment, but also in delaying subsequent pregnancies, completing high school, and attending college (Britner and Reppucci 1997).

Child-Centered Programs

There are two relatively common types of mental health promotion programs targeted on young children. First, Spivack and Shure's (1974) theory that problem-solving skills are an important part of adjustment has influenced the development of interpersonal problem-solving programs. The general aim is to instruct children in the use of cognitive strategies to identify interpersonal problems and develop effective means of resolving such difficulties. Based on six studies, the effect size for these programs for children aged 2–7 was 0.93. However, these approaches tended to increase competencies (ES = 1.11) rather than ameliorate problems (ES = 0.41). Maladjustment was not significantly reduced and the increase in competencies was largely attributable to better problem-solving. This program is argued to be more effective when combined with other program elements under the broader framework of social competence training (Weissberg and Bell 1997). The teaching of multiple competencies such as self-control, stress management, responsible decision making, and communication training within one program are underway (Consortium on the School-Based Promotion of Social Competence 1994).

The second category of programs offered affective education to young children with the aim of increasing their awareness and expression of feelings and their ability to understand the possible causes of behavior. These studies (n = 46) assume that children's social and behavioral adjustment will improve if they learn to have a greater awareness of feelings and behavioral attributions. Affective education programs range from brief interventions to lesson plans lasting an entire school year and may combine stories, puppet play, music, and exercises appropriate for the child's age. Three quarters (76%) of young children who had the benefit of the program were better off than untreated controls (ES = 0.7). The program was also successful in reducing problems (ES = 0.85) and somewhat less successful in enhancing competencies (ES = 0.69). These programs were far less effective for older children, indicating the possibility that a critical period exists for the acquisition of mental state attributions under seven years of age. Preventative initiatives using affective education are either insufficiently intensive or inappropriate once children's strategies become enduring.

Features of Successful Programs

Effective programs have been shown to have a number of features in common (Dryfoos 1990): (a) comprehensiveness, (b) system orientation, (c) relatively long duration, (d) proactive orientation, (e) early commencement, and (f) specificity to particular risk factors.

As no single program component can prevent multiple high risk behavior, a package of coordinated collaborative strategies is necessary for successful outcome. For example, the Consortium of School-Based Promotion of Social Competence (Elias and Tobias 1996) includes in its package (a) the teaching of families, (b) phasing in new competencies at developmentally appropriate times, (c) the provision of "booster shots" to reinforce learning, and (d) changes to the school environment consistent with the assumptions of the program.

Simultaneous focus on the system or context within which the child lives (e.g., school, family, community), as well as on the child, is more likely to be successful than programs that focus on the child alone. *The Child Development Project* (CDP - Battistich et al. 1989), for example, endeavors to cover the course of the entire elementary school period. It aims to engineer a total school environment designed to promote wellness by enhancing the child's sense of autonomy, competence, and relatedness. Measures include students setting and upholding discipline standards, cooperative learning formats, buddy systems, and problem-solving and conflict resolution strategies that embody democratic values and stress the value of helping others. Partnerships involving parents, teachers, and children, designed to incorporate all facets of the child's life in a coherent, goal-oriented way, form the core of CDP. Benefits of the program are seen in some areas of academic attainment (reading comprehension) as well as major social improvements (e.g., dealing with conflict, peer competence, empathy and sensitivity to others, self-esteem, and sense of community) (Battistich et al. 1995).

Short-term programs have, at best, time-limited benefits, especially with at-risk groups. Programs over several years (e.g. Johnson and Walker 1987b; Seitz, Rosenbaum, and Apfel 1985) tend to impact on more risk factors and have more lasting effects. *Head Start* offers only one year preschool experience, which may be too short to have a lasting effect with multi-risk families. Preventative efforts need to be titrated to the severity of the disorder they are intended to prevent. Previous preventative efforts were only partial when the net was cast too wide; the prevention of serious disturbance requires a long-term and intensive enterprise.

Risk and protective factors require the focus, rather than problem behaviors. In this way, multiple adverse outcomes may be addressed within a single program. Developmental psychopathology offers a framework for focusing on the mediators on the developmental paths leading to mental disorders and social maladaptation (National Institute of Mental Health 1995). This approach was used in the Baltimore prevention research studies (e.g., Kellam et al. 1994) and in the work of the *Conduct Problems Prevention Group*. Generic, unstructured approaches such as the provision of counseling or group discussion are less effective than focused proactive programs.

Early commencement of preventative interventions is agreed to be essential. Additionally, intervention during pregnancy brings additional benefits (e.g., Larson 1980). Spivack and Shure's (1974) prevention strategy, involving the teaching of interpersonal problem-solving skills, was more effective in preschoolers than in older children (Shure and Spivack 1988). There is, nonetheless, a need to sustain any improvements brought about by early intervention (Cox 1993b).

It is possible that the impact of early intervention on both intellectual development and parent-child relationships is greater because of so-called "sensitive periods," which may make later attempts at prevention more challenging, if not impossible (Ramey, Yeates, and Short 1984; Rutter 1990).

The era of generic therapies is over. Every disorder requires particular modifications to treatment regimens. Similarly, it is unrealistic to hope that a single generic preventative intervention will be able to reduce the risk for all psychological disorders. In the Durlak and Wells meta-analysis, there was a significant heterogeneity revealed in the outcomes of primary prevention programs. Developmental level, type of program, and target group all affected outcome. Thus the homogeneity assumption ("one size fits all"), implicitly held by some preventionists, should be abandoned (Lorion 1990). As with treatment, prevention will need to be adjusted to disorder, context, and objective. We should therefore address our efforts to those disorders where longitudinal studies have given us sufficient clues about identifying "at risk" populations. The very generality of universal prevention, however desirable, mitigates against any particular individual experiencing it as relevant to them. To design a program so that it is perceived to be of equal relevance to all groups would be a major challenge (McGuire and Earls 1991).

The literature on the qualifications required to perform preventative work has not reached a consensus. In the UK, most studies use health visitors—nurses who have a statutory obligation to visit young children and their caregivers. Preventative programs added to health visitors' training by providing extra didactic seminars, back-up consultation (Hewitt and Crawford 1988), support groups and joint case work (Thompson and Bellenis 1992), and a combination of didactic, supervisory and mutual support case discussion formats (Bellenis and Thompson 1992). Despite the highly trained nature of this group and their excellent integration with the statutory services, no striking results either from the point of view of the caregiver or the child (Stevenson, Bailey, and Simpson 1988) or from the point of view of reduced referral on to secondary services have been reported (Bellenis and Thompson 1992; Thompson and Bellenis 1992). A disappointingly low uptake of the preventative service (less than 15%) was found in one study (Stevenson et al. 1988). Interestingly, although not formally compared, the outcomes from volunteer-based schemes seem more promising (Cox 1993a). In the latter studies, there was no expert helper and the distinction between befriender/volunteer and the befriended mother was not stressed (Pound and Mills 1985). These minimally trained volunteers were shown to be effective in bringing about improvements not only in the mother's mental state but also some degree of improvement in mother-child relations as revealed by blind rating of video recordings (Cox, Pound, and Puckering 1992). Experts have not been shown to be more effective than non-experts in delivering preventative interventions.

Supportive interventions have their roots in nursing, social work, and community psychology. Intervention improves parents' (normally mothers') access to resources such as housing, child-care, and welfare benefit (see Booth et al. 1987; Minde et al. 1983). The role of support, however, goes beyond this. Such interventions aim to activate the young mother's attachment system through the provision of a stable, safe, non-exploitative relationship with the home visitor (Minde et al. 1983). A subsidiary goal of prevention programs may be the provision of information concerning child development (e.g., Belsky 1985; Pfannenstiel and Honig 1995). It is hard to conceive of such information directly impacting on the child's relation to the caregiver and an implicit goal must include the enhancement of parental sensitivity to the child. The establishment of a good relationship with the individual involved in prevention must form an important component of such programs.

Conclusions

The promise of preventative intervention is considerable. Taken together from the studies we have referred to and others, we may conclude that early preventative interventions have the potential to improve in the short-term the child's health and welfare (including better nutrition and physical health, fewer feeding problems, low birthweight, accidents and emergency room visits and reduced potential for maltreatment) while the parents can also expect to benefit in significant ways (including educational and work opportunities, better use of services, improved social support, enhanced self-efficacy as parent, and improved relationship with both their child and partner). In the long-term children may further benefit in critical ways behaviorally (less aggression, distractibility and delinquency), educationally (better attitudes to school, higher achievement), and in terms of social functioning and attitudes (increased prosocial attitudes) while the parents can benefit in terms of employment, education, and mental well-being.

These conclusions should be qualified substantially in the following ways, however. First, outcomes are selective—no study achieved all these effects together. Second, many of the studies reported unacceptable rates of refusal, which threatens generalizability. For example, even in the highly successful Rochester nurse home visitation program, only 80% of the pregnant women invited to participate agreed to become involved (Olds et al. 1986b). Unfortunately, it is most likely those in greatest need who decline the invitation to take part. Third, attrition is high in most studies, making conclusions from long-term follow-ups doubtful; the low self-perceived risk of adverse outcome may account for the low uptake and high rates of attrition observed in many prevention studies. For example, three of the most influential studies, the *Houston Parent-Child Development Center Program* (Johnson and Walker 1987a; Johnson 1990, 1991), the *Parent-*

Child Interaction Training Project (Strayhorn and Weidman 1991) and the "*I Can Problem Solve: An Interpersonal Cognitive Problem-Solving Program*" (Shure and Spivack 1982, 1988) had attrition rates of around 50%. Fourth, results are generally poorer with, what appear to be, higher risk samples. Fifth, the theoretical models of prevention studies are less sophisticated than for treatment interventions. Finally, the heterogeneity of the studies does not permit clear recommendations about the effective preventative intervention program. Nevertheless, in the final section of this chapter, we make some suggestions for action in Kansas.

WHAT COULD BE DONE IN KANSAS

1. In the light of the evidence reviewed it may seem advisable to develop a statutory home visiting program with the following features:

(a) Working with mothers before the birth of their child.

(b) Designing a structured program of proven efficacy.

(c) Giving priority to single young mothers with a history of childhood maltreatment.

(d) Home visitors training to include special training in child management techniques.

(e) Working within a keyworker framework where one home visitor is assigned and aims to maintain contact with a specific family.

2. Experimental trials should be established for early parent training with high-risk urban families with the following key features:

(a) A focus on child behavior management.

(b) Children recruited from within day-care programs based on reports of aggression and disruptiveness.

(c) Parent training should be community rather than clinic based, and offered in groups rather than to individuals.

(d) The program should be accompanied by system-level interventions in the schools and communities.

3. Experimental trials should be undertaken in parent training, focused on sensitivity enhancement. These could be:

(a) A broader brief voluntary program to mothers in high-risk groups.

(b) Initiated within the first six months of the child's life.

(c) Administered by specialist trainer.

(d) Offered with the objective of enhancing attachment security.

4. An experimental trial could be undertaken to integrate affective training with the preschool curriculum. This intervention would be:

(a) Focused on high-risk groups in urban areas.

(b) Be delivered by specially trained preschool teachers.

(c) Aimed at reducing the risk of behavioral disorders, including conduct problems and delinquency.

5. Statutory programs for children and parents negotiating separation and divorce could be offered in the context of current voluntary services. Its critical features might be:

(a) Assisting parents in the management of conflict in order to reduce the child's exposure to marital disharmony.

(b) Attempting to maximize the child's contact with both parents following the divorce.

(c) Focusing on low SES groups in order to avoid increasing social inequalities by selective take-up amongst middle class parents.

(d) Integration of these services with school-based counseling services for children of divorce.

6. This review of evidence suggested certain possibilities not yet empirically explored in the literature, which may help focus or enhance strategies for reducing the effects of social inequalities:

(a) It is conceivable that the socialization of middle class children equips them better for the task of parenting than lower SES groups. If this is confirmed, modification of educational programs to incorporate parenting education may help in addressing these anomalies.

(b) The quality of preschool child care is clearly variable, but no criteria are available to evaluate the performance of these services. It may be helpful to establish systematic criteria for the performance of day care based on the emotional as well as the cognitive development of the child. More attention should be given to issues of socialization and emotional development in designing preschool curricula.

(c) There is a dearth of research on the relationship between early emotional development and health outcomes. The association of the use of social support and health outcomes suggests that the child's capacity to form bonds may be critical, not just in behavioral outcomes, but also directly or indirectly in terms of physical health. Existing cohort studies could be expanded to explore this possibility.

REFERENCES

Ackerman, S. (1980). Early life events and peptic ulcer susceptibility: An experimental model. *Brain Research Bulletin*, 5 (suppl.), 43–49.

Alpert-Gillis, L. J., Pedro-Carroll, J. L., and Cowen, E. L. (1989). The children of divorce intervention program: Development, implementation, and evaluation of a program for young urban children. *Journal of Consulting and Clinical Psychology*, 57, 583–589.

Andersson, B. (1989). Effect of public day-care: A longitudinal study. *Child Development*, 60, 857–866.

Andersson, B. (1992). Effects of day-care on cognitive and socioemotional competence of thirteen-year-old Swedish schoolchildren. *Child Development*, 63, 20–36.

Arbuthnot, J., and Gordon, D. A. (1996). Does mandatory divorce education for parents work? A six-month outcome evaluation. *Family and Conciliation Courts Review*, 34, 60–81.

Barth, R. P. (1991). An experimental evaluation of in-home child abuse prevention services. *Child Abuse and Neglect*, 15, 363–375.

Barton, M., and Schwarz, J. (1981). *Day care in the middle class: Effects in elementary school*. Paper presented at the American Psychological Association Annual Convention, Los Angeles, CA.

Bassuk, E. L., Weinreb, L. F., Dawson, R., Perloff, J. N., and Buckner, J. C. (1997). Determinants of behavior in homeless and low-income housed preschool children. *Pediatrics*, 100, 92–100.

Battistich, V., Solomon, D., Kim, D. I., Watson, M., and Schaps, E. (1995). Schools as communities, poverty levels of student populations, and students' attitudes, motives and performance: A multi-level analysis. *American Educational Research Journal*, 32, 627–658.

Battistich, V., Solomon, D. S., Watson, M., Solomon, J., and Schaps, E. (1989). Effects of an elementary school program to enhance prosocial behavior and children's cognitive social problem solving skills and strategies. *Journal of Applied Developmental Psychology*, 10, 147–169.

Baydar, N., and Brooks-Gunn, J. (1991). Effects of maternal employment and child care arrangements on preschoolers' cognitive and behavioral outcomes: Evidence from the children of the national longitudinal survey of youth. *Developmental Psychology*, 27, 932–945.

Beeghly, M., and Cicchetti, D. (1994). Child maltreatment, attachment, and the self system: Emergence of an internal state lexicon in toddlers at high social risk. *Development and Psychopathology*, 6, 5–30.

Bellenis, C., and Thompson, M. J. J. (1992). A joint assessment and treatment service for the under fives—work with health visitors in a child guidance clinic—part 2: Work done and outcome. *Newsletter of the Association for Child Psychology and Psychiatry*, 14, 262–266.

Belsky, J. (1984). The determinants of parenting: A process model. *Child Development*, 55, 83–96.

Belsky, J. (1985). Experimenting with the family in the newborn period. *Child Development*, 56, 376–391.

Belsky, J. (1996). Parent, infant, and social-contextual antecedents of father-son attachment security. *Developmental Psychology*, 32, 905–913.

Belsky, J. (1998). Quantity of nonmaternal care and boys' problem behavior/adjustment at 3 and 5: Exploring the mediating role of parenting (manuscript in preparation, Pennsylvania State University).

Belsky, J., and Rovine, M. (1988). Nonmaternal care in the first year of life and the security of infant-parent attachment. *Child Development*, 59, 157–167.

Belsky, J., Woodworth, S., and Crnic, K. (1996). Trouble in the second year: Three questions about family interaction. *Child Development*, 67, 556–578.

Benoit, D., and Parker, K. (1994). Stability and transmission of attachment across three generations. *Child Development*, 65, 1444–1457.

Biondi, E. D. (1996). Legal implementation of parent education programs for divorcing and separating parents. *Family and Conciliation Courts Review*, 34, 82–92.

Booth, C. L., Barnard, K. E., Mitchell, S., and Spieker, S. J. (1987). Successful intervention with multiproblem mothers: Effects on the mother-infant relationship. *Infant Mental Health Journal*, 8, 288–306.

Borge, A., and Mehuish, E. (1995). A longitudinal study of childhood behavior problems, maternal employment, and day care in a rural Norwegian community. *International Journal of Behavioral Development*, 18, 23–42.

Bowlby, J. (1988). *A Secure Base: Clinical Applications of Attachment Theory*. London: Routledge.

Bradley, R., and Caldwell, B. (1984). The HOME Inventory and family demographics. *Developmental Psychology*, 20, 315–320.

Bradley, R. H., Whiteside, L., Mundfrom, D. J., Casey, P. H., Caldwell, B., and Barrett, K. (1994a). Impact of the infant health and development program (IHDP) on the home environments of infants born prematurely and with low birthweight. *Journal of Educational Psychology*, 86, 531–541.

Bradley, R. H., Whiteside, L., Mundfrom, D. J., Casey, P. H., Kelleher, K. J., and Pope, S. (1994b). Early indications of resilience and their relation to experiences in the home environments of low birthweight, premature children living in poverty. *Child Development*, 65, 346–360.

Braver, S. L., Salem, P., Pearson, J., and DeLuse, S. R. (1996). The content of divorce education programs: Results of a survey. *Family and Conciliation Courts Review*, 34, 41–59.

Brazelton, T. B. (1985). *Working and Caring*. New York: Basic Books.

Britner, P. A., and Reppucci, N. D. (1997). Prevention of child maltreatment: Evaluation of a parent education program for teen mothers. *Journal of Child and Family Studies*, 6, 165–175.

Bronfenbrenner, U. (1979). *The Ecology of Human Development: Experiments by Nature and Design*. Cambridge, Mass.: Harvard University Press.

Brooks-Gunn, J., McCarton, C. M., Casey, P. H., McCormick, M. C., Bauer, C. R., Bernbaum, J. C., Tyson, J., Swanson, M., Bennett, F. C., Scott, D. T., Tonascia, J., and Meinert, C. L. (1994). Early intervention in low-birth-weight premature infants. Results through age 5 years from the infant health and development program. *Journal of the American Medical Association*, 272, 1257–1262.

Broussard, E. R. (1995). Infant attachment in a sample of adolescent mothers. *Child Psychiatry and Human Development*, 25, 211–219.

Bruvold, W. H. (1993). A meta-analysis of adolescent smoking prevention programs. *American Journal of Public Health*, 83, 872–880.

Burchinal, M. R., Follmer, A., and Bryant, D. M. (1996). The relations of maternal social support and family structure with maternal responsiveness and child outcomes among African American families. *Developmental Psychology*, 32, 1073–1083.

Campbell, S. B., Cohn, J. F., and Meyers, T. (1995). Depression in first-time mothers: Mother-infant interaction and depression chronicity. *Developmental Psychology*, 31, 349–357.

Carlson, J., Cicchetti, D., Barnett, D., and Braunwald, K. G. (1989). Finding order in disorganization: Lessons from research on maltreated infants' attachments to their caregivers. In D. Cicchetti and V. Carlson (Eds.), *Child Maltreatment: Theory and Research on the Causes and Consequences of Child Abuse and Neglect*. Cambridge: Cambridge University Press.

Cherny, S. S., Fulker, D. W., Corley, R. P., Plomin, R., and DeFries, J. C. (1994). Continuity and change in infant shyness from 14–20 months. *Behavioral Genetics*, 24, 365–379.

Christmas, A. L., Wodarski, J. S., and Smokowski, P. R. (1996). Risk factors for physical abuse: A practical theoretical paradigm. *Family Therapy*, 23, 233–248.

Cicchetti, D., and Barnett, D. (1991). Attachment organisation in preschool aged maltreated children. *Development and Psychopathology*, 3, 397–411.

Cicchetti, D., and Cohen, D. J. (1995). Perspectives on developmental psychopathology. In D. Cicchetti and D. J. Cohen (Eds.), *Developmental Psychopathology, Vol. 1: Theory and Methods* (pp. 3–23). New York: John Wiley and Sons.

Cicchetti, D., and Toth, S. L. (1995). A developmental psychopathology perspective on child abuse and neglect. *Journal of the American Academy of Child and Adolescent Psychiatry*, 34, 541–565.

Clarke-Stewart, K. A. (1989). Infant day-care: Maligned or malignant? *American Psychologist*, 44, 266–273.

Clarke-Stewart, K. A., Gruber, C., and Fitzgerald, L. (1994). *Children at Home and in Day Care*. Hillsdale, NJ: Erlbaum.

Coll, C. G., Vohr, B. R., Hoffman, J., and Oh, W. (1986). Maternal and environmental factors affecting developmental outcome of infants of adolescent mothers. *Journal of Developmental and Behavioral Pediatrics*, 7, 230–235.

Consortium on the School-Based Promotion of Social Competence. (1994). The school-based promotion of social competence: Theory, research, practice, and policy. In R. J. Haggerty, L. R. Sherrod, N. Garmezy, and M. Rutter (Eds.), *Stress, Risk, and Resilience in Children and Adolescents: Processes, Mechanisms, and Interventions* (pp. 268–316). New York: Cambridge University Press.

Cowen, E. L. (1986). Primary prevention in mental health: Ten years of retrospect and ten years of prospect. In M. Kessler and S. E. Goldston (Eds.), *A Decade of Progress in Primary Prevention* (pp. 3–45). Hanover, NH: University Press of New England.

Cowen, E. L. (1997). The coming of age of primary prevention: Comments on Durlak and Wells's Meta-Analysis. *American Journal of Community Psychology*, 25, 153–167.

Cox, A. D. (1993a). Befriending young mothers. *British Journal of Psychiatry*, 163, 6–18.

Cox, A. D. (1993b). Preventive aspects of child psychiatry. *Archives of Disease in Childhood*, 68, 691–701.

Cox, A. D., Pound, A., and Puckering, C. (1992). Newpin: A befriending scheme and therapeutic network for carers of young children. In J. Gibbons (Ed.), *The Children Act 1989 and Family Support* (pp. 37–47). London: HMSO.

Cox, M. J., Owen, M. T., Lewis, J. M., and Henderson, V. K. (1989). Marriage, adult adjustment, and early parenting. *Child Development*, 60, 1015–1024.

Crittenden, P. M. (1995). Attachment and risk for psychopathology—the early years. Rose F. Kennedy Center's Conference: Young children with developmental delays and psychopathology: Issues in diagnosis and treatment (1994, Bronx, New York). *Journal of Developmental and Behavioral Pediatrics*, 16 (supplement), S12–S16.

Crittenden, P. M., Partridge, M. F., and Clausen, A. H. (1991). Family patterns of relationship in normative and dysfunctional families. *Development and Psychopathology*, 3, 491–513.

Crockenberg, S., and Litman, C. (1991). Effects of maternal employment on maternal and two-year-old child behavior. *Child Development*, 62, 930–953.

Culp, R. E., Appelbaum, M. I., Osofsky, J. D., and Levy, J. A. (1988). Adolescent and older mothers: Comparison between prenatal, maternal variables and newborn interaction measures. *Infant Behavior and Development*, 11, 353–362.

Cummings, E. M., Ianotti, R. J., and Zahn-Waxler, C. (1985). The influence of conflict between adults on the emotions and aggression of young children. *Developmental Psychology*, 21, 495–507.

Cummings, E. M., Zahn-Waxler, C., and Radke-Yarrow, M. (1981). Young children's responses to expressions of anger and affection by others in the family. *Child Development*, 52, 1274–1282.

Das Eiden, R., Teti, D. M., and Corns, K. M. (1995). Maternal working models of attachment, marital adjustment, and the parent-child relationship. *Child Development*, 66, 1504–1518.

Dawson, G., Klinger, L. G., Panagitodes, H., Hill, D., and Spieker, S. (1992). Frontal lobe activity and affective behavior of infants and mothers with depressive symptoms. *Child Development*, 63, 725–737.

Department of Health and Human Services. (1994). *The Statement of the Advisory Committee on Services for Families with Infants and Toddlers.*

Dodge, K. A., Pettit, G., and Bates, J. E. (1994). Socialization mediators of the relation between socioeconomic status and child conduct problems. *Child Development*, 65, 649–665.

Dryfoos, J. G. (1990). *Adolescents at Risk: Prevalence and Prevention.* New York: Oxford University Press.

Durlak, J. A., and Wells, A. M. (1997). Primary prevention mental health programs for children and adolescents: A meta-analytic review. *American Journal of Community Psychology*, 25, 115–152.

Easterbrooks, M. A., Cummings, E. M., and Emde, R. N. (1994). Young children's responses to constructive marital disputes. *Journal of Family Psychology*, 8, 160–169.

Easterbrooks, M. A., and Emde, R. N. (1986). *Marriage and infant: Different systems' linkages for mothers and infants.* Paper presented at the International Conference on Infant Studies, Beverly Hills, CA.

Egeland, B., Jacobovitz, D., and Sroufe, L. A. (1988). Breaking the cycle of abuse. *Child Development*, 59, 1080–1088.

Elder, G. H., and Rockwell, R. C. (1979). Economic depression and post-war opportunity in men's lives: A study of life patterns and health. *Research in Community and Mental Health*, 1, 249–303.

Elias, M. J., and Tobias, S. E. (1996). *Social Problem Solving: Interventions in the Schools.* New York: Guilford Press.

Farrington, D. P., and West, D. J. (1981). The Cambridge study in delinquent development. In S. A. Mednick and A. E. Baert (Eds.), *Prospective Longitudinal Research* (pp. 137–145). New York: Oxford University Press.

Field, T. (1991). Quality infant day-care and grade school behavior and performance. *Child Development*, 62, 863–870.

Field, T. (1995). Infants of depressed mothers. *Infant Behavior and Development*, 18, 1–13.

Field, T., Fox, N., Pickens, J., and Nawrocki, T. (1995). Relative right frontal EEG activation in 3- to 6-month-old infants of depressed mothers. *Developmental Psychology*, 31, 358–363.

Field, T., Healy, B., Goldstein, S., and Guthertz, M. (1990). Behavior-state matching and synchrony in mother-infant interactions of nondepressed vs. depressed dyads. *Developmental Psychology*, 26, 7–14.

Fonagy, P., Steele, H., and Steele, M. (1991). Maternal representations of attachment during pregnancy predict the organization of infant-mother attachment at one year of age. *Child Development*, 62, 891–905.

Fonagy, P., and Target, M. (1997). Attachment and reflective function: Their role in self-organization. *Development and Psychopathology*, 9, 679–700.

Fox, N., and Fein, G. (1990). *Infant Day-Care: The Current Debate.* Norwood, NJ: Ablex.

Fox, R. A., Platz, D. L., and Bentley, K. S. (1995). Maternal factors related to parenting practices, developmental expectations, and perceptions of child behavior problems. *Journal of Genetic Psychology*, 156, 431–441.

Gordon, R. (1983). An operational classification of disease prevention. *Public Health Reports*, 98, 107–109.

Gray, J. D., Cutler, C. A., Dean, J., and Kempe, C. H. (1979a). Prediction and prevention of child abuse. *Seminars in Perinatology*, 3, 85–90.

Gray, J. D., Cutler, C. A., Dean, J., and Kempe, C. H. (1979b). Prediction and prevention of child abuse and neglect. *Journal of Social Issues*, 35, 127–139.

Grych, J. H., and Fincham, F. D. (1990). Marital conflict and children's adjustment: A cognitive-contextual framework. *Psychological Bulletin*, 108, 267–290.

Haller, D. L., Knisely, J. S., Dawson, K. S., and Schnoll, S. H. (1993). Perinatal substance abusers: Psychological and social characteristics. *Journal of Nervous and Mental Disease*, 181, 509–513.

Halpern, R. (1993). Poverty and infant development. In C. H. Zeanah (Ed.), *Handbook of Infant Mental Health* (pp. 73–86). New York: Guilford.

Hamilton, C. (1994). *Continuity and discontinuity of attachment from infancy through adolescence*. Unpublished doctoral dissertation, UC-Los Angeles, Los Angeles.

Hardy, J., and Streett, R. (1989). Family support and parenting education in the home: An effective extension of clinic- based preventive health care services for poor children. *Journal of Pediatrics*, 115, 927–931.

Harnish, J. D., Dodge, K. A., Valente, E., and the Conduct Problems Prevention Group. (1995). Mother-child interaction quality as a partial mediator of the roles of maternal depressive symptomatology and socioeconomic status in the development of child behavior problems. *Child Development*, 66, 739–753.

Hart, C. G., DeWolf, M., Wozniak, P., and Burts, D. C. (1992). Maternal and paternal disciplinary styles: Relations with preschooler's playground behavioral orientations and peer status. *Child Development*, 63, 879–892.

Hart, J., Gunnar, M., and Cicchetti, D. (1995). Salivary cortisol in maltreated children: Evidence of relations between neuroendocrine activity and social competence. Special issue: Emotions in developmental psychopathology. *Development and Psychopathology*, 7, 11–26.

Haskins, R. (1985). Public school aggression among children with varying day-care experience. *Child Development*, 56, 689–703.

Hechtman, L. (1989). Teenage mothers and their children: Risks and problems. A review. *Canadian Journal of Psychiatry*, 34, 569–575.

Herrenkohl, E. C., Herrenkohl, R. C., Rupert, L. J., Egolf, B. P., and Lutz, J. G. (1995). Risk factors for behavioral dysfunction: The relative impact of maltreatment, SES, physical health problems, cognitive ability, and quality of parent-child interaction. *Child Abuse and Neglect*, 19, 191–203.

Hetherington, E. M., Cox, M., and Cox, R. (1982). *Effects of divorce on parents and children*. Hillsdale, NJ: Erlbaum.

Hewitt, K., and Crawford, W. V. (1988). Resolving behaviour problems in pre-school children. Evaluation of a workshop for health visitors. *Child Care, Health and Development*, 14, 1–9.

Hofer, M. A. (1996). On the nature and consequences of early loss. *Psychosomatic Medicine*, 58, 570–581.

Howes, C., and Olenick, M. (1986). Family and child care influences on toddler's compliance. *Child Development*, 57, 202–216.

Howes, C., Phillips, D., and Whitebook, M. (1992). Thresholds of quality: Implications for the social development of children in center-based child care. *Child Development*, 63, 449–460.

Howes, P., and Markman, H. J. (1989). Marital quality and child functioning: A longitudinal investigation. *Child Development*, 60, 1044–1051.

Johnson, D., and Walker, T. (1987a). Primary prevention of behavior problems in Mexican-American children. *American Journal of Community Psychology*, 15, 375–385.

Johnson, D. L. (1990). The Houston Parent-Child Development Center Project: Disseminating a viable program for enhancing at-risk families. *Prevention in Human Services*, 7, 89–108.

Johnson, D. L. (1991). Primary prevention of behavior problems in young children: The Houston Parent-Child Development Center. In R. Price, E. L. Cowen, R. P. Lorion, and J. Ramos-McKay (Eds.), *Fourteen Ounces of Prevention: A Casebook for Practitioners* (pp. 44–52). Washington, DC: American Psychological Association.

Johnson, D. L., and Walker, T. (1987b). Primary prevention of behavior problems in Mexican-American children. *American Journal of Community Psychology*, 15, 375–385.

Jouriles, E. N., Murphy, C. M., Farris, A. M., Smith, D. A., Richter, J. E., and Waters, E. (1991). Marital adjustment, parental disagreements about childrearing, and behavior problems in boys: Increasing the specificity of the marital assessment. *Child Development*, 62, 1424–1433.

Kagan, J., Reznick, J. S., and Snidman, N. (1988). Biological bases of childhood shyness. *Science*, 240, 167–173.

Kagan, J., and Snidman, N. (1991). Temperamental factors in human development. *American Psychologist*, 46, 856–862.

Karen, R. (1994). *Becoming Attached*. New York: Warner.

Karoly, L. A., Greenwood, P. W., Everingham, S. S., Houbé, J., Kilburn, M. R., Rydell, C. P., Sanders, M., and Chiesa, J. (1998). *Investing in Our Children: What We Know and Don't Know About the Costs and Benefits of Early Childhood Interventions*. Santa Monica, CA: RAND Corp.

Kellam, S. G., Rebok, G. W., Ialongo, N., and Mayer, L. S. (1994). The course and malleability of aggressive behavior from early first grade into middle school: Results of a developmental epidemiologically-based preventive trial. *Journal of Child Psychology and Child Psychiatry*, 35, 259–281.

Kitzman, H., Olds, D., Henderson Jr., C. R., Hanks, C., Cole, R., Tatelbaum, R., McConnochie, K. M., Sidora, K., Luckey, D. W., Shaver, D., Engelhardt, K., James, D., and Barnard, K. (1997). Effect of prenatal and infancy home visitation by nurses on pregnancy outcomes, childhood injuries, and repeated childbearing: A randomized controlled trial. *Journal of the American Medical Association*, 278, 644–652.

Klerman, L. V. (1991). The health of poor children: Problems and programs. In A. C. Huston (Ed.), *Children in Poverty: Child Development and Public Policy* (pp. 136–157). Cambridge, MA: Cambridge University Press.

Koblinsky, S. A., Morgan, K. M., and Anderson, E. A. (1997). African-American homeless and low-income housed mothers: Comparison of parenting practices. *American Journal of Orthopsychiatry*, 67, 37–47.

Kochanska, G., and Aksan, N. (1995). Mother-child mutually positive affect, the quality of child compliance to requests and prohibitions, and maternal control as correlates of early internalization. *Child Development*, 66, 236–254.

Koretz, D. S., and Moscicki, E. K. (1997). An ounce of prevention research: What is it worth? *American Journal of Community Psychology*, 25, 189–195.

Korner, A. F., Stevenson, D. K., Kraemer, H. C., Spiker, D., Scott, D. T., Constantinou, J., and Duivcek, S. (1993). Prediction of the development of low birth weight preterm infants by a new neonatal medical index. *Journal of Developmental and Behavioral Pediatrics*, 14, 106–111.

Kuczynski, L., and Kochanska, G. (1995). Function and content of maternal demands: Developmental significance of early demands for competent action. *Child Development*, 66, 616–628.

Lally, J. R., Mangione, P., and Honig, A. S. (1988). The Syracuse University family development research program: Long-range impact of an early intervention with low-income children and their families. In D. Powell (Ed.), *Parent Education as Early Childhood Intervention: Emerging Directions in Theory, Research and Practice* (pp. 79–104). Norwood, NJ: Ablex.

Lamb, M., and Sternberg, K. (1990). Do we really know how day-care affects children? *Journal of Applied Developmental Psychology*, 11, 351–379.

Larson, C. P. (1980). Efficacy of prenatal and postpartum home visits on child health and development. *Pediatrics*, 66, 191–197.

Laucht, M., Esser, G., and Schmidt, M. H. (1994). Parental mental disorder and early child development. *European Child and Adolescent Psychiatry*, 3, 124–137.

Lempers, J., Clarke-Lempers, D., and Simons, R. (1989). Economic hardship, parenting, and distress in adolescence. *Child Development*, 60, 25–49.

Lester, B. M., and Tronick, E. Z. (1994). The effects of prenatal cocaine exposure and child outcome. *Infant Mental Health Journal*, 15, 107–120.

Levenstein, P. (1992). The Mother-Child Home Program: Research methodology and the real world. In J. McCord and R. E. Tremblay (Eds.), *Preventing Antisocial Behavior: Interventions from Birth Through Adolescence* (pp. 43–66). New York: Guilford Press.

Lipsey, M. W. (1990). *Design Sensitivity: Statistical Power for Experimental Research*. Newbury Park, CA: Sage.

Loeber, R., and Stouthamer-Loeber, M. (1986). Family factors as correlates and predictors of juvenile conduct problems and delinquency. In M. Tonry and N. Morris (Eds.), *Crime and Justice: An Annual Review of Research*, Vol. 7 (pp. 29–150). Chicago: University of Chicago Press.

Lojkasek, M., Cohen, N. J., and Muir, E. (1994). Where is the infant in infant intervention? A review of the literature on changing troubled mother-infant relationships. *Psychotherapy*, 31, 208–220.

Lorion, R. P. (1990). Evaluation of HIV risk-reduction efforts: Ten lessons from psychotherapy and prevention outcome strategies. *Journal of Community Psychology*, 18, 325–336.

Lyons-Ruth, K. (1996). Attachment relationships among children with aggressive behavior problems: The role of disorganized early attachment patterns. *Journal of Consulting and Clinical Psychology*, 64, 64–73.

Lyons-Ruth, K., Connell, D. B., and Grunebaum, H. U. (1990). Infants at social risk: Maternal depression and family support services as mediators of infant development and security of attachment. *Child Development*, 61, 85–98.

MacMillan, H. L., MacMillan, J. H., Offord, D. R., Griffith, L., and MacMillan, A. (1994a). Primary prevention of child physical abuse and neglect: A critical review. Part I. *Journal of Child Psychology and Psychiatry*, 35, 835–856.

MacMillan, H. L., MacMillan, J. H., Offord, D. R., Griffith, L., and MacMillan, A. (1994b). Primary prevention of child physical abuse and neglect: A critical review. Part II. *Journal of Child Psychology and Psychiatry*, 35, 857–876.

Main, M. (1997). *Attachment narratives and attachment across the lifespan.* Paper presented at the Fall Meeting of the American Psychoanalytic Association, New York.

Main, M., and Hesse, E. (1990). Parents' unresolved traumatic experiences are related to infant disorganized attachment status: Is frightened and/or frightening parental behavior the linking mechanism? In M. Greenberg, D. Cicchetti, and E. M. Cummings (Eds.), *Attachment in the Preschool Years: Theory, Research and Intervention* (pp. 161–182). Chicago: University of Chicago Press.

Main, M., and Solomon, J. (1990). Procedures for identifying infants as disorganized/disoriented during the Ainsworth Strange Situation. In D. C. M.Greenberg and E. M. Cummings (Eds.), *Attachment in the Preschool Years: Theory, Research and Intervention* (pp. 121–160). Chicago: University of Chicago Press.

Marlowe, H. A., and Weinberg, R. B. (1983). *Primary Prevention: Fact or Fallacy.* Tampa, FL: University of South Florida.

Maynard, R. A. (1997). *Kids Having Kids.* New York: The Urban Institute.

McAdoo, H. P. (1988). *Black Families* (2nd edition). Newbury Park, CA: Sage.

McCartney, K., Scarr, S., Phillips, D., Grajik, S., and Schwarz, C. J. (1982). Environmental differences among day care centres and their effects on children's development. In E. Zigler and E. Gordon (Eds.), *Day Care: Scientific and Social Policy Issues.* Boston: Auburn House.

McCord, J. (1986). Instigation and insulation: How families affect antisocial aggression. In J. Block, D. Olweus, and M. Radke-Yarrow (Eds.), *Development of Antisocial and Prosocial Behavior* (pp. 343–357). San Diego, CA: Academic Press.

McGuire, J., and Earls, F. (1991). Prevention of psychiatric disorders in early childhood. *Journal of Child Psychology and Psychiatry,* 32, 129–154.

McLoyd, V. C. (1990). The impact of economic hardship on black families and children: Psychological distress, parenting, and socioemotional development. *Child Development,* 61, 311–346.

Miller, S. M., and Lewis, M. (1990). *Handbook of Developmental Psychopathology.* New York: Plenum.

Minde, K., Shosenberg, N., Thompson, J., and Marton, P. (1983). Self-help groups in a premature nursery— follow-up at one year. In J. D. Call, E. Galenson, and R. L. Tyson (Eds.), *Frontiers of Infant Psychiatry* (pp. 264–272). New York: Basic Books.

Moffitt, T. E. (1997). Helping poor mothers and children. Editorial. *Journal of the American Medical Association,* 278, 680–681.

Moss, E., Parent, S., Gosselin, C., Rousseau, D., and Stlaurent, D. (1996). Attachment and teacher-reported behavior problems during the preschool and early school-age period. *Development and Psychopathology,* 8, 511–525.

Mrazek, P., and Haggerty, R. J. (Eds.). (1994). *Reducing risks for mental disorders. Frontiers for preventive intervention research.* Washington, DC: National Academy Press.

Murray, L., and Cooper, P. J. (1997). The role of infant and maternal factors in postpartum depression, mother-infant interactions and infant outcome. In L. Murray and P. J. Cooper (Eds.), *Postpartum Depression and Child Development* (pp. 111–135). New York: Guilford Press.

Murray, L., Fiori-Cowley, A., Hooper, R., and Cooper, P. (1996). The impact of postnatal depression and associated adversity on early mother-infant interactions and later infant outcome. *Child Development,* 67, 2512–2526.

Nachmias, M., Gunnar, M. R., Mangelsdorf, S., Parritz, R. H., and Buss, K. (1996). Behavioral inhibition and stress reactivity: Moderating role of attachment security. *Child Development,* 67, 508–522.

National Institute of Mental Health. (1993). *The Prevention of Mental Disorders: A National Research Agenda.* Rockville, MD: National Institute of Mental Health.

National Institute of Mental Health. (1995). *A Plan for Prevention Research for the National Institute of Mental Health: A Report to the National Advisory Mental Health Council.* Rockville, MD: National Institute of Mental Health.

NICHD Early Child Care Network. (1997). Mother-child interaction and cognitive outcomes associated with early child care: Results of the NICHD study. *Poster symposium presented at the biennial meetings of the Society for Research in Child Development, Washington, DC.*

NICHD Early Child Care Research Network. (1996). Characteristics of infant child care: Factors contributing to positive caregiving. *Early Childhood Research Quarterly,* 11, 269–306.

NICHD Early Child Care Research Network. (1997). The effects of infant child care on infant-mother attachment: security: Results of the NICHD study of early child care. *Child Development,* 68, 860–879.

NICHD Early Child Care Research Network. (1998). Early child care and self-control, compliance, and problem behavior at 24 and 36 months. *Child Development,* 69, 1145–70.

Oda, D. S., Heilbron, D., and Taylor, H. J. (1995). A preventive child health program: The effect of telephone and home visits by public health nurses. *American Journal of Public Health*, 85, 854–855.

Olds, D., Henderson, C., Phelps, C., Kitzman, H., and Hanks, C. (1993). Effects of prenatal and infancy nurse home visitation on government spending. *Medical Care*, 31, 156–174.

Olds, D., and Kitzman, H. (1993). Review of research on home visiting for pregnant women and parents of young children. *Future of Children*, 3, 63–92.

Olds, D. L., Eckenrode, J., Henderson Jr., C. R., Kitzman, H., Powers, J., Cole, R., Sidora, K., Morris, P., Pettitt, L. M., and Luckey, D. (1997). Long-term effects of home visitation on maternal life course and child abuse and neglect: Fifteen-year follow-up of a randomized trial. *Journal of the American Medical Association*, 278, 637–643.

Olds, D. L., Henderson, C., and Kitzman, H. (1994a). Does prenatal and infancy nurse home visitation have enduring effects on qualities of parental caregiving and child health from 25 to 50 months of life. *Pediatrics*, 93, 89–98.

Olds, D. L., Henderson, C., and Tatelbaum, R. (1994b). Prevention of intellectual impairment in children of women who smoke cigarettes during pregnancy. *Pediatrics*, 93, 228–233.

Olds, D. L., Henderson, C. R., Chamberlin, R., and Tatelbaum, R. (1986a). Preventing child abuse and neglect: A randomized trial of nurse home visitation. *Pediatrics*, 78, 65–78.

Olds, D. L., Henderson, C. R., Tatelbaum, R., and Chamberlin, R. (1986b). Improving the delivery of prenatal care and outcomes of pregnancy: A randomized trial of nurse home visitation. *Pediatrics*, 77, 16–28.

Olds, D. L., Henderson, C. R., Tatelbaum, R., and Chamberlin, R. (1988). Improving the life course development of socially disadvantaged mothers: A randomized trial of nurse home visitation. *American Journal of Public Health*, 78, 1436–1445.

Osofsky, J. D., Hann, D. M., and Peebles, C. (1993). Adolescent parenthood: Risks and opportunities for mothers and infants. In C. H. Zeanah (Ed.), *Handbook of Infant Mental Health* (pp. 106–119). New York: Guilford.

Paneth, N. S. (1995). The problem of low birth weight. In R. E. Behrman (Ed.), *The Future of Children: Low Birthweight* (pp. 11–34). Los Altos, CA: David and Lucille Packard Foundation.

Parker, S., Greer, S., and Zuckerman, B. (1988). Double jeopardy: The impact of poverty on early child development. *Pediatric Clinics of North America*, 35, 1227–1240.

Passino, A. W., Whitman, T. L., Borkowski, J. G., Schellenbach, C. J., Maxwell, S. E., Keogh, D., and Rellinger, E. (1993). Personal adjustment during pregnancy and adolescent parenting. *Adolescence*, 28, 97–122.

Patterson, G. R. (1986). Performance models for antisocial boys. *American Psychologist*, 41, 432–444.

Perry, B. (1997). Incubated in terror: Neurodevelopmental factors in the "cycle of violence." In J. Osofsky (Ed.), *Children in a Violent Society* (pp. 124-149). New York: Guilford Press.

Pfannenstiel, A., and Honig, A. S. (1995). Effects of a prenatal 'Information and Insights about Infants' program on the knowledge base of first-time low-education fathers one month postnatally. *Early Child Development and Care*, 111, 87–105.

Phillips, D., McCartney, K., and Scarr, S. (1987). Child care quality and children's social development. *Developmental Psychology*, 23, 537–543.

Plomin, R. (1994). The Emanuel Miller Memorial Lecture 1993: Genetic research and identification of environmental influences. *Journal of Child Psychology and Psychiatry and Allied Disciplines*, 35, 817–834.

Plomin, R., Emde, R. N., Braungart, J. M., and Campos, J. (1993). Genetic change and continuity from fourteen to twenty months: The MacArthur Longitudinal Twin Study. *Child Development*, 64, 1354–1376.

Pollitt, E. (1994). Poverty and child development: Relevance of research in developing countries to the United States. *Child Development*, 65, 283–295.

Pound, A., and Mills, M. (1985). A pilot evaluation of Newpin. *Newsletter of the Association of Child Psychology and Psychiatry*, 70, 13–15.

Power, T. G., and Chapieski, M. (1986). Child-rearing and impulse control in toddlers: A naturalistic investigation. *Developmental Psychology*, 22, 271–275.

Price, R. H. (1986). Education for prevention. In M. Kessler and S. E. Goldston (Eds.), *A Decade of Progress in Primary Prevention* (pp. 289–306). Hanover, NH: University Press of New England.

Pulkkinen, L. (1983). Search for alternatives to aggression in Finland. In A. P. Goldstein and M. H. Segall (Eds.), *Aggression in Global Perspective* (pp. 104–144). Elmsford, NY: Pergamon Press.

Ramey, C. T., and Campbell, F. A. (1991). Poverty, early childhood education, and academic competence: The Abecedarian experiment. In A. C. Huston (Ed.), *Children in Poverty: Child Development and Public Policy* (pp. 190–221). Cambridge, MA: Cambridge University Press.

Ramey, C. T., Yeates, K. O., and Short, E. J. (1984). The plasticity of intellectual development: Insights from preventive intervention. *Child Development*, 55, 1913–1925.

Reiss, D., Hetherington, E. M., Plomin, R., Howe, G. W., Simmens, S. J., Henderson, S. H., O'Connor, T. J., Bussell, D. A., Anderson, E. R., and Law, T. (1995). Genetic questions for environmental studies. Differential parenting and psychopathology in adolescence. *Archives of General Psychiatry*, 52, 925–936.

Roberts, I., and Pless, B. (1995). Social policy as a cause of childhood accidents: The children of lone mothers. *British Medical Journal*, 311, 925–928.

Robinson, J., Zahn-Waxler, C., and Emde, R. N. (1998). Moderators of individual differences in empathic development: Mothers and examiners in distress. The transition from infancy to early childhood: Genetic and environmental influences in the MacArthur Longitudinal Twin Study (manuscript in preparation).

Robinson, J. L., Kagan, J., Reznick, J. S., and Corley, R. (1992). The heritability of inhibited and uninhibited behavior: a twin study. *Developmental Psychology*, 28, 1–8.

Rutter, M. (1979). Protective factors in children's responses to stress and disadvantage. In M. W. Kent and J. E. Rolf (Eds.), *Primary Prevention of Psychopathology*: Vol. 3. *Social Competence in Children* (pp. 49–74). Hanover, NH: University Press of New England.

Rutter, M. (1981). Socioemotional consequences of day-care for preschool children. *American Journal of Orthopsychiatry*, 51, 4–28.

Rutter, M. (1987). Psychosocial resilience and protective mechanisms. *American Journal of Orthopsychiatry*, 57, 316–331.

Rutter, M. (1990). Psychosocial resilience and protective mechanisms. In J. Rolf, A. S. Masten, D. Cicchetti, and S. Weintraub (Eds.), *Risk and protective factors in the development of psychopathology*. New York: Cambridge University Press.

Schneider-Rosen, K., and Cicchetti, D. (1991). Early self-knowledge and emotional development: Visual self-recognition and affective reactions to mirror self-image in maltreated and non-maltreated toddlers. *Developmental Psychology*, 27, 481–488.

Seifer, R., and Dickstein, S. (1993). Parental mental illness and infant development. In C. H. Zeanah (Ed.), *Handbook of Infant Mental Health* (pp. 120–142). New York: Guilford.

Seifer, R., Sameroff, A. J., Anagnostopolou, R., and Elias, P. K. (1992). Child and family factors that ameliorate risk between 4 and 13 years of age. *Journal of the American Academy of Child and Adolescent Psychiatry*, 31, 893–903.

Seitz, V., and Apfel, N. H. (1994). Parent-focused intervention: Diffusion effects on siblings. Special Issue: Children and poverty. *Child Development*, 65, 677–683.

Seitz, V., Rosenbaum, L. K., and Apfel, N. H. (1985). Effects of family support intervention: A ten-year follow-up. *Child Development*, 56, 376–391.

Shaw, D. S., and Vondraa, J. I. (1993). Chronic family adversity and infant attachment security. *Journal of Child Psychology and Psychiatry*, 34, 1205–1215.

Shure, M., and Spivack, G. (1982). Interpersonal problem-solving in young children: A cognitive approach to prevention. *American Journal of Community Psychology*, 10, 341–356.

Shure, M., and Spivack, G. (1988). Interpersonal cognitive problem-solving. In R. Price, E. L. Cowen, R. P. Lorion, and J. Ramos-McKay (Eds.), *Fourteen Ounces of Prevention: A Casebook for Practitioners* (pp. 69–82). Washington, DC: American Psychological Association.

Singh, G. K. (1998). Maternal and infant health. In G. K. Singh, A. V. Wilkinson, and F. F. Song (Eds.), *Health and Social Factors in Kansas: A Data and Chartbook, 1997-8*. Topeka, KA: Kansas Health Institute.

Smith, J. R., and Brooks-Gunn, J. (1997). Correlates and consequences of harsh discipline for young children. *Archives of Pediatric and Adolescent Medicine*, 151, 777–786.

Socolar, R. (in press). Conceptualization of discipline: Type, mode of administration, context. *Aggression and Violent Behavior Review Journal*.

Solomon, J., George, C., and Dejong, A. (1995). Children classified as controlling at age six: Evidence of disorganized representational strategies and aggression at home and at school. *Development and Psychopathology*, 7, 447–463.

Spangler, G., and Grossman, K. E. (1993). Biobehavioral organization in securely and insecurely attached infants. *Child Development*, 64, 1439–1450.

Spieker, S. J., and Bensley, L. (1994). Roles of living arrangements and grandmother social support in adolescent mothering and infant attachment. *Developmental Psychology*, 30, 102–111.

Spieker, S. J., and Booth, C. L. (1988). Maternal antecedents of attachment quality. In J. Belsky and T. Nezworski (Eds.), *Clinical Implications of Attachment* (pp. 95–135). Hillsdale, NJ: Erlbaum.

Spivack, G., and Shure, M. B. (1974). *Social Adjustment of Young Children*. San Francisco, CA: Jossey-Bass Publications.

Sroufe, L. A. (1988). A developmental perspective on daycare. *Early Childhood Research Quarterly*, 3, 283–291.

Steele, H., Steele, M., and Fonagy, P. (1996). Associations among attachment classifications of mothers, fathers, and their infants: Evidence for a relationship-specific perspective. *Child Development*, 67, 541–555.

Sternberg, K., Lamb, M., Hwang, C., Broberg, A., Ketterlinus, R., and Bookstein, B. (1991). Does out-of-home care affect compliance in preschoolers? *International Journal of Behavioral Development*, 14, 45–65.

Stevenson, J., Bailey, V., and Simpson, J. (1988). Feasible intervention in families with parenting difficulties: A primary prevention perspective on child abuse. In K. Browne (Ed.), *The Prediction and Prevention of Child Abuse and Neglect* (pp. 121–138). Chichester: Wiley.

Strayhorn, J. M., and Weidman, C. S. (1991). Follow-up one year after parent-child interaction training: Effects on behavior of preschool children. *Journal of the American Academy of Child and Adolescent Psychiatry*, 30, 138–143.

Sucheki, D., Nelson, D. Y., VanOers, H., and Levine, S. (1995). Activation and inhibition of the hypothalamic-pituitary-adrenal axis of the neonatal rat: Effects of maternal deprivation. *Psychoneuroendocrinology*, 20, 169–182.

Thompson, M. J. J., and Bellenis, C. (1992). A joint assessment and treatment service for the under fives. *Newsletter of the Association for Child Psychology and Psychiatry*, 14, 221–227.

Tobler, N. S. (1992). Drug prevention programs can work: Research findings. *Journal of Addictive Diseases*, 11, 1–28.

Tronick, E. Z., Frank, D. A., Cabral, H., and Zuckerman, B. S. (in press). A dose-response effect of in utero cocaine exposure on infant neurobehavioral functioning. *Pediatrics*.

van IJzendoorn, M. H. (1995). Adult attachment representations, parental responsiveness, and infant attachment: A meta-analysis on the predictive validity of the Adult Attachment Interview. *Psychological Bulletin*, 117, 387–403.

van IJzendoorn, M. H., Goldberg, S., Kroonenberg, P. M., and Frenkel, O. J. (1992). The relative effects of maternal and child problems on the quality of attachment: A meta-analysis of attachment in clinical samples. *Child Development*, 59, 147–156.

Vandell, D. L. (1979). The effects of a playgroup experience on mother-son and father-son interaction. *Developmental Psychology*, 15, 379–385.

Varin, D., Crugnola, C., Ripamonti, C., and Molina, P. (1994). *Critical periods in the growth of attachment and the age of entry into day care*. Paper presented at the Annual Conference of the Developmental Section of the British Psychological Society, University of Portsmouth, UK.

Villar, J., Farnot, U., Barros, F., Victora, C., Langer, A., and Belizan, J. M. (1992). A randomized trial of psychosocial support during high-risk pregnancies. *New England Journal of Medicine*, 327, 1266–1271.

Volling, B., and Feagans, L. (1995). Infant day care and children's social competence. *Infant Behavior and Development*, 18, 177–188.

Wakschlag, L. S., Lahey, B. B., Loeber, R., Green, S. M., Gordon, R. A., and Leventhal, B. L. (1997). Maternal smoking during pregnancy and the risk of conduct disorder in boys. *Archives of General Psychiatry*, 54, 670–676.

Waters, E., Merrick, S., Albersheim, L., Treboux, D., and Crowell, J. (1995, May). *From the strange situation to the Adult Attachment Interview: A 20-year longitudinal study of attachment security in infancy and early adulthood*. Paper presented at the Society for Research in Child Development, Indianapolis.

Watson, J. E., Kirby, R. S., Kelleher, K. J., and Bradley, R. H. (1996). Effects of poverty on home environment: An analysis of three-year outcome data for low birth weight premature infants. *Journal of Pediatric Psychology*, 21, 419–431.

Weiner, H. (1996). The use of animal models in peptic ulcer disease. *Psychosomatic Medicine*, 58, 524–545.

Weiss, B., Dodge, K. A., Bates, J. E., and Pettit, G. S. (1992). Some consequences of early harsh discipline: Child aggression and a maladaptive social information processing style. *Child Development*, 63, 1321–1335.

Weissberg, R. P., and Bell, D. N. (1997). A meta-analytic review of primary prevention programs for children and adolescents: Contributions and caveats. *American Journal of Community Psychology*, 25, 207–214.

Werner, E. E., and Smith, R. S. (1982). *Vulnerable, but Invincible: A Longitudinal Study of Resilient Children and Youth.* New York: McGraw-Hill.

Whipple, E. E., and Wilson, S. R. (1996). Evaluation of a parent education and support program for families at risk of physical child abuse. *Families in Society, 77,* 227–239.

Whitman, T. L., Borkowski, J. G., Schellenbach, C. J., and Nath, P. S. (1987). Predicting and understanding developmental delay of children of adolescent mothers: A multidimensional approach. *American Journal of Mental Deficiency, 92,* 40–56.

Wise, P. H., and Meyers, A. (1988). Poverty and child health. *Pediatric Clinics of North America, 35,* 1169–1186.

Wolchik, S. A., West, S. G., Westover, S., Sadler, I. N., Martin, A., Lustig, J., Tein, J., and Fisher, J. (1993). The Child of Divorce Parenting Intervention: Outcome evaluation of an empirically based program. *American Journal of Community Psychology, 21,* 292–331.

Yogman, M. W., Kindlon, D., and Earls, F. (1995). Father involvement and cognitive/behavioral outcomes of preterm infants. *Journal of the Academy of Child and Adolescent Psychiatry, 34,* 58–66.

Seven

EARLY DEVELOPMENT IN MONKEYS

Stephen J. Suomi

INTRODUCTION

A BASIC theme recurrent throughout this volume is that the well-being of a society is ultimately dependent on the physical and mental well-being of its children. Children, especially infants, are particularly sensitive to certain aspects of the environments they are experiencing as they grow up. They generally react with more pronounced behavioral, emotional, and physiological responses to changes in their physical and social worlds than do adults, and some of these responses, in turn, can have long-lasting effects on their physical and mental health, sometimes extending well into their adult years. Moreover, there appear to be major differences among children not only in the manner in which they respond to common features of their respective environments but also in the likely long-term consequences for their health and well-being. Some of these response differences might be attributed in part to age and gender differences, while others might be linked to factors such as income gradients or life-style changes. Identifying and understanding the basis for such differences among children represents an important challenge for scientists, clinicians, and public policy makers alike. The challenge is not only important but formidable, as noted by several other contributors to this volume.

Over the past four decades numerous insights regarding the well-being of children, some of them surprising if not revolutionary, have come from developmental studies of our closest biological relatives, the nonhuman primates. This chapter will summarize some of this research, focusing on aspects of biobehavioral development that are common to most primates, as well as characterizing some specific developmental patterns that lead to vastly different long-term health and well-being outcomes and identifying factors that help shape such patterns.

PRIMATE COMMUNITY LIFE

A FUNDAMENTAL feature of primates is their inherent sociality. Like humans, most monkeys and apes spend virtually all of their lives as members of distinctive communities, each typically characterized by complex kinship and status-defined social relationships.[1] These primate communities often encompass three or more generations within individual family units and usually retain their basic identity long beyond the lifespan of any one community member or generation of members. In most primate species the relationships between individual family members, between families within a given community, and even between different

Much of the research described in this manuscript was supported by the Division of Intramural Research, National Institute of Child Health and Human Development, National Institutes of Health.

communities are far from static, and dramatic changes in each type of relationship can and do occur, often with long-term consequences for all involved. Yet even after events or episodes that result in major social disruption, most surviving individuals, families, and communities quickly return to species-normative patterns of social interactions, relationships, and overall group organization.[2]

An illustrative example of the complex and dynamic nature of primate social group life is provided by rhesus monkeys (*Macaca mulatta*). Although rhesus monkeys are not our closest phylogenetic relatives (that role falls to chimpanzees and bonobos), in evolutionary terms they are probably our most *successful* primate relatives. Next to humans, rhesus monkeys live over a wider geographic range, encompassing a broader mix of climatic and habitat variation, than any other primate species, with one or two possible exceptions. While the majority of nonhuman primate species are currently classified as endangered or threatened, some with rapidly dwindling natural populations that forecast almost certain extinction in the near future, rhesus monkeys are actually expanding local populations in certain parts of their extensive range. They also thrive in a wide variety of captive environments and have long had a reputation for being unusually robust laboratory subjects.[3]

Although rhesus monkey communities in nature vary widely in size, ranging from a few dozen to several hundred individuals, the basic social structure of each of these distinctive communities—termed "troops"—is remarkably similar from setting to setting. Rhesus monkey troops are always organized around multigenerational matrilines, i.e., female-headed extended families. Each troop is comprised of several different matrilines, each encompassing multiple generations of close female kin. The long-term stability of these matrilines (and indeed, of the troop as a distinctive whole) derives from the fact that every female spends her entire life in her natal troop, whereas virtually all males emigrate around the

time of puberty.[4] After leaving home, most adolescent males first briefly congregate in all-male gangs, then attempt to join other established troops. Some of the males who are successful in these efforts remain in their "new" troop for the rest of their lives, whereas others stay no more than a few years and then leave to seek membership in other established troops, sometimes repeating this pattern several times throughout their adult years.[5]

It is thus the adult females and their female progeny who provide the long-term foundation for rhesus monkey communities. To be sure, every rhesus monkey troop contains numerous males of all ages—but troop membership for any one male is typically transitory, while it is always lifelong for all females. This is not to say that males play insignificant roles in rhesus monkey social group life; to the contrary, their presence is essential for the long-term survival of the troop as a whole. Nevertheless, it is the female matrilines around which most of the social activities of the troop are organized and the underlying social structure of the troop is defined and maintained.

A second feature characteristic of all rhesus monkey troops is their multiple dominance hierarchies.[6] There is one clear-cut linear hierarchy among the troop's different matrilines, such that all members of the highest ranking matriline, including infants, are socially dominant over all members of the second-ranking matriline, including adults, who in turn outrank all members of the third-ranking matriline, etc. Such a hierarchy can be maintained only as long as all members of a matriline consistently support any member who is challenged by someone from a lower-ranking matriline, as when adult members of a high-ranking matriline come to the immediate defense of one of their infants whenever it is threatened or attacked by a non-family member. Another hierarchy can be found within each matriline; it follows the general rule that younger sisters outrank older sisters. Such status differences among female siblings most likely have their origin in the mother's consistent preferential defense of her female infant in the face of harassment by jealous older sisters; curiously, such status differences tend to remain remarkably stable throughout the rest of the sisters' respective lifetimes. A third hierarchy exists among the males that immigrate into the troop. Although male status superficially seems related to relative tenure (i.e., the longer a male has been in a troop, the more likely he is to be high in rank), in fact it appears to be more a function of the male's skills in joining and maintaining coalitions, not only with other males but with high-ranking females in the troop as well.

Rhesus monkeys are status seekers by nature, and a substantial proportion of their social activity is directed toward efforts to advance or at least maintain their current status within the troop's various hierarchies. However, it seems clear that social status in a rhesus monkey troop is less a function of an individual's relative size or strength than who its friends and relatives happen to be. Indeed, the complex familial and dominance relationships that characterize every rhesus monkey troop seemingly require any functioning troop member to have some knowledge of most if not all other members' specific kinship and dominance status—and to utilize such knowledge—in order to survive, let alone thrive, in everyday troop life. How might such knowledge be acquired, maintained, and utilized in generation after generation of monkeys born into the troop? An impressive body of both laboratory and field data strongly suggests that it is an emergent property of the species-normative pattern of socialization that rhesus monkey infants experience as they grow up in their natal troop.[7] A description of this species-normative pattern follows.

DEVELOPMENTAL ASPECTS OF RHESUS MONKEY SOCIALIZATION

RHESUS monkey infants spend virtually all of their first weeks of life in physical contact with or within arm's reach of their biological mother, who provides them with nourishment, physical and psychological warmth, and protection from the elements, potential predators, and other troop members, including pesky older siblings. During this time a strong and enduring social bond inevitably develops between mother and infant, recognized by Bowlby[8] to be homologous with the mother-infant attachment relationship universally seen in all human cultures, most likely representing the product of diverse evolutionary pressures over millions of years.

Rhesus monkey infants are also inherently curious, and like human infants, once they have become attached to their mother they quickly learn to use her as a secure base from which to organize the exploration of their physical and social environment.[9] Unlike human infants, rhesus monkey infants are sufficiently precocious in their locomotor capabilities to be able to wander considerable distances away from their mother before the end of their first month of life (by comparison, weaning typically takes place during the fourth and fifth postnatal month). They are therefore physically capable of stumbling into potentially life-threatening situations from their second month on, and initially most monkey mothers spend considerable time and effort monitoring and often physically restricting their infant's early exploratory efforts.[10,11] However, in succeeding weeks the rhesus monkey equivalent of human stranger anxiety emerges in the infants' behavioral repertoire,[12] and thereafter it is the infant who is largely responsible for maintaining proximity to its mother.[13]

The usual result of this sequence—attachment formation, emerging exploratory tendencies (curiosity), and maturation of the capacity for developing social fears—is that rhesus monkey infants come to use their mothers as a home base for virtually all of their environmental exploration. As they grow older these young monkeys are able and willing to spend increasing amounts of time at increasing distances from their mother, secure in the knowledge that whenever they become frightened or tired, they will be able to return to her protective care without interruption or delay on her part. The presence of such a psychologically secure base clearly promotes exploration of both physical and social aspects of their immediate environment. On the other hand, when rhesus monkey infants develop less than optimal attachment relationships with their mothers, their subsequent exploratory behavior is inevitably compromised, just as Bowlby and other attachment theorists have described for human infants and young children.[14]

During the course of their early exploratory forays away from their mother, rhesus monkey youngsters frequently come into contact with other troop members, including same-aged infants from other matrilines who have comparable physical, cognitive, and social capabilities to themselves. Interactions with these agemates begin to occur with increasing frequency in the third and fourth months of life, such that by the time of weaning most rhesus monkey youngsters are typically spending several hours each day playing with peers.[15] These peer interactions continue to increase in both frequency and complexity throughout the rest of the monkeys' first year, and they tend to remain at high levels until the onset of puberty.[16] During this time the play patterns that dominate peer interactions become increasingly gender specific and sex segregated (i.e., males tend to play more with males and females with females.[17]) Moreover, as the young monkeys get older, these extended play bouts begin to include behavioral sequences that resemble prototypical adult social interaction patterns. As a result, by the end of their third year most rhesus monkey juveniles have had ample opportunity to develop, practice, and perfect activities that will be crucial for normal functioning when they become adults. Among the most important lessons learned through such play with peers is the appropriate expression—and control—of emerging aggressive capabilities, as well as knowledge about and respect for the various dominance hierarchies within the troop.[18]

The onset of puberty usually occurs for females near the end of their third year, when they have their initial menses (and regular 28-day menstrual cycles thereafter), and the beginning of the fourth year for males, when their testes enlarge and begin producing viable sperm. Adolescence in rhesus monkeys is associated not only with a pronounced growth spurt and altered hormonal activity but also with major social changes for both sexes. The biggest change occurs for males: during adolescence, they sever all ties with their matriline and emigrate out of their natal troop. Most of these males soon join "gangs" comprised of other adolescent and young adult males, and they typically remain in these all-male groups for at least several months before attempting to join another established rhesus monkey troop. Field data have clearly shown that the process of natal troop emigration represents an exceedingly dangerous transition period for adolescent males: the mortality rate for these males from the time they leave their natal troop until they have successfully joined another one approaches 50 percent.[19] Recent field studies have also revealed major individual differences in both the timing of male emigration and the basic strategy followed in attempting to enter an unfamiliar troop. Moreover, once they have successfully joined a new troop, some males stay in that troop for the rest of their life, whereas others subsequently switch troops, often several times, although even these males never go back to their natal troop.[20]

Females, by contrast, never leave their natal troop. Puberty for rhesus monkey females is instead associated with increases in social activities directed toward their matrilinear kin, generally at the expense of interactions with peers. Kin-directed interactions are heightened even more when these young females begin to have offspring of their own. Indeed, the birth of a new infant (especially to a new mother) has the effect of invigorating the rest of the matriline, drawing its members closer both physically and socially and, conversely, providing a buffer from external threats and stressors for the new mother and infant. As they age, rhesus monkey adult females continue to be actively involved in family social affairs, even after they cease having infants of their own.[21]

INDIVIDUAL DIFFERENCES
IN RHESUS MONKEY
BIOBEHAVIORAL DEVELOPMENT

WHILE the pattern of behavioral development described above is generally characteristic of rhesus monkeys growing up both in natural troops in the wild and in social groups maintained in captivity, there are nevertheless substantial differences among individual monkeys in the precise timing and relative ease with which they make major developmental transitions, as well as how they manage the day-to-day challenges and stresses that are an inevitable consequence of complex social group life. In particular, recent research has identified two subgroups of individuals who tend to follow aberrant developmental trajectories that can potentially result in increased long-term risk for behavioral pathology and even mortality. Members of one subgroup, comprising approximately 15–20% of both wild and captive populations, consistently respond to novel and/or mildly challenging situations with extreme behavioral disruption and pronounced physiological arousal. Whereas most other monkeys typically find novel stimuli interesting and will readily explore them, usually with minimal physiological arousal, "high-reactive" individuals instead prefer to avoid such stimuli and, if that is not possible, they usually exhibit obvious behavioral expressions of fear and anxiety and experience significant (and often prolonged) activation of the hypothalamic-pituitary-adrenal (HPA) axis, sympathetic nervous system arousal, and increased noradrenergic turnover.[22]

High-reactive monkeys can be readily identified in their first few months of life. Most begin leaving their mothers later chronologically and spend less time exploring their physical and social environment than the other infants in their birth cohort. High-reactive youngsters also tend to be shy and withdrawn in their initial encounters with peers—laboratory studies have shown that they exhibit significantly higher and more stable heartrates and greater secretion of cortisol in such interactions than do their less reactive cohorts. However, when these individuals are in familiar and stable settings they tend to be indistinguishable, both behaviorally and physiologically, from others in their peer group. On the other hand, when high-reactive monkeys encounter extreme and/or prolonged stress, their behavioral and physiological differences from others in their social group usually become exaggerated.[23]

For example, virtually all rhesus monkey juveniles growing up in naturalistic settings experience functional maternal separations during the 2-month-long annual breeding season when their mothers repeatedly leave the troop for brief periods to consort with selected males.[24] The departure of its mother clearly represents a major social stressor for any young monkey and, not surprisingly, virtually all youngsters initially react to their mother's departure with short-term behavioral agitation and physiological arousal, much as Bowlby[25,26] has described for human infants experiencing involuntary maternal separation. However, whereas most juvenile monkeys soon begin to adapt to the separation and readily seek out the company of others in their social group, high-reactive individuals typically lapse into a behavioral depression characterized by increasing lethargy, lack of apparent interest in social stimuli, eating and sleeping difficulties, and a characteristic hunched-over, fetal-like posture.[27] Laboratory studies simulating these naturalistic maternal separations have shown that relative to their like-reared peers, high-reactive individuals not only are more likely to exhibit depressive-like behavioral reactions to short-term social separation but also tend to show greater and more prolonged HPA activation, more dramatic sym-

pathetic arousal, more rapid central noradrenergic turnover, and greater immunosuppression.[28]
These differential patterns of biobehavioral response to separation tend to remain remarkably
stable throughout prepubertal development and
may even be maintained in adolescence and
adulthood.[29] An increasing body of evidence has
demonstrated significant heritability for these
differences.[30]

Recent field studies have shown that high-
reactive rhesus monkey males usually emigrate
from their natal troop at significantly older ages
than the rest of their adolescent male cohort and,
when they do finally leave their home troop, they
typically employ more conservative strategies for
entering a new troop than do their less-reactive
peers.[31] Laboratory research has shown that
high-reactive young females are significantly
more likely to exhibit inadequate care of their
first-born offspring than are other primiparous
mothers. This risk for inadequate parenting is
exacerbated under conditions of environmental
stress and/or social instability, especially in the
absence of matrilineal social support.[32]

A recent study comparing accident and injury
rates among captive high- and low-reactive
rhesus monkeys living in a 5-acre outdoor enclo-
sure has demonstrated an intriguing relationship
between biobehavioral reactivity and environmental stress.[33] During periods of relatively low
stress high-reactive monkeys tend to have significantly *lower* rates of accidents and physical
injuries than low-reactive members of their social group. However, when the physical and social environment becomes more stressful and/or
less predictable, accident and injury rates sky-
rocket for high-reactive individuals of all ages
but remain surprisingly stable for low-reactive
individuals. These findings suggest that high reactivity in rhesus monkeys can represent a significant *protective factor* for individuals living in
benign environments, but under conditions of
increased stress high reactivity can become a significant *risk factor* for increased morbidity and
even mortality.

A second subgroup of rhesus monkeys, comprising approximately 5–10% of the population,
tend to be highly impulsive in their social interactions, especially those that involve aggression.
These impulsive individuals, male and female
alike, also tend to have chronically low central
serotonin metabolism, as reflected in unusually
low cerebrospinal fluid (CSF) concentrations of
the primary central serotonin metabolite
5-hydroxyindoleacetic acid (5-HIAA). These behavioral and neurochemical characteristics
emerge early in life and are notably stable
throughout development, as was the case for
high-reactive monkeys. Impulsive individuals,
especially males, seem unable to moderate their
behavioral responses to rough-and-tumble play
initiations from peers, and they often escalate
initially friendly play bouts into full-blown,
tissue-damaging aggressive exchanges, disproportionately at their own expense.[34] Impulsive
juvenile males also show a propensity for making
dangerous leaps from treetop to treetop, sometimes with disastrous outcomes.[35]

Recent field studies have found that the most
impulsive males are permanently expelled from
their natal troop a year or more prior to puberty,
long before the rest of their male cohort begins
the normal emigration process.[36] These males
tend to be grossly incompetent socially and, lacking the requisite social skills necessary for successful entrance into another troop or even an all-
male gang, most of them become solitary and
typically perish within a year.[37] Hence, few if any
of these males are likely to contribute to any
troop's gene pool. Young females who have
chronically low CSF levels of 5-HIAA also tend
to be rather incompetent socially. However, unlike the males, they are not expelled from their
natal troop (or even from their matriline) at any
point during their lifetime, although studies of
captive rhesus monkey groups suggest that these
females usually remain at the bottom of their respective dominance hierarchies.[38] While most
soon become mothers, recent research suggests
that their maternal behavior often leaves much to

be desired. In sum, rhesus monkeys who exhibit excessive impulsive and aggressive behavior (and who have low central serotonin turnover) early in life tend to follow developmental trajectories that typically result in premature death for males and chronically low social status and poor parenting for females.

EFFECTS OF DIFFERENTIAL
EARLY SOCIAL EXPERIENCE
ON RHESUS MONKEY
DEVELOPMENTAL TRAJECTORIES

ALTHOUGH considerable evidence from both field and laboratory studies has shown that individual differences among rhesus monkeys in stress reactivity and impulsivity tend to be quite stable from infancy to adulthood and are at least in part heritable, this does not mean that these behavioral and physiological features are necessarily fixed at birth or are immune to subsequent environmental influence. To the contrary, an increasing body of experimental evidence has repeatedly demonstrated that prototypical patterns of biobehavioral response to environmental novelty and stress can be modified substantially by certain early experiences, particularly those involving early social attachment relationships.

One set of studies has focused on rhesus monkey infants raised only with peers for their initial 6 months of life. These infants are hand-reared in a neonatal nursery for their first month of life, housed with same-aged, like-reared peers for the rest of their first 6 months, and then moved into larger social groups containing both peer-reared and mother-reared agemates. Peer-reared infants readily develop strong social attachment bonds to each other, much like mother-reared infants develop attachment relationships with their own mothers.[39] However, because peers are not nearly as effective as most monkey mothers in reducing fear in the face of novelty or stress, or in providing a "secure base" for exploration, the attachment relationships that these peer-reared infants develop are almost always "anxious" in nature. While peer-reared monkeys show completely normal physical and motor development, their early exploratory behavior is usually somewhat limited. They seem reluctant to approach novel objects, and they tend to be shy in initial encounters with unfamiliar peers. Moreover, even when they interact with their same-aged cagemates in familiar settings, their emerging social play repertoires are usually retarded both in frequency and complexity. One explanation for their relatively poor play performance is that their cagemates must serve both as attachment objects and playmates, a dual role that neither mothers nor mother-reared peers have to serve. It is also difficult, if not impossible, to develop sophisticated play repertoires with basically incompetent play partners. Perhaps as a result, peer-reared youngsters typically drop to and remain at the bottom of their respective dominance hierarchies when they are grouped with mother-reared monkeys their own age.[40]

In addition, throughout development peer-reared monkeys consistently exhibit more extreme behavioral, adrenocortical, and noradrenergic reactions to social separations than do their mother-reared cohorts, even after they have been living in the same social groups for extended periods.[41] Such differences in prototypical biobehavioral reactions to separation persist from infancy to adolescence, if not beyond. Interestingly, the general nature of the separation reactions of peer-reared monkeys seems to mirror that of "naturally occuring" high-reactive mother-reared subjects.[42]

Early peer-rearing has another long-term developmental consequence for rhesus monkeys—they tend to become excessively aggressive, especially if they are males. Like the previously described impulsive monkeys growing up in the wild, peer-reared males begin to exhibit inappropriate aggressive behavior in the context of juvenile play, and as they approach puberty the frequency and severity of their aggressive episodes typically exceed those of mother-reared group members of similar age. Peer-reared fe-males tend to groom (and be groomed by) others in their social group less frequently and for shorter durations than their mother-reared counterparts and, as before, they usually stay at the bottom of their respective dominance hierar-chies. These differences between peer-reared and mother-reared agemates in aggression, grooming, and dominance remain relatively ro-bust when the monkeys are subsequently moved into newly formed social groups, and they gen-erally are quite stable throughout the preadoles-cent and adolescent years.[43] Peer-reared monkeys also consistently show lower CSF con-centrations of 5-HIAA than their mother-reared counterparts. These group differences in 5-HIAA concentrations appear well before 6 months of age, they persist during the transition to mixed-group housing, and they remain stable at least throughout adolescence and into early adulthood. Thus, peer-reared monkeys as a group resemble the impulsive subgroup of wild-living (and mother-reared) monkeys not only be-haviorally but also in terms of decreased serotonergic functioning.[44]

An additional risk that peer-reared females carry into adulthood concerns their maternal be-havior. Peer-reared mothers are significantly more likely to exhibit neglectful and/or abusive treatment of their first-born offspring than are their mother-reared counterparts, although their risk for inadequate maternal care is not nearly as great as is the case for females reared in social isolation; moreover, their care of subsequent offspring tends to improve dramatically.[45] Nev-ertheless, most multiparous mothers who expe-rienced early peer-rearing continue to exhibit nonnormative patterns of ventral contact with their offspring throughout the whole of their re-productive years.[46]

In summary, early peer-rearing seems to make rhesus monkey infants both more highly reactive and more impulsive, and their resulting develop-mental trajectories not only resemble those of naturally occurring subgroups of rhesus monkeys growing up in the wild but also persist in that vein long after their period of exclusive exposure to peers has been completed and they have been living in more species-typical social groups. In-deed, some effects of early peer-rearing may well be passed on to the next generation via aberrant patterns of maternal care, as appears to be the case for both high-reactive and impulsive moth-ers rearing infants in their natural habitat.[47] As noted by Bowlby and other attachment theorists for the human case, the effects of inadequate early social attachments may be both lifelong and cross-generational in nature.

What about the opposite situation—are there any consequences, either short- or long-term, of enhanced early social attachment relationships for rhesus monkeys? A recent series of studies at-tempted to address this question by rearing rhesus monkey neonates selectively bred for dif-ferences in temperamental reactivity with foster mothers who differed in their characteristic ma-ternal "style," as determined by their patterns of care of previous offspring. In this work specific members of a captive breeding colony were se-lectively bred to produce offspring who, on the basis of their genetic pedigree, were either un-usually high-reactive or within the normal range of reactivity. These selectively bred infants were then cross-fostered to unrelated multiparous fe-males preselected to be either unusually nur-turant with respect to attachment-related behavior or within the normal range of maternal care of previous offspring. The selectively bred infants were then reared by their respective foster mothers for their first 6 months of life, after which they were moved to larger social groups containing other cross-fostered agemates, as well as those reared by their biological mother.[48]

During the period of cross-fostering, control infants (i.e., those whose pedigrees suggested normative patterns of reactivity) exhibited essen-tially normal patterns of biobehavioral develop-ment, independent of the relative nurturance of their foster mother. In contrast, dramatic differ-ences emerged among genetically high-reactive infants as a function of their type of foster mother: whereas high-reactive infants cross-fostered by control females exhibited expected deficits in early exploration and exaggerated responses to minor environmental perturbations, high-reactive infants cross-fostered to nurturant females actually appeared to be behaviorally precocious. They left their mothers earlier, explored their environment more, and displayed less behavioral disturbance during weaning than not only the high-reactive infants cross-fostered to control mothers but even the control infants reared by either type of foster mother. Their attachment relationships with their nurturant foster mothers thus appeared to be unusually secure.

When these monkeys were permanently separated from their foster mothers and moved into larger social groups at 6 months of age, an additional advantage for those high-reactive youngsters who had been reared by nurturant foster mothers became apparent. These individuals turned out to be especially adept at recruiting and retaining other group members as allies during agonistic encounters and, perhaps as a consequence, most of them rose to and maintained top positions in their group's dominance hierarchy. In contrast, high-reactive youngsters who had been foster-reared by control females tended to drop to and remain at the bottom of the same hierarchies.[49]

Finally, some of the cross-fostered females from this study have since become mothers themselves, and their maternal behavior toward their first-born offspring has been assessed. It appears that these young mothers have adapted the general maternal style of their foster mothers, independent of both their own original reactivity profile and the type of maternal style shown by their biological mother. Thus, the apparent benefits accrued by high-reactive females raised by nurturant foster mothers can seemingly be transmitted to the next generation of offspring, even though the mode of transmission is nongenetic in nature.[50] Clearly, high-reactivity need not al-

ways be associated with adverse outcomes. Instead, following certain early experiences high-reactive infants appear to have relatively normal, if not actually optimal, long-term developmental trajectories which, in turn, can be amenable to cross-generational transmission. Whether the same possibilities exist for genetically impulsive rhesus monkey infants is currently the focus of ongoing research.

These and other findings from studies with monkeys demonstrate that differential early social experiences can have major long-term influences on an individual's behavioral and physiological propensities over and above any heritable predispositions. The nature of early attachment experiences appears to be especially relevant: whereas insecure early attachments tend to make monkeys more reactive and impulsive, unusually secure early attachments seem to have essentially the opposite effect, at least for some individuals. In either case, how a rhesus monkey mother rears her infant can markedly affect its biobehavioral developmental trajectory, even long after its interactions with her have ceased.

IMPLICATIONS FOR THE STUDY OF HUMAN DEVELOPMENT

THIS chapter has summarized findings from many years of studies investigating biobehavioral development in rhesus monkeys. These studies have described species-normative patterns of development that unfold across a wide range of field and captive environments, characterized variations in developmental trajectories that appear to persist across multiple generations, and demonstrated the influence of early social experiences on both short- and long-term outcomes of these different developmental trajectories. What implications might these findings have for advancing our understanding of human development as well as the well-being of children?

One must begin with the caveat that rhesus monkeys are clearly not furry little humans with tails but instead are only close phylogenetic relatives who share much of our genetic heritage but lack certain capabilities, e.g., spoken and written language, that make us uniquely human. It is therefore unlikely that specific findings from studies with rhesus monkeys or any other non-human primates will generalize across all levels of analysis to specific aspects of human development. On the other hand, two general principles can be gleaned from studies involving this highly successful primate species that arguably can provide meaningful insights to our general understanding of basic human developmental phenomena.

First and foremost is the general principle that early social experiences, especially those with primary attachment figures, can have profound consequences for both behavioral and physiological functioning throughout the lifespan. Freud and Bowlby, among others, always emphasized the long-term importance of the initial relationship with one's mother, but the primate data clearly demonstrate that the impact of that first important social relationship encompasses not only social, emotional, and cognitive domains but also affects specific aspects of a remarkably wide range of physiological functioning throughout the lifespan. These early experience effects occur in the absence of any apparent linguistic capabilities or specific cultural traditions among the individuals involved. It is hard to believe that most humans would not be at least as sensitive to differences in their initial attachment relationships as are most rhesus monkeys, and one could easily argue that the unique linguistic and memory capabilities of humans might even enhance the long-term impacts of specific early social experiences over those found for rhesus monkeys.

Second, both short- and long-term consequences of specific events that occur in a social context are seldom (if ever) uniform across all individuals experiencing those particular events. Rather, some individuals, owing to heritable predispositions, previous experiences, or (most likely) both, may be more sensitive behaviorally and/or physiologically to the fallout from such events than are others. Not all young monkeys respond in a depressive manner to their mother's brief departures that are specifically devoted to the conception of their next sibling, and not all infants blessed with unusually nurturant (foster) mothers subsequently exhibit obvious enhancement of their respective biobehavioral developmental trajectories. These differential effects of early experiences are readily expressed without the benefit of self-reflecting capabilities that are universal among humans but apparently lacking in rhesus monkeys. One might surmise that self-reflection could well enhance differential perceptions of the same or similar events, such that the range of different long-term consequences for particular events experienced early in life might actually be greater (and perhaps even more stable) for developing humans than for developing monkeys.

NOTES

1. Novak, M.A., and Suomi, S. J. (1991). Social interaction in nonhuman primates: An underlying theme for primate research. *Laboratory Animal Science, 41*: 308–314.

2. Suomi, S. J. (in press). Conflict and cohesion in rhesus monkey family life. In: Cox, M., and Brooks-Gunn, J. (Eds.), *Conflict and Cohesion in Families*. Mahwah, N.J.: Lawrence Erlbaum Associates, Inc.

3. Novak, M. A., and Suomi, S. J. (1991). *Op cit.*

4. Lindburg, D. G. (1971). The rhesus monkey in North India: An ecological and behavioral study. In: Rosenblum, L. A. (Ed.), *Primate behavior: Developments in field and laboratory research* (Vol. 2). New York: Academic Press, pp. 1–106.

5. Berard, J. (1989). Male life histories. *Puerto Rico Health Sciences Journal, 8*: 47–58.

6. Sade, D. S. (1967). Determinants of social dominance in a group of free-ranging rhesus monkeys. In: Altmann, S. A. (Ed.), *Social communication among primates*. Chicago: University of Chicago Press, pp. 99–114.

7. Sameroff, A. J., and Suomi, S. J. (1996). Primates and persons: A comparative developmental understanding of social organization. In: Cairns, R. B., Elder, G. H., and Costello, E. J. (Eds.), *Developmental Science*. Cambridge: Cambridge University Press, pp. 97–120.

8. Bowlby, J. (1969). *Attachment*. New York: Basic Books.

9. Harlow, H. F., and Harlow, M. K. (1965). The affectional systems. In: Schrier, A. M., Harlow, H. F., and Stollnitz, F. (Eds.), *Behavior of nonhuman primates* (Vol. 2). New York: Academic Press, pp. 287–334.

10. Hansen, E. W. (1966). The development of maternal and infant behavior in the rhesus monkey. *Behaviour, 27*: 107–149.

11. Hinde, R. A., and Spencer-Booth, Y. (1967). The behaviour of socially living rhesus monkeys in their first two and a half years. *Animal Behaviour, 15*: 169–196.

12. Sackett G. P. (1966). Monkeys reared in isolation with pictures as visual input: Evidence for an innate learning mechanism. *Science, 154*: 1468–1472.

13. Hinde, R. A., and White, L. E. (1974). The dynamics of a relationship—rhesus monkey ventro-ventro contact. *Journal of Comparative and Physiological Psychology, 86*: 8–23.

14. Suomi, S. J. (1995). Influence of Bowlby's Attachment Theory on research on nonhuman primate biobehavioral development. In: Goldberg, S., Muir, R., and Kerr, J. (Eds.), *Attachment theory: Social, developmental, and clinical perspectives*. Hillsdale, N.J.: The Analytic Press, pp. 185–201.

15. Harlow, H. F., and Harlow, M. K. (1965). *Op cit.*

16. Ruppenthal, G. C., Harlow, M. K., Eisele, C. D., Harlow, H. F., and Suomi, S. J. (1974). Development of peer interactions of monkeys reared in a nuclear family environment. *Child Development, 45*: 670–682.

17. Harlow, H. F., and Lauersdorf, H. E. (1974). Sex differences in passion and play. *Perspectives in Biology and Medicine, 17*: 348–360.

18. Suomi, S. J. (1979). Peers, play, and primary prevention in primates. In: Kent, M. W., and Rolf, J. E. (Eds.), *Primary prevention in psychopathology* (Vol. 3). Hanover, N.H.: University Press of New England, pp. 127–149.

19. Dittus, W. P. J. (1979). The evolution of behaviours regulating density and age specific sex ratios in a primate population. *Behaviour, 69*: 265–302.

20. Suomi, S. J., Rasmussen, K. L. R., and Higley, J. D. (1992). Primate models of behavioral and physiological change in adolescence. In: McAnarney, E. R., Kriepe, R. E.,

Orr, D. P., and Comerci, G. D. (Eds.), *Textbook of adolescent medicine*. Philadelphia: Saunders, pp. 135–139.

21. Suomi, S. J. (1995). *Op cit.*

22. Suomi, S. J. (1986). Anxiety-like disorders in young primates. In: Gittelman, R. (Ed.), *Anxiety disorders of childhood*. New York: Guilford Press, pp. 1–23.

23. Suomi, S. J. (1991a). Up-tight and laid-back monkeys: Individual differences in the response to social challenges. In: Brauth, S., Hall, W., and Dooling, R. (Eds.), *Plasticity of development*. Cambridge, Mass.: MIT Press, pp. 27–56.

24. Berman, C. M., Rasmussen, K. L. R., and Suomi, S. J. (1994). Responses of free-ranging rhesus monkeys to a natural form of social separation: I. Parallels with mother-infant separation in captivity. *Child Development, 65*: 1028–1041.

25. Bowlby, J. (1960). Grief and mourning in infancy and early childhood. *Psychoanalytic Study of the Child, 15*: 9–52.

26. Bowlby, J. (1973). *Separation: anger and anxiety*. New York: Basic Books.

27. Suomi, S. J. (1991b). Primate separation models of affective disorders. In: Madden, J. (Ed.), *Neurobiology of learning, emotion, and affect*. New York: Raven Press, pp. 195–214.

28. Suomi, S. J. (1991a). *Op cit.*

29. Suomi, S. J. (1995) *Op cit.*

30. Higley, J. D., Thompson, W. T., Champoux, M., Goldman, D., Hasert, M. F., Kraemer G. W., Scanlan, J. M., Suomi, S. J., and Linnoila, M. (1993). Paternal and maternal genetic and environmental contributions to CSF monoamine metabolites in rhesus monkeys (*Macaca mulatta*). *Archives of General Psychiatry, 50*: 615–623.

31. Suomi, S. J., Rasmussen, K. L. R., and Higley, J. D. (1992). *Op cit.*

32. Suomi, S. J., and Ripp, C. (1983). A history of motherless mother monkey mothering at the University of Wisconsin Primate Laboratory. In: Reite, M., and Caine, N. (Eds.), *Child abuse: the nonhuman primate data*. New York: Alan R. Liss, pp. 49–77.

33. Boyce, W. T., O'Neill-Wagner, P. L., Price, C. S., Haines, M., and Suomi, S. J. (1998). Crowding stress and violent injuries among behaviorally inhibited rhesus macaques. *Health Psychology, 17*, 285–289.

34. Higley, J. D., Linnoila, M., and Suomi, S. J. (1994). Ethological contributions. In: Ammerman, R. T. (Ed.), *Handbook of aggressive behavior in psychiatric patients*. New York: Raven Press, pp. 153–167.

35. Mehlman, P. T., Higley, J. D., Faucher, I., Lilly, A. A., Taub, D. M., Vickers, J., Suomi, S. J., and Linnoila, M. (1994). Low cebrospinal fluid 5-hydroxyindoleacetic acid concentrations are correlated with severe aggression and reduced impulse control in free-ranging primates. *American Journal of Psychiatry, 151,* 1485–1491.

36. Mehlman, P. T., Higley, J. D., Faucher, I., Lilly, A. A., Taub, D. M., Vickers, J., Suomi, S. J., and Linnoila, M. (1995). CSF 5-HIAA concentrations are correlated with sociality and the timing of emigration in free-ranging primates. *American Journal of Psychiatry, 152,* 901–913.

37. Higley, J. D., Mehlman, P. T., Taub, D. M., Higley, S., Fernald, B., Vickers, J., Lindell, S. G., Suomi, S. J., and Linnoila, M. (1996b). Excessive mortality in young free-ranging nonhuman primates with low CSF 5-HIAA concentrations. *Archives of General Psychiatry, 53:* 537–543.

38. Higley, J. D., King, S. T., Hasert, M. F., Champoux, M., Suomi, S. J., and Linnoila, M. (1996a). Stability of interindividual differences in serotonin function and its relationship to severe aggression and competent social behavior in rhesus macaque females. *Neuropsychopharmacology, 14:* 67–76.

39. Harlow, H. F. (1969). Age-mate or peer affectional system. In: Lehrman, D. H., Hinde, R. A., and Shaw, E. (Eds.), *Advances in the study of behavior* (Vol. 2). New York: Academic Press, pp. 333–383.

40. Suomi, S. J. (1995). *Op cit.*

41. Higley, J. D., and Suomi, S. J. (1986). Parental behaviour in primates. In: Sluckin, W., and Herbert, M. (Eds.), *Parental behaviour.* Oxford: Blackwell, pp. 152–207.

42. Suomi, S. J. (1997). Early determinants of behaviour: evidence from primate studies. *British Medical Bulletin, 53:* 170–184.

43. Higley, J. D., Suomi, S. J., and Linnoila, M. (1996). A nonhuman primate model of Type II alcoholism? (Part 2): Diminished social competence and excessive aggression correlates with low CSF 5-HIAA concentrations. *Alcoholism: Clinical and Experimental Research, 20:* 643–650.

44. Suomi, S. J. (1997). *Op cit.*

45. Ruppenthal, G. C., Arling, G. L., Harlow, H. F., Sackett, G. P., and Suomi, S. J. (1976). A 10-year perspective of motherless mother monkey behavior. *Journal of Abnormal Psychology, 85:* 341–439.

46. Champoux, M., , Byrne, E., Delizio, R. and Suomi, S. J. (1992). Rhesus maternal behavior and rearing history. *Primates, 33:* 251–25.

47. Suomi, S. J., and Levine, S. (In press). Psychobiology of intergenerational effects of trauma: Evidence from animal studies. In: Daniele, Y. (Ed.), *International handbook of multigenerational legacies of trauma.* New York: Plenum Press.

48. Suomi, S. J. (1987). Genetic and maternal contributions to individual differences in rhesus monkey biobehavioral development. In: Krasnagor, N., Blass, E., Hofer, M., and Smotherman, W. (Eds.), *Perinatal development: A psychobiological perspective.* New York: Academic Press, pp. 397–420.

49. Suomi, S. J. (1991a). *Op cit*

50. Suomi, S. J., and Levine, S. (In press). *Op cit.*

Eight

EARLY CHILD DEVELOPMENT
IN THE CONTEXT OF POPULATION HEALTH

Clyde Hertzman

INTRODUCTION

THIS chapter approaches early child development from the perspective of the socioeconomic gradient in health status. It describes how a focus on early child development emerges as a corollary of the characteristics of the gradient. The focus on the gradient also points to the need to understand the biology of early childhood and the interplay of individual human development with the socioeconomic and psychosocial conditions the individual encounters day-to-day throughout life. The chapter finishes by identifying generic "policy challenges" which arise from these insights; that a modern society needs to take a large measure of collective responsibility for the quality of the early experiences of its children if it expects to maintain and improve the health and well-being of its population over time.

THE CHARACTER OF THE GRADIENT

WHY does health status vary with income distribution in wealthy countries? No one has a precise answer to this question, but it is clear that it has something to do with the way in which different wealthy societies handle the tendency for socioeconomic and psychosocial inequality to emerge. There is a large fact which

supports this observation: health status increases with increasing socioeconomic status[1,2] in every wealthy society on earth. The pattern is not, typically, a simple difference between the healthy rich and the unhealthy poor. Rather, the health status of each class within the population seems to be better than the classes below and worse than the classes above. In other words, middle class people may live longer and healthier lives than the poor, as we would expect, but they also live shorter, less healthy lives than the rich. The pattern just described is remarkably consistent across OECD countries, regardless of whether the classes are defined by levels of income, education, or occupation; so much so that it has been canonized as the "socioeconomic gradient" in health status.

The socioeconomic gradient in health status is not new. It has remained largely unchanged since the beginning of the twentieth century, *despite the fact that the principal causes of death have changed completely*. In fact the socioeconomic gradient in health status seems to be able to replicate itself on the principal diseases of each era, despite the fact that their pathologic basis varies greatly. For instance, at the turn of the century the gradient was found among the infectious diseases which were the principal causes of death at the time. By late in the century, the socioeconomic gradient had replicated itself in heart disease, injuries, and almost all prevalent cancers; the current major causes of death. This observation undermines the belief that socioeconomic factors affected health through the consumption of items such as food, housing, and medical care. It is now clear that there is much more at stake, and that the socioeconomic effect is not confined to those too poor to buy health-enhancing goods. The prospect is that socioeconomic gradient functions tap attributes which are deeply embedded in the psychosocial character of human societies.

EXPLAINING SOCIOECONOMIC GRADIENTS IN HEALTH STATUS

THE life cycle is fundamental to the study of health status because it is the basis of biological change in all individual organisms. Early in life there is a socioeconomic gradient in infant mortality and low birth weight; during childhood and adolescence there is a gradient in injurious deaths, as well as in cognitive and socioemotional development; in early adulthood the gradient is found among deaths from injuries and mental health problems; in late middle age early chronic disease mortality and morbidity show a gradient; and in late life a similar pattern is seen for dementia and other degenerative conditions.

The largest component of the socioeconomic gradient in health status is differential mortality and morbidity at one specific stage of the life cycle: the period of premature chronic degenerative disease. But this is not the time at which the principal determinants of differential mortality and morbidity begin to have their biological effect. It is necessary to work backward in time to find their origin. This issue has been framed by a conceptual framework which accounts for "sources of heterogeneity" across the life cycle; wherein sources of heterogeneity are defined as the basic types of causal pathways or mechanisms that might lead to the differences in health status

which are observed across population partitions and stages of the life cycle. Each type of causal pathway has radically different implications for how we think about the origins of health and disease, and about policies to address them.

Six mechanisms encompass all the relevant pathways. The first two of these explain away the gradient as an artefact; and the latter four are causal explanations. The artefactual explanations are health selection (or reverse causality) and differential susceptiblity (those with healthy constitutions are upwardly mobile and *vice versa*). The causal explanations are:

Individual lifestyle—That is, the health habits and behaviors of those in different sub-groups lead them to have different risks of particular life-threatening and/or disabling conditions. In particular, health promoting behaviors may tend to be practiced more frequently among those in higher socioeconomic groups, and health damaging behaviors, the reverse.

Physical environment—That is, differential exposures to physical, chemical, and biological agents at home, at work, and in the community lead to differences in health status. This category would include all the diverse influences of the built environment on health.

Socioeconomic and psychosocial (SEP) conditions per se—This includes the "grand interaction" between the developing human and factors such as access to material resources, social isolation, responsiveness of civil society, income distribution, and the panoply of psychosocial stresses of daily living.

Differential access to/response to health care services—This encompasses differences in health status that are related to differences in care seeking behavior, the quality of health services and access to them, and to differential outcomes for a given treatment.

The evidence regarding the socioeconomic gradient in health status has been evaluated according to this framework, and can be summarized as follows. The reverse causality hypothesis is refuted by the fact that the socioeconomic gradient is as strong when social class is based upon education as when it is based upon income or occupation. After all, educational status does not decline with health status, as is possible with the income or occupational category. Differential susceptiblity can only be evaluated through evidence from longitudinal studies. When this has been done, as it was in a series of longitudinal studies in Britain, it turns out that factors such as height, which are developmental markers of future health, are also markers for upward social mobility. However, these factors' contribution to the gradient is not large, and also partially reflect the quality of the SEP environment.[3]

Similarly, those in lower socioeconomic groups are exposed, on average, to more toxic chemicals and more unsafe physical environments than those in higher socioeconomic groups. However, the proportion of deaths in wealthy countries that can be attributed to the physical and chemical environment is small, and does not explain a large percentage of the gradient.[4] The same thing can be said for access to/response to health care services. Even in countries like Canada and the United Kingdom, where universal access to "medically necessary" services is the rule, there are social/economic differences in how individuals use the system. There are also differences in survival following treatment. But "medically avoidable death," that is, life threatening disease for which there is effective *life saving* treatment, represents a small proportion of all deaths, and, also, a small proportion of the overall gradient in health status.

By exclusion, this leaves lifestlye and SEP conditions per se. There is no question that lifestyle factors play a significant role in the socioeconomic gradient in health status. Mortality from diseases with a large lifestyle/behavioral component, such as lung cancer, does have a steep socioeconomic gradient. But the socioeconomic gradient is not confined to diseases with a lifestyle or behavioral component. When multivariable models are contructed, most of the gradient in mortality survives after the contribution of social class differences in the behavior of interest has been taken into account.

A detailed understanding of how the socioeconomic gradient comes about depends upon an understanding of the complex mixture of psychosocial and material influences operating at various levels of social aggregation, and a series of biological responses whose character and significance vary from stage to stage across the life cycle. Moreover, the explanation must account for the fact that the gradient cuts across a wide range of pathological outcomes.

Biological Embedding

By invoking insights into primate and human biology, it is possible to offer an hypothesis which could account for the gradient: spending one's early years in an unstimulating, emotionally and physically unsupportive environment will affect the sculpting and neurochemistry of the central nervous system in adverse ways, and lead to cognitive and socioemotional deficits (which may or may not be wholly reversible). The problems that children so affected will display early in school will lead them to experience much more acute and chronic stress than others, which will have both physiological and life path consequences. Because the central nervous system, which is the center of human consciousness, "talks to" the immune, hormone, and clotting systems, systematic differences in the experience of life will increase or decrease levels of resistance to disease. This will change the long-term function of vital organs of the body and, in conjunction with the differential stresses of daily living, lead to socioeconomic differentials in morbidity and mortality. This hypothesis, which suggests how human experience affects the healthfulness of life across the life cycle, has come to be known as "biological embedding."[5]

Insights into biological embedding come from a variety of sources, including primate studies, studies of critical periods in brain development, and psychoneuroimmunology and psycho-neuroendocrinology. For instance, the observation that the neurological system can talk to the immune and endocrine systems provides a modicum of biological plausibility to the notion that the conditions of life, filtered through a perceptual screen, could affect vitality through a wide variety of pathological mechanisms.

An Animal Model of the Determinants of Health in Whole Societies

IN humans, the study of the determinants of health across the whole life cycle is limited by money, time, and the supply of instructive experiments of nature. But these limitations do not apply as much to studies of certain other primate populations which, nevertheless, show remarkable similarities to humans. Their usefulness derives from the fact that the investigators are able to juxtapose measurements of well-being against a detailed understanding of the developmental histories of individual primates; and the social dynamics and living conditions of the primate population "in the wild." One of the most useful of these has been the study of free-ranging baboon populations in the Serengeti.[6] Four observations come from this study that may be useful in understanding the complex interplay of individual development and social dynamics in human societies.

1. *Rank*—When all other factors are held constant, higher rank in a (baboon) society means higher levels of well-being.
2. *Social stability and its enforcement*—When (baboon) societies are stable, those in dominant positions have higher levels of well-being than they do during periods of instability. When stability is imposed by high levels of violence and coercion the non-dominant members of society will have lower levels of well-being than when it is maintained with low levels of violence and coercion.
3. *The individual experience of rank, stability, and enforcement*—When social instability occurs, some non-dominant baboons will actually experience increases in well-being. This is because their relation-

ships with those higher in the hierarchy are traditionally stressful. These relationships may be interrupted by the preoccupations the more dominant baboons have with each other during fights for supremacy. Other low ranked baboons, however, will do worse if they become the victims of displaced aggression from the losers in the fight for social dominance.
4. *Personality and coping styles*—Individual characteristics matter, too. The ability to distinguish seriously threatening situations from ruses; to distinguish winning from losing a fight; to relieve stress by displacing aggression; and to be able to develop friendships and strategic alliances all lead to increased well-being. Each of these characteristics has a component that is related to circumstances of upbringing and mentorship.

With one eye on primates and the other on people, it has been possible to identify analogous elements of human society and use the above insights to build a preliminary model of society and health.

To begin with, the baboon model suggests that all levels of societal aggregation need to be considered simultaneously. Hierarchy and social stability are, fundamentally, characteristics of whole societies, although they may be encrypted either within society as a whole (social stability) or within the individual (place in hierarchy). There is a parallel between the pattern of increased well-being in baboon communities with low levels of violence and coercion, and the findings in wealthy human societies which show that relative income equality[7,8] and shallow social class gradients in health[9] are determinants of longevity. The experience of hierarchy, stability, and enforcement (e. g., the day-to-day stresses of good times, such as a positive workplace and home life, and bad times, for example loss of control at work, layoffs or long-term unemployment) are, by current terminology, "civil society" functions that reside in an intermediate zone between the individual and the state. Personality and coping styles are embedded in the individual, but have both a social network aspect and a longitudinal, developmental aspect.

These relationships are summarized by the

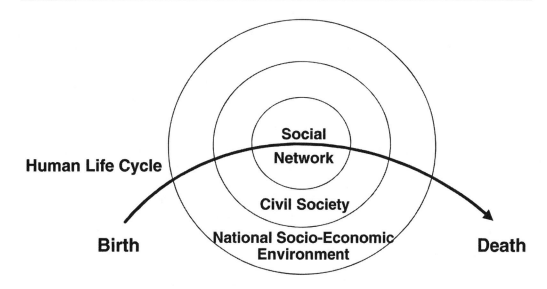

Figure 1
Human Development and the Social Determinants of Health

model in Figure 1, which represents the individual life cycle as an arrow, piercing a bull's eye, which represents society. Society is shown to have three classes of factors, represented by three concentric circles, which represent determinants of health and well-being at three levels of social aggregation. At the most intimate level are the factors associated with social support. At the intermediate level are the factors associated with "civil society" which can buffer or exacerbate the stresses of daily living. Finally, at the broadest level of aggregation are state factors, in particular, national wealth, income distribution, and the structure of opportunity created by history, geography, and fortune that support or undermine health and well-being.

The picture that emerges is of a lifelong interaction between the cognitive and socioemotional capabilities of the *developing* individual and SEP conditions as they present themselves at the in-

timate, civic, and state level. The dimension of human development emerges as one of the principal components of the SEP conditions that determine health throughout the life cycle. A developmental perspective that begins at the very beginning of life would seem indispensable here. In practice, this means paying particularly close attention to insights gleaned from longitudinal studies, especially those which begin at birth and follow large population samples for decades into the future.

LATENT AND PATHWAY EFFECTS

TWO different, and sometimes conflicting explanatory models emerge of this interactive relationship. The first, called the "latency" model, emphasizes the prospect that SEP conditions very early in life will have a strong effect later in life *independent of intervening experience.*

The second, called the "pathways" model, emphasizes the *cumulative* effect of life events and the ongoing importance of SEP conditions throughout the life cycle.

Latency Model

The essence of the latency model can be illustrated with an example from animal research. A series of studies has been carried out that examined the lifelong impact of "handling" newborn rats.[10] Handling involves removing the mother from the litter, placing individual pups into a new cage for fifteen minutes, then returning both mother and pups to their cage. This is done once per day for the first three weeks of life. When compared to non-handled pups, this simple intervention was associated with improved function of the "stress system" throughout the life cycle (i.e. lower basal corticosterone concentrations and faster physiological recovery in stressful situations). These changes reduced the total lifetime exposure of the brain to corticosterone, which is toxic to nerve cells in a brain structure known as the hippocampus, and thus the rate of loss of nerve cells in the hippocampus was reduced in the handled rats over their life span.

Cognitive functions are sensitive to relatively small degrees of hippocampal damage, and so by twenty-four months of age, elderly by rat standards, the handled rats had been spared some of the cognitive deterioration typical of aging. The significance of this was demonstrated by performance on a learning task wherein rats had to find a submerged platform in a pool of opaque water, relying entirely upon visuospatial cues from the surrounding room. Nonhandled rats had a progressive deterioration in their performance with age; in contrast, no deterioration occurred in aged handled rats. *Most relevant in this context is the final observation: the handling phenomenon could not be induced by carrying out the handling paradigm at a later age.*[10]

This example clearly illustrates the notion of a critical period in development. For the purposes of understanding the latency model, its essence is an opportunity to develop a competence which occurs at a discrete and unique time in (early) life, and has a lifelong impact on well-being, independent of intervening experience. For instance, the risk of death from heart disease in the fifth decade of life is strongly associated with the size of an individual's placenta at birth and weight gain during the first year of life.[11-19] Certain early childhood stimulation programs have been effective in improving the life trajectories of disadvantaged children[20-21] even without any attempt to provide them with ongoing support. The common theme here is the notion of a discrete time, early in life, when the right things must happen, or else it is "all over."

Pathways Model

The hypothesis underlying the pathways model is that, over time, the physiological aspects of less than optimal neurophysiological development, chronic stress and its physiological impacts, a sense of powerlessness and alienation, and a "social support" network made up of others who have been marginalized, will create a vicious cycle with implications for education, criminality, drug use, and teen pregnancy in the first two decades of life; and later life implications for psychosocial working conditions, social support, chronic disease in mid life, and degenerative conditions in late life. It is most closely associated with the findings from long-term follow-up studies of newborns, adolescents, working populations, and the elderly. These studies can be put together in a time sequence to reconstruct the life cycle. A pattern then emerges that highlights the enduring impact of SEP conditions on health, well-being, and competence from cradle to grave. In highly abbreviated form, it goes something like this:

Status differences at birth are associated with

Percent

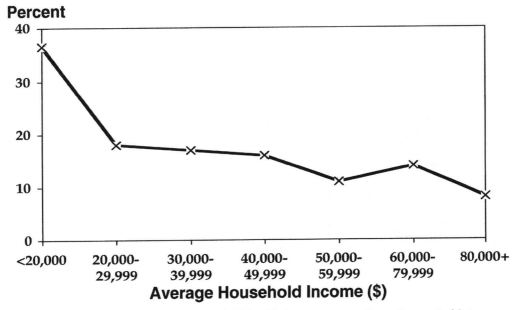

Ross DP, Roberts P. (1999) Income and child well-being: a new perspective on the poverty debate. Canadian Council on Social Development: Ottawa, p 25.

Figure 2
Kindergarten Children with Delayed Vocabulary
Development in Canada

different levels of stability and security in early childhood, which are, in turn, associated with different levels of readiness for schooling.[22] Lack of school readiness leads to an increased risk of behavioral problems in school and ultimate school failure.[23] These patterns have been demonstrated among the school age subsample of the National Longitudinal Study of Children and Youth in Canada (NLSCY).[31] The NLSCY is a random sample of 22,000 children who were 0–11 years old in 1994/95 and are being followed on a biennial basis. These data are presented in Figure 2. Furthermore, by early high school, international comparisons show that socioeconomic gradients in educational achievement have emerged, such that countries with steep gradients (such as the United States) are doing

less well, on average, than those with shallower gradients (Figure 3). This pattern of "the flatter the gradient the higher the mean" is similar to what happens for health outcomes.

Continuing with the pathways story; behavioral problems and failure in school lead to low levels of mental well-being in early adulthood.[23] Meanwhile, the status of one's parents helps to determine the community where one grows up, which, by the early school years, starts to influence the child's life chances through the social networks, community values, and opportunities which present themselves.[24]

By early adulthood individuals start to define their own status. Already, differences begin to emerge wherein those who are doing better report higher levels of well-being. As adulthood

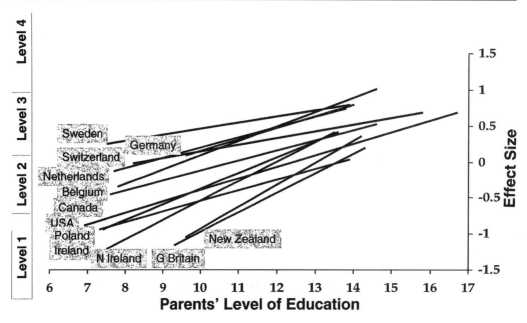

Organisation for Economic Co-operation and Development and Statistics Canada. (1995) Literacy, economy, and society: results of the first international adult literacy survey. OECD/Ministry of Industry Canada, p 151.

Figure 3
Quantitative Literacy Scores for Youth Ages 16–25.
International Adult Literacy Study, 1994.

unfolds, lower status individuals tend to end up in jobs that make relatively high demands on them, but that offer low levels of control of the pace and character of the work.[25] (A good example of this is bus driving, which could be contrasted with conducting an orchestra.) By the fifth decade of life, those who are stuck in such jobs first develop high rates of disability and absenteeism[26,27] and then begin to die prematurely, and from the full range of major causes of death.[28] This general pattern, which is more pronounced among those who are also socially isolated, persists into the eighth decade of life.[29]

The latency and pathway models complement one another. After all, there is no reason to suppose that latent factors act only independently, because any early life event which could exert a latent effect could also be the first step along a lifelong pathway which might have implications for health, well-being, or competence in the future. Conversely, any early childhood intervention designed to improve health and well-being in the long run will occur within a specific context which will provide a mixture of opportunities or barriers. Indeed, the closer the correlation between early life events and subsequent lifelong pathways, the more difficult the statistical problem of estimating the partial contribution of each.

The relative contribution of latent versus pathway effects in explaining long-term socioeconomic gradients in health and well-being can only be elucidated with detailed information on individuals followed over time. Longitudinal studies (both observational and intervention) are indispensable in this endeavor. Given that it is particularly in relation to development in utero and in infancy that latency models have been proposed, it is also of importance that follow-up studies commence at birth, if not before. Thus longitudinal studies starting at birth, namely birth cohorts, are of particular importance, especially when follow-ups extend far enough into adult life to include the chronic and degenerative conditions of middle and late life. Typically intervention studies have had shorter periods of follow-up, but their importance lies in their ability to demonstrate long-term impacts through altered life trajectories.

THE 1958 BIRTH COHORT STUDY

THE task defined by the above observations is, in essence, to measure the effects on health, well-being, and competence of the dimensions presented in Figure 1 while simultaneously disentangling latent and pathway effects. Yet, there are few studies that allow concurrent investigation of individual lifecourse and societal influences as the model in Figure 1 requires. However, a notable exception is the 1958 British birth cohort study, which is especially useful for the purpose of investigating latency and pathway effects because of its large sample size. Over 17,000 subjects were included in the original study population of all births in one week in 1958 (3rd-9th March) in England, Scotland and Wales.[3] Subsequent follow-up of survivors has been undertaken at ages 7, 11, 16, 23 and, most recently in 1991, at 33 years. At ages 7, 11 and 16 immigrants to Britain born during the same week were included in the study. 11,407 subjects (69% of the target) remained in the study at the most recent follow-up at age 33.

The 1958 birth cohort data base has information that can help characterize each of the dimensions in Figure 1. Lifecourse influences which have been identified as predictors of adult health, and are available in the 1958 cohort,

include birth weight and rate of physical development; early cognitive and behavioral development; socioeconomic circumstances of the family; quality of the home environment from the standpoint of stimulation and support; academic success; behavior in school; age of school leaving; and neighborhood conditions in childhood. In terms of societal effects, socioeconomic status, social trust and participation, marital status, and quality of social support are all available for analysis. In addition, the 1958 cohort includes factors that emerge from the interaction of the lifecourse and social environment, such as job insecurity and life control.

Health status in early adulthood is represented by a range of measures (mainly self-reported) that fulfill two criteria. They are particularly prevalent among young adults and, also, they predict future disease risk. Measures include: self-assessed health rating, longstanding conditions that limit activities of daily life, psychological distress (as indicated by the Malaise Inventory symptom check list), back pain, respiratory symptoms (cough and phlegm), and obesity, as derived from the body mass index (>30 for men and >28.6 for women).

LATENCY AND PATHWAY EFFECTS IN THE 1958 COHORT

A preliminary look at latent and pathway effects in the 1958 cohort study is given by the comparison of Table 1 and Table 2. Table 1 shows the relationship between social class at birth (as defined by father's occupation in 1958) and selected health measures at age 33. The relationships are summarized as odds ratios of classes IV and V (lowest) versus classes I and II. It is evident that the lowest social classes at birth have elevated risks for almost all health measures, especially for psychiatric distress and poor self-health rating for both sexes. The table suggests a latent effect of social circumstances at birth and health in early adulthood.

Table 1.

Gradients in Health Outcome, Age 33,
by Social Class at Birth (1958 British Birth Cohort)

	Men	Women
Fair/Poor Self-rated Health	2.67 *	3.22
Limiting Illness	1.58 (n.s.)	2.14
Respiratory Symptoms (≥)	1.88	2.56
High Malaise Score	2.10	2.97
BMI—Obese	2.19	1.99

*Odds ratio, based on slope index
Source: Reference 32

Table 2.

Gradients in Health Outcome, Age 33, by Educational
Qualifications (1958 British Birth Cohort)

	Men	Women
Fair/Poor Self-rated Health	5.58 *	6.11 *
Limiting Illness	3.33	2.19
Respiratory Symptoms (≥)	4.21	5.08
High Malaise Score	5.17	9.54
BMI—Obese	2.82	2.38

*Odds ratio, based on slope index
Source: Reference 33

However, a latent effect of early life social circumstances is difficult to establish from this information alone, and a latency model may be an incomplete explanation because there is no representation of intervening experience in the table. It is possible that social class at birth predisposes the individual to a series of social and biological events that evolve over time, and which are similarly related to social position. If so, social class at birth would be a marker for subsequent experience and the data in Table 1 could, instead, be explained by a pathway model.

For example, if the pathway model were important, then adult health risk would be more strongly related to factors which accumulate over time than to social class at birth. One test of this is provided by a comparison of the relationships for educational attainment and adult health (Table 2) with those for social class at birth and adult health (Table 1). It appears that gradients of health outcome, at this stage in the lifecourse, are stronger in general in relation to educational attainment than to social class at birth.

Educational attainment is strongly influenced by social background, but it is not equivalent to it. Indeed, social measures such as occupational class and education may be related but they are theoretically distinct, with occupation representing working and living conditions, and education representing cultural, or human capital. This distinction is validated by the observation that health behaviors such as smoking and diet are more closely associated with education than they are with income and occupation.[30] In the present context, educational attainment is likely to be representing aspects of readiness for school, social and behavioral adjustment, social investment opportunities made available, social stability, and health-related behaviors. Thus, it is an excellent marker of the "healthfulness" of accumulated childhood experience. That educational attainment is more strongly associated with adult health status than class at birth suggests that pathway effects may be operating, but it does not rule out latent effects because educational attainment may merely be an indicator of the quality of early life circumstances.

A PRELIMINARY WORKING
OF THE MODEL IN FIGURE 1

THIS previous work dealt only with the lifecourse and did not include societal factors as conceived in Figure 1. The current analysis extends this by operationalizing the socioeconomic environment with individual cohort member's reports of their circumstances; the civil society with their organizational participation, social trust, and job control; their social support with marital status and perceived emotional and practical support; and intersecting factors with job insecurity and life control. Self-rated health was used as the outcome of interest, because of its predictive validity for subsequent mortality.

Commencing with early life variables, 8 of 13 were significant determinants of self-rated health at age 33: height at age 7, behavior at age 7, teacher's rating of parental interest at age 7, parental reading to child at age 7, teacher's rating of reading ability at age 7, teacher's rating of oral ability at age 7, ratio of age 7 height to adult height, and walking alone by 1.5 years. Birthweight, creativity, and three of the developmental variables—talking by 2 years, enuresis by day after 3 years, and enuresis by night after 5 had no significant impact on self-rated health. With respect to pathway variables, cumulative social class at ages 0, 7, 11, and 16; behavior scores at 11 and 16; qualifications at school leaving; and edu-

cational qualifications by age 33 were all associated with self-rated health at age 33.

With respect to current time social factors, two socioeconomic items, material circumstances and social class at age 33, were associated with self-rated health. Self-reported social trust and self-reported level of control at work were the two civil society variables which were associated with self-rated health, whereas organizational membership and access to multiple sources of financial assistance were not. Two social support factors, marital status and self-rated emotional support at age 33, were associated with self-rated health. Finally, two factors which are "emergent functions" of the interaction between the individual and society, job insecurity and life control, were both associated with self-rated health.

Table 3.

Best Fit Model: Explaining Self-Rated Health at Age 33

Variable	β	SE (β)	(p)	r(r²)
Latent Variables				
behavior score age	.015939	.006649	.0165	
parents read to child at age 7	−.022430	.006309	.0004	
height age 7/height age 33	.005665	.002262	.0123	
Pathway Variables				
social class, age 0, 7, 11, 16	.010701	.002492	.0000	
behavior scores, 11 and 16	.013056	.004327	.0026	.30(.09)
qualif'ns at school leaving	.041638	.009068	.0000	
Economic Environment				
material circumstances at 33	.065538	.011908	.0000	
Civil Society				
most people can be trusted	.053844	.018116	.0030	
level of control at work	.025448	.009366	.0066	
Emergent Functions				
job insecurity at age 33	.033491	.007880	.0000	
level of control in life	.126961	.011617	.0000	

Source: Reference 34

From these analyses, the variables that contributed significantly to explaining self-rated health were entered as blocks into a multiple regression analysis designed to test the model in Figure 1. This included the 21 variables which were associated with self-rated health in the above analyses, as well as gender. Among these variables, gender, height at age 7, parental interest, oral ability, reading ability, creativity, walking alone by age 1.5, educational qualifications, social class at age 33, marital status, and emotional support did not achieve statistical significance (p>.05), and were excluded from further analysis.

The final and best fit model for explaining self-rated health at age 33 was achieved with 11 variables, and is displayed in Table 3. Apparent from this table is the loss of the social support block of variables, with the remaining 5 being represented. All 11 variables in this model are significant, with life control, material circumstances and end of school qualifications having the strongest impact (standardized regression coefficients not shown). Importantly, longitudinal early life, pathway/cumulative, and current factors are all shown to contribute to explaining self-rated health. Over time, model testing can be improved by including more early life variables in the 0–7 year period; and variables which characterize the socioeconomic environment and civil society using community-level information to supplement the individual level data included here.

For the purposes of the balance of this chapter, the most important outcome is that the effect of early childhood (latent) variables is not removed by including the other dimensions. A Canadian policy response to our new understandings about the importance of early childhood is presented here. It is relevant because it is currently serving as a template for wide-ranging policy and program initiatives at the local community, provincial and national level in Canada. It deserves consideration as a model to adapt to the realities of Kansas, too.

THE POLICY RESPONSE IN CANADA

IN Canada, the role of early child development as a determinant of health, well-being, and competence throughout the life course has gained acceptance in policy circles. This is reflected in the National Strategy on Healthy Child Development (the Strategy), created by the Federal/Provincial/Territorial Advisory Committee on Population Health.[35] The cornerstone of the Strategy is the recognition of society's *collective* responsibility to create access to the conditions for optimal development for all children. Accordingly, the goal of the Strategy is to improve the overall health and well-being of Canadians throughout the lifecourse by focusing government, non-governmental "social sector," and private sector policies on those conditions most relevant to optimal developmental outcomes.

The Strategy designates the period from preconception to age 5 as the "investment phase" of healthy child development, in recognition of the fact that it is an extremely sensitive and critically important time in mental and emotional development. The Strategy states:

> During the investment phase children develop language skills, the ability to learn, to cope with stress, to have healthy relationships with others, and to have a sense of self. Good mental, physical, and social health also has roots in the earliest experiences in life, and, through the parents, in the period before conception. Failure to provide optimum conditions for development during this time makes the developing brain physically different from those of children who have been well-nurtured. This can have lifelong consequences for their health, well-being and coping skills.

The period between ages 6 to 18 is referred to as the "enhancement" or "remediation phase." The Strategy states:

> If the period from conception to five years has not gone well, children may enter school unready to learn, either because their cognitive skills will be lacking or because their emotions and behaviour will interfere with learning. The tendency is for

schools, families and communities to react to such children, and label them as problems. Improving child development in this period means strengthening family, community and school capacities to help children overcome developmental lags and deficits. While it can require considerably more effort and resources than does early investment, investment during this period is worthwhile and can prevent problems later on in adulthood.

In other words, the Strategy implicitly recognizes latent and pathway effects, makes the facts of child development explicit, and writes them into policy. It goes on to identify six "policy challenges" that arise from new understandings of the importance of child development. These are, in effect, the rallying points for government, social sector, and private sector initiative:

- Investing in early child development—The Strategy recognizes that the first priority for investment is the period from preconception to age five. Most importantly, it recognizes that we have a *collective responsibility* to ensure that every child has adequate prenatal care and support; adequate nutrition; and warm, secure, trusting relationships early in life. Moreover, it emphasizes a collective responsibility to address family stress and help the child develop social skills.
- Supporting families—The Strategy recognizes that balancing work and family is an increasing concern of family life, making it difficult for families to provide stable, predictable and nurturing environments for children. Also, with increased numbers of lone-parent and dual-income families, family capacity to care for children has become an issue in daily life. Family difficulties are reflected in developmental outcomes, so collective responsibility must be taken to devise comprehensive, coordinated and collaborative policies that benefit families; including strategies that provide financial support for families, quality child care arrangements, parental leaves, flexible working arrangements, reduced hours at work, benefits and vacations.
- Reducing inequities—The Strategy explicitly recognizes the notion, arising from the work of Wilkinson[8] and Kaplan[7] with respect to health outcomes, and with respect to educational outcomes (Figure 3), that the flatter the socioeconomic gradient (in a particular outcome of human well-being), the higher the mean level of that outcome in the population as a whole. It states:

It is clear from international and interprovincial comparisons of child development, that improving the conditions of the least well off does not have a negative effect on the most well-off. In fact, improving conditions at the low end of the socioeconomic spectrum helps improve them at the upper end as well . . . The challenge is to provide access for all children to conditions that provide adequate income, nutrition, support, stimulation, care, advocacy and safety. At present, access to these factors differs with socioeconomic status.

- Reporting on outcomes and impacts—The Strategy recognizes the need to develop a system to report on the progress of child development in communities in Canada. There is a need for an outcome-oriented approach, particularly with respect to socioemotional development and academic performance, since these are predictors of later health status. It is recommended that monitoring take place over time at the community, provincial, territorial and national levels. The National Longitudinal Survey of Children and Youth will provide the baseline data with which to compare future outcomes. Readiness to learn, measured at kindergarten age, is emerging as the leading indicator since it is perceived as a valid reflection of the quality of experiences in early childhood and a valid predictor of future health, well-being, and competence.
- Investing in research—It is recognized that, unlike in the health sector, there has never been an organized system to diffuse best practices in early child development in Canada. Such an infrastructure must be developed. The policy states:

Research is critical to self-correcting, evidence-based decision making and should be geared to inform public policy. Analyses of findings, at both the individual and community level, can assist in determining best practices and serve to enlighten investment decisions . . . [therefore we must] build dissemination/uptake capacity of research findings throughout all sectors of the child-serving community . . . Use research to create a more knowledgeable public on issues of child development.

- Working in partnership and across sectors—Widespread social and economic conditions influence health; therefore, improving child development requires a broad, conscious, and collective effort to engage multiple stakeholders. This means that stakeholders, many of which have not traditionally been viewed as relevant, need to be made aware of how their sector relates to healthy child development; to actively consider the impacts of their policies on child health outcomes; and to collaborate with others to improve the impact of what they do on healthy child development. The policy recognizes a collective responsibility to build intersectoral alliances that will establish and coordinate policies and programs to improve opportunities for healthy child development.

NOTES

1. Kunst, A. E., and Mackenbach, J. P. *An International Comparison of Socio-economic Inequalities in Mortality.* Erasmus University, Rotterdam (1992).

2. Kunst, A. E., Guerts, J. J. M., and Berg, J. *International Variation in Socio-economic Inequalities in Self-reported Health.* Netherlands Central Bureau of Statistics, The Hague (1992).

3. Power, C., Manor, O., and Fox, J. *Health and class: the early years.* Chapman & Hall, London (1991).

4. Hertzman, C. *Environment and Health in Central and Eastern Europe.* World Bank, Washington D.C. (1995).

5. Hertzman, C. and Wiens, M. Child development and long-term outcomes: a population health perspective and summary of successful interventions. *Social Sciences and Medicine* 43, 1083–95 (1996).

6. Sapolsky, R. M. *Stress, the aging brain, and the mechanisms of neuron death.* The MIT Press, Cambridge (1992).

7. Kaplan, G. A., Pamuk, E. R., Lynch, J. W., Cohen, R. D., and Balfour, J. L. Inequality in income and mortality in the United States: analysis of mortality and potential pathways. *British Medical Journal* 312, 999–1003 (1996).

8. Wilkinson, R. G. Income distribution and life expectancy. *British Medical Journal* 304, 165–8 (1992).

9. Vagero, D. and Lundberg, O. Health Inequalities in Britain and Sweden. *Lancet* ii, 35–6 (1989).

10. Meaney, M., Aitken, D., Bhatnager, S., van Berkel, C., and Sapolsky, R. Effect of neonatal handling on age-related impairments associated with the hippocampus. *Science* 239, 766 (1988).

11. Barker, D. and Osmond, C. Infant mortality, childhood nutrition, and ischaemic heart disease in England and Wales. *The Lancet* May 10, 1077–1081 (1986).

12. Barker D., Osmond C., Golding J., Kuh, D. and Wadsworth, M. Growth in utero, blood pressure in childhood and adult life, and mortality from cardiovascular disease. *British Medical Journal* 298, 564–567 (1989).

13. Barker, D., Osmond, C., Winter P., Margetts, B. and Simmonds, S. Weight in infancy and death from ischaemic heart disease. *The Lancet* September 9, 577–580 (1989).

14. Barker, D., Bull, A., Osmond, C. and Simmonds, S. Fetal and placental size and risk of hypertension in adult life. *British Medical Journal* 301, 259–262 (1990).

15. Barker, D. The intrauterine environment and adult cardiovascular disease. In *The Childhood Environment and Adult Disease*, Ciba Foundation Symposium 156, 3–16, Wiley, Chichester, (1991).

16. Barker, D. and Martyn, C. The maternal and fetal origins of cardiovascular disease. *Journal of Epidemiology and Community Health* 46, 8–11 (1992).

17. Barker, D., Godfrey, K., Osmond, C. and Bull, A. The relation of fetal length, ponderal index and head circumference to blood pressure and the risk of hypertension in adult life. *Pediatric and Perinatal Epidemiology* 6, 35–44 (1992).

18. Barker, D., Meade, T., Fall, C., Lee, A., Osmond, C., Phipps, K. and Stirling, Y. Relation of fetal and infant growth to plasma fibrinogen and factor VII concentrations in adult life. *British Medical Journal* 304, 148–152 (1992).

19. Barker, D., Osmond, C., Simmonds, S. and Wield, G. The relation of small head circumference and thinness at birth to death from cardiovascular disease in adult life. *British Medical Journal* 306, 422–426 (1993).

20. Schweinhart, L. J., Barnes, H. V. and Weikart, D. P. Significant benefits: the High/Scope Perry preschool study through age 27. *Monographs of the High/Scope Educational Research Foundation* 10 (1993).

21. Palmer, F. H. Long-term gains from early intervention: findings from longitudinal studies. In *Project Head Start: A Legacy of the war on poverty* (Zigler, E. and Valentine, J. eds), The Free Press, New York (1979).

22. Case, R. and Griffin, S. Rightstart: An early intervention program for insuring that children's first formal learning of arithmetic is grounded in their intuitive knowledge of numbers. *Report to the James S. McDonnell Foundation* (1991).

23. Pulkkinen, L. and Tremblay, R. E. Patterns of boys' social adjustment in two cultures and at different ages: a longitudinal perspective. *International Journal of Behavioural Development* 15, 527–553 (1992).

24. Haan, M., Kaplan, G. A. and Camacho, T. Poverty and health: prospective evidence from the Alameda County Study. *American Journal of Epidemiology* 125, 989–997 (1987).

25. Karasek, R. and Theorell, T. *Healthy work: stress, productivity, and the reconstruction of working life.* Basic Books, New York (1990).

26. Marmot, M. Explaining Socioeconomic differences in sickness absence: The Whitehall II Study. *Canadian Institute for Advanced Research*. Toronto (1993).

27. Marmot, M., Smith, G., Stansfeld, S., Patel, C., North, F., Head, J., White, L., Brunner, E. and Feeney, A. Health inequalities among British Civil Servants: the Whitehall II Study. *The Lancet* 337, 1387–1393 (1991).

28. Marmot, M., Kogevinas, M. and Elston, M. Social/economic status and disease. *Annual Review of Public Health* 8, 111–135 (1987).

29. Wolfson, M., Rowe, G., Gentleman, J. and Tomiak, M. Career earnings and death: A longitudinal analysis of older Canadian men. *Canadian Institute for Advanced Research, Population Health Working Paper, 12*, Toronto (1991).

30. Winkleby, M. A. Socioeconomic status and health: how education, income, and occupation contribute to risk factors for cardiovascular disease. *American Journal of Public Health* 82, 816–820 (1992).

31. Human Resources Development Canada. Growing up in Canada: National Longitudinal Survey of Children and Youth. *HRDC*, Ottawa, 1996.

32. Power, C., Hertzman, C., Matthews, S., Manor, O. Social differences in health: life-cycle effects between ages 23 and 33 in the 1958 British birth cohort. *American Journal of Public Health* 87, 1499–1503 (1997).

33. Power, C. and Hertzman, C. Social and biological pathways linking early life and adult disease. *British Medical Bulletin* 53, 210–221 (1997).

34. Hertzman, C., Power, C., Matthews, S. and Manor, O. Using an interactive framework of society and lifecourse to explain self-rated health in early adulthood, upcoming.

35. Working Group on the National Strategy on Healthy Child Development. Building a national strategy for healthy child development. *Federal/Provincial/Territorial Advisory Committee on Population Health*, Minister of Public Works and Government Services Canada, Ottawa, 1998.

Part Three

ADULT HEALTH AND FACTORS
THAT INFLUENCE IT

Nine

THE SOCIAL CONTEXT OF SMOKING, NUTRITION, AND SEDENTARY HEALTH BEHAVIOR IN KANSAS

Manuella Adrian and Anna Wilkinson

WE studied the prevalence, in Kansas at the individual county level, of three health behaviors known to be risk factors for cardiovascular disease, i.e. sedentary lifestyle (excluding employment-related physical work), tobacco smoking, and one measure of diet, the consumption of fruits and vegetables. We related the prevalence of these health behaviors to individual level variables (such as age, race, marital status, educational level, employment status, family income, and health insurance coverage) and to community contextual features (average education, average household income, unemployment rate, and population density for each county). Although these measures of community are crude and certainly do not comprise a full assessment of the context within which life is organized in the individual county, we found that, at least for smoking in men and fruit and vegetable consumption in both men and women, the community features studied did exert an independent effect on the adoption of health behaviors that have a detrimental impact on health. These findings, among the first to formally assess community context and health, suggest that both individual person level characteristics as well as community characteristics, acting independently and perhaps interactively, exert important influences on the adoption of health behaviors important to health outcomes. These findings have implications for the development of strategies to improve population health.

INTRODUCTION

HEALTH behaviors are those behaviors that have a positive or negative impact on health either in the short or long term. A health behavior can affect the health of the individual who behaves in a given manner or it can affect the health of others who, while themselves not behaving in that fashion, are nevertheless influenced by the behavior of another person. The person who drinks and drives may risk having a drunk driving accident and also exposes other drivers on the road to the risk of being in a car crash with a drunk driver. The person who smokes may experience coughing in the short-term and possibly lung cancer after many years of smoking. The non-smoker who breathes the smoker's secondhand smoke may also cough and can also face the long-term risks of cancer. Health behaviors can have effects not only on the individual person who exhibits that behavior but also on the population at large and, thus, may be said to affect population health.

Personal behaviors are determined by a variety of factors including biological, psychological, and societal factors—factors that interact with one another to both shape and constrain human behavior.

BIOLOGICAL FACTORS

Biology provides us with a human body and the physiological mechanisms that allow behavior to occur. Biological characteristics of the organism set general limits on the kinds of behaviors that can manifest. No matter how much a young child may want to fly by leaping off a rooftop, it is not possible given the laws of physics and the shape of the human body with its lack of wings and weight-to-size ratio. Heredity and genetic endowment can predispose certain persons toward certain types of behaviors and make persons more or less susceptible to develop certain (ill-) health conditions[1,2] while some have hypothesized a genetic predisposition to certain behaviors.[3]

PSYCHOLOGICAL FACTORS

Psychological factors are important in determining human behavior; they provide the desire and the impetus to action as well as setting limits to action by what we can conceive of doing or how we feel about it. A number of theories and mechanisms have been proposed to account for the link between behavior and individual psychological characteristics. In classical *behavioral conditioning* positive (or negative) feedback is considered to encourage (or discourage) the acquisition and maintenance of specific behaviors. Freud, Adler, and Piaget's theories emphasize that the occurrence of certain types of behaviors is linked to *developmental stages*, which people pass through in a typically pre-determined order as they grow older. Other models emphasize that *personality types* can account for the lesser or greater occurrence of certain types of behaviors. Thus, so-called type "A" personalities have been

described as driven and impatient, and more prone to heart disorders,[4,5] whereas risk aversive persons are generally less likely to become professional rodeo bull-riders or race car drivers. Cognitive psychology emphasizes the importance of *social learning* as well as the individual's interpretation and response to the social situation, in determining behaviors. For example, a person's behavior is considered to reflect modeled behaviors to which they have been exposed and that they are capable of reproducing if they perceive or believe the behavior will lead to beneficial consequences.[6] The psychological characteristics of the individual are important in determining human behavior in relation to the social environment. Many psychological theories recognize a mutual interdependence between individual psychological factors and the social environment. For example, the type of conditioning cues, personality development, the range of modeled behavior, the meaning assigned to selected events or behaviors, and the very behaviors available to the person are themselves socially determined.[6,7] Personal temperament, interests, and drives are socially mediated: the social environment acts as a factor leading to their existence and as a means, a forum, and a context in which they may be expressed.

SOCIETAL FACTORS

The effect of the social environment is particularly important. The social environment includes both the immediate micro-level social context environment, as well as the larger macro-level societal environment. The immediate social environment can include family, friends, school, and work settings. Their impact on health behaviors can be easily demonstrated as when early childhood family experiences influence life-long food preferences,[8] or peer groups influence adolescents' sexual behavior.[9,10]

The pervasive effect of the larger social environment operates through the individual's socioeconomic and demographic characteristics as well as the socioeconomic and demographic characteristics of the community in which the person lives. Most studies that recognize the importance of societal influences on health and health behaviors tend to focus on the effect of the social characteristics of the individual. This approach is frequently used to segment populations in terms of identifying the characteristics of those persons who have a specific health condition or health behavior. Data that identify the very young, and especially young males, as well as the very old as being more likely to be involved in certain types of automobile crashes result in special driving education classes directed to these groups through school-based driver education for teens or "Fifty-Five Alive" driving refresher courses for older drivers. This approach is particularly important in identifying potential at-risk groups in order that special attention can be directed to them, including early detection in at-risk groups, targeted community-based health education programs, and other narrowly focused prevention or remediation activities and interventions.[11] When particular high-risk groups have been identified, programs can be directed to afford them the opportunity to alter their behavior and improve their health status. Programs directed at high-risk groups need to meet the special needs of at-risk communities, whether this be increasing educational levels, or providing culturally appropriate prenatal care.

However, the larger social environment also operates through the socioeconomic and demographic characteristics of the community in which the person lives. The life experiences of persons within a societal context depend not only on their individual or personal characteristics, but also on the social characteristics of the communities in which they live. The community's socioeconomic and demographic environment determines the opportunities available to a person. Community characteristics, such as the average per capita income or the rate of unemployment within a county—characteristics which themselves may reflect availability of high paying jobs on the one hand or plant closings and seasonal employment patterns on the other

hand—will affect the opportunities available to people in a community, their behavioral choices within their community opportunity structure, and their health. For example, during economic boom times, when the unemployment in a community is low, poorly trained people, members of minority groups, married women, and handicapped persons will all be drawn into the labor force to fill job vacancies. Community socioeconomic conditions determine the individual's socioeconomic position. A key element is the "role of the social environment in conditioning the behaviors and 'choices' of individuals and in doing so, shifting the focus of health determinants from the individual to groups and their socioeconomic and sociocultural contexts."[12, p.11]

Our understanding of the mechanisms that make specific societal groups more (or less) vulnerable to deleterious health behaviors is developing. Macro-level social forces such as the national (or international) business cycle[13] or political conditions such as war result in greater or lesser scarcity for the population due to changes in the level of employment, the wage rate, consumption patterns, and the standard of living. Improved economic conditions and economic well-being are postulated to have an impact on improving psychophysiological functioning due to perceptions of increased self-worth as a result of improved access to job and income security as well as higher consumption of "socially valued goods, services, and symbols that signify comfort, pleasure, intellectual stimulation, and participation in cultural life."[13, p.215] Such conditions allow the person to feel a "sense of mastery" over potential life problems and invulnerable to stress or threat. Conversely, poor economic circumstances generate feelings of social and economic deprivation, chronic stress, frustration and tension, and negative self-esteem.

To reduce the level of stress in their lives, people can use a variety of behaviors that are available to them and which they believe will help them cope. Some of these behaviors, such as smoking or drinking, may be deleterious to their health, whereas others, such as moderate exercise, are considered to be beneficial. Persons who, through societally-mediated circumstances, experience low levels of self-determination and autonomy in their lives due to occupational or economic circumstances, or who live in communities where poor socioeconomic conditions are stress inducing, are expected to exhibit more stress relieving behavior than are persons living in less stressful environments or persons who have a higher degree of control over their lives. Persons who are in high stress situations due to their individual- or community-level socioeconomic and demographic characteristics and who choose stress relieving behaviors that are detrimental to health, are at high risk for deleterious health behaviors and their health consequences. It is precisely this relationship that we propose to investigate in Kansas in the current study.

This is not to imply, however, that impersonal social forces act on persons as passive objects. People are active agents exerting varying degrees of control over their own life. A person's reflexive action in response to life events affects not only their own life but also that of others within their social networks. Because of the link between behavior and health, changes in behaviors can lead to changes in the health status of a person, as well as resulting in changes in the average level of health of a whole community. Because health behaviors are linked to socioeconomic and demographic factors, changes in socioeconomic circumstances influence people's health behaviors and can lead to improvements in both the individual's health and their community's health. The result is to reduce the effect of social disparities and improve opportunities for health for all.

RESEARCH QUESTION

THE leading causes of disease and death in Kansas are related to health behaviors such as smoking, nutrition, and physical activity. The leading causes of death in Kansas were diseases of the circulatory system, which accounted for 45%

of all deaths,[14] with heart disease, stroke, and atherosclerosis alone accounting for 40.4% of all deaths;[15, Table IV.8] in addition, neoplasms account for another 23% of all deaths.[14, 15, Table IV.8] Diseases of the circulatory system accounted for 6.4% of all hospital discharges, including heart failure and shock, percutaneous cardiovascular procedures, cerebrovascular disease (except transient ischemic attack), and angina pectoris,[15, Table VI.2] while 24.6% of adults in Kansas aged 18 years and over reported they had hypertension,[15, Table IV.6] and 5% reported diabetes.[15, Table IV.7]

In this study, we examine the impact of socioeconomic and demographic factors on health behaviors in Kansas. First, we describe the socioeconomic and demographic profiles of Kansans involved in selected health behaviors—smoking, nutrition, and exercise, which have been linked to heart disease. The results of these bivariate analyses were used to inform the development of the multivariate models that account for health behaviors in Kansas. Then we examined the effect of individual socioeconomic and demographic characteristics of Kansans in determining these health behaviors. Finally, we examined the concurrent effect of community socioeconomic and demographic characteristics in addition to individual socioeconomic and demographic characteristics in determining these health behaviors. This comparison of results obtained with individual socioeconomic and demographic characteristics, and with both individual and community socioeconomic and demographic characteristics allowed us to determine the effect of community conditions on health behaviors.

RESEARCH METHODS

Data Sources

We used individual data on health behaviors in Kansas, collected through the Kansas Behavioral Risk Factor Surveillance System (BRFSS) survey. This omnibus survey conducted by the Kansas Department of Health and Environment

(KDHE) is based on an instrument developed by the Centers for Disease Control and Prevention (CDC) used to monitor health in Kansas as part of the Healthy People 2000 program.[16] The BRFSS data were not gathered specifically to study the effects of community environment and socioeconomic factors on health. Results from analyses using such general-purpose data tend to be robust, so that our findings represent relationships that are likely to be valid and generalizable to the total population. The effect of community variables was measured through the inclusion of community data prepared by KDHE.

We analyzed data collected over the four-year period 1992–95, yielding a sample size of n = 6,122. A number of the participants chose not to respond to some of the questions on the BRFSS. In terms of the demographic and socioeconomic items, completeness in the data ranged from 100% with gender, to 89% reporting their household income. The sample used for the bivariate analysis included approximately six thousand (n = 6,000) respondents depending on the specific health behavior. In the multivariate analysis, the deletion of records with missing demographic and socioeconomic information resulted in a sample size of n = 5,497. A subsequent 227 observations were deleted due to missing information on the dependent variables, resulting in a sample size of n = 5,270 used in the current multivariate analysis. The Kolmogrov-Smirnov statistic[17] showed that the deletion of these cases did not systematically change the data set in terms of the frequency distribution of each of the socioeconomic and demographic variables.

Each year, survey data were collected throughout the year using a simple random dialing sampling method to ensure that all noninstitutionalized persons aged 18 or older, living in a household with a telephone, have an equal likelihood of being asked to participate in the survey. According to the U.S. Bureau of the Census, 4% of households in Kansas do not have a telephone. Therefore, the data may underrepresent certain risk factors associated with low socioeconomic status, assuming that telephone ownership is associated with income and other socioeconomic factors. Data used in this report are based on unweighted data; prevalence estimates in the current report do not differ materially from those presented by KDHE and CDC, whose estimates are based on data using a CDC-designed weighting procedure that accounts for the number of telephone numbers in a household and the over- or underrepresentation of certain subgroups in the sample.

For the multivariate analysis, we created an augmented data set by appending three additional measures from the Kansas Primary Care data, compiled by the Bureau of Local and Rural Health Systems at KDHE, to the record of every individual in the BRFSS data set. The three variables, measured at the county level, represent the percent of people with a four-year college degree in the county, the percent unemployed in the county, as well as the median household income for the county.

Bivariate Analysis: Descriptive Profiles
Initial results were published in *Health and Social Factors in Kansas: A Data and Chartbook, 1997-98.*[15] We describe health behaviors in Kansas by age, sex, marital status, race/ethnicity, educational attainment, employment status, income level$_1$, and population density: frontier, rural, densely-settled rural, semi-urban, and urban$_2$.

---

1. An unknown category was included for income, in all bivariate tabulations, due to a substantial percentage of respondents who chose not to report their annual household income.

2. Frontier (less than 6 persons per square mile), rural (between 6 and 20 persons per square mile), densely-settled rural (between 20 and 50 persons per square mile), semi-urban (between 50 and 150 persons per square mile), and urban (greater than or equal to 150 persons per square mile). (Definitions are based on a 1997 memorandum entitled Definition of Rural and Urban, from Richard Morrissey, Office of Local and Rural Health Systems, KDHE.)

The results from the bivariate analysis were used to inform the multivariate analysis.

Multivariate Analysis

Our objective was then to determine if we could find a significant effect for the community socioeconomic and demographic characteristics in addition to, or in interaction with, the individual socioeconomic and demographic characteristics, which are usually included in these kinds of studies. Because of the strong effect of gender on socially mediated health behaviors,[18] models were developed separately for men and women as well as for the total population.

THE DEPENDENT VARIABLES

We examined the relationship between three health behaviors, smoking, nutrition, and sedentariness, which have been linked to heart disease, and the socioeconomic and demographic factors using multiple logistic regression techniques. Health behaviors were taken as the dependent variables, and were measured as dichotomous variables consisting of 1) smoking or not smoking, 2) eating the recommended five or more fruits or vegetables a day or not, and 3) living a sedentary lifestyle or not.

THE EXPLANATORY VARIABLES

In addition to the explanatory variables used in the descriptive profiles, we also included health insurance status, since persons may be more prone to undertake high-risk activities if they have health insurance to cover the cost of treatment of any subsequent ill-health conditions that may develop as a result of risky behavior.

We used nominal (qualitative), or ordinal (quantitative) variables. Age was measured as the actual years of age. Household income and educational attainment were ranked from one to five (1 = lowest level and 5 = highest).

Dummy variables were measured relative to the "best" health behavior group or the charac-

teristic of the majority of the cases. The category with the "best" health behavior was based on the results of the descriptive profiles. Women are more likely to consume the recommended five or more fruit or vegetables a day than men, so women served as the "best" behavior gender comparison group. Because the majority of participants are non-Hispanic white (roughly 92%), non-Hispanic whites served as the reference for the race/ethnicity variables. Dummy variables allow us to compare how a specific category of a variable (for example the effect of a 4-year college diploma relative to that of having a high school diploma or any other educational level) differs from the other categories with respect to the dependent variable.

Following a methodology outlined by Birch, Stoddart, and Beland (1997)[12] for modeling aspects of "community" as a determinant of health in conjunction with individual level data, we used the community level variables as well as the interaction of the community variable with each corresponding individual level variable. With regards to education, for example, the following variables were included in the model: a) the individual's educational attainment; b) the percent of people with a four-year college degree in each county; and c) the interaction between the individual's educational attainment and the percentage of people with a four-year college degree in the individual's county.

The appropriateness of each model's ability to account for smoking, sedentariness, and nutritional behavior was based on regression results using the Hosmer and Lemeshow goodness-of-fit statistic at the 0.05 probability level.[19] We also considered the extent to which our model explained the observations (R^2) and the relative importance of each factor, holding all other factors constant (odds ratio). Although the results we report here show only the best-fit model for each behavior and gender, the results of the other models, which generally showed the same trends for the explanatory variables, helped clarify our understanding of the health behaviors of Kansans.

PROFILES OF KANSANS AT-RISK: RESULTS FROM THE BIVARIATE ANALYSES

Description of Health Behaviors in Kansas

USE OF TOBACCO

The rate of current smokers, people who smoke daily, among adults in Kansas is comparable to the national rate (22%). On a per capita basis Kansans smoke an estimated 88.4 packs of cigarettes annually (compared to 80.5 packages nationally). Kansan men (24.6%) are more likely to smoke than women (21%). Only 10.4% of Kansans aged 65 and older are current smokers. Older Kansans are more likely than younger persons to have ever smoked: between 45.5% and 58.1% of Kansans aged 45 and older have ever smoked whereas for those aged 18–24 years, only 31.3% said they had ever smoked. The percentage of smokers decreases as household income increases: 29.6% of those with income below $10,000 are current smokers, in contrast to the 15.7% of adults living in households with income greater than $50,000. Similarly, the percentage of smokers decreases as the level of education increases: among those with grade 9–11 education 33% are current smokers compared to 12.6% current smokers among those with a 4-year college education or more. Current smoking is lowest in rural counties (18.7% compared to 23.3 and 23.6% in urban and mixed urban-rural counties respectively).[15, Table V.2]

SEDENTARY LIFE STYLE

In comparison to the national average, more Kansans report that they have no leisure time physical activity (34.4% of Kansans compared to 28.8% nationally).[15, Table V.1] Of adult Kansans, 57.6% lead sedentary lives, that is, other than their typical work-related activities, they engage in no recreational physical activity or they exercise less than three times a week for less than twenty minutes each time. Men and women are almost equally sedentary (57.2% for men and 57.9% for women). The proportion of the population leading sedentary lives increases with increasing age: 47.7% of people aged 18–24 lead a sedentary lifestyle compared to 64.6% among those aged 65 and older. The proportion who are sedentary decreases with increasing education: 75.9% of those with less than grade 9 education are sedentary whereas this figure drops down to 45.9% among those with a college education or more. People with less than grade 9 education are 3.4 times more likely to be sedentary when compared to those with the highest educational level, even after taking into account the effect of the different age composition of the two groups. The rate of the population that is sedentary decreases with increasing income: 63.8% of people whose household income is less than $10,000 are sedentary, whereas only 40.1% of those with household income of $50,000 and over are sedentary. People who are unable to work have the highest rate of sedentariness (71%), followed by retirees (64.5%), and the self-employed (63.7%). Men are more likely to be sedentary if they live in rural counties (62.7%) or in mixed urban-rural counties (59.9%) than in urban counties (53%). There is no significant difference in the rates of sedentariness among women regardless of their place of residence.[15, Table V.7]

NUTRITION

Adult Kansans consume an average 3.8 fruits and vegetables daily. Only 25.6% consume the recommended quantity of five or more a day. Women (28.5%) are more likely to consume the recommended amount than men (21.9%). Consumption increases with increasing age, with less than 20% of those aged 18 to 24 consuming the recommended amount of 5 or more fruit and vegetables daily, with this rate rising with increasing age until it reaches 38.4% in those aged 65 and older. More of the retired (38.4%) consume the recommended amount of fruits and vegetables, while those who are unemployed are the least likely to do so (15.3%).[15, Table V.4]

Multivariate Analysis

A descriptive profile of the characteristics of persons who exhibit specific behaviors allows us to identify the population at-risk for these behaviors and it also allows us to predict in broad terms the likelihood of a person with those characteristics exhibiting that behavior. Given information on a Kansan's gender, age, educational attainment, income, and place of residence, we can determine his or her risk for selected health behaviors. This information can be used when identifying at-risk groups and tailoring subsequent health interventions to fit the specific group's needs.

However, people have more than one characteristic. For example, each of us is a person of a certain age and gender, and each of these characteristics contributes to the extent to which we will exhibit certain behaviors. The question arises as to how much each of these characteristics contributes to a behavior. The importance of this can be illustrated in the case of young women, whose gender makes them more likely to be sedentary, but whose age makes them less likely to be sedentary.

Similarly, communities can have multiple characteristics. Urban communities with a higher population density are more likely to have both high unemployment and high per capita income, more people with a 4-year college degree or a high school diploma, and more households without a vehicle, and more public transportation. The combination of these characteristics is, to a greater or lesser extent, typical of the greater heterogeneity found in more geographically compact urban spaces.

The question arises as to which of these opposing tendencies will determine whether young women will be more, or less, likely to be sedentary, or whether it is community levels of income

or population density that account best for the observed variations in health behaviors. Such questions can be answered through the use of multivariate techniques, such as multiple regression, which we discuss in the following section.

RESULTS FROM THE REGRESSION ANALYSIS

WE used multiple regression techniques to investigate the concurrent effect of multiple factors that can influence smoking, nutrition, and sedentary lifestyle in order to determine the relative importance of each factor. We found that regardless of the behavior examined, the addition of community socioeconomic and demographic characteristics into the model improved the explanatory power of our model, due primarily to the inclusion of additional explanatory variables, as did the inclusion of dummy variables.

Sedentary Lifestyle

Men and women are about equally likely to be sedentary, unlike smoking and nutrition, for which men are more likely to exhibit negative behavior. For both men and women, regardless of the type of variable chosen, the models that included individual socioeconomic and demographic variables alone consistently offered a superior fit to those incorporating community variables.

Sedentary lifestyle is intended to capture people who, outside of their regular work activities, do no leisure time recreational physical activity or exercise less than three times a week for less than twenty minutes each time.[22] Compared to married men, both single and divorced/separated men are less likely to lead a sedentary lifestyle, as are men who have health care coverage when compared to men who are uninsured. Men aged 45–54 are also more likely to be sedentary when compared to young men aged 18–24. Men with less than a college education, when compared to men with a four-year college degree, are more likely to lead a sedentary lifestyle. Men whose annual household income is $20,000–$34,999, when compared to men whose annual household income is greater than $50,000, as well as men who are self-employed when compared to men who work for wages, are more likely to lead a sedentary lifestyle.

In the case of women, the likelihood of not leading a sedentary lifestyle increases as both income and years of education increase. In addition, single women, when compared to married women, are less likely to lead a sedentary lifestyle. Black women are more likely to be sedentary than white women, as are women who are self-employed when compared to those who work for wages.

Smoking

In the case of smoking, we obtained better fitting models, as measured by the Hosmer and Lemeshow[19] goodness-of-fit statistic, with the inclusion of community socioeconomic and demographic characteristics in all cases but one. Specifically, in the case of women, the model based on individual socioeconomic and demographic characteristics alone using all dummy measures provided the best fit. The model for both sexes combined, based solely on the individual level data (entered as dummies) was misspecified (goodness-of-fit statistic=16.5, df=8. P<0.02).

For men, the best fitting model included community as well as individual variables (See Table 1). Having health care insurance, being self-employed or retired increased the likelihood of being a male non-smoker, as did residing in a less populated area (although this latter did not achieve statistical significance). On the other hand, being younger, single, divorced/separated, or widowed, or having less than a high-school education increased the likelihood of smoking among men.

In the best model for women a similar pattern emerged. Women with health insurance were 71

percent more likely to be non-smokers compared to women who lacked health care coverage. Similar to men, younger women, divorced/separated women, and women who are self-employed or who are unable to work, were more likely to be smokers than women over the age of 65, married women, and women who work for wages, respectively. In contrast to the situation for men, all women with less than a four-year college degree were more likely to smoke than women with 16 or more years of education, as were women whose household income fell between $35,000 and $49,999 when compared to women in the highest household income category.

Nutrition: Consumption of Fruit and Vegetables

For men, the better fitting model incorporated community socioeconomic and demographic characteristics. For women, the goodness-of-fit statistic[19] appears to be dependent on the type of variable used in each model: thus, with dummy variables the model incorporating individual socioeconomic and demographic characteristics appears to have a better fit, whereas with mixed ordinal and dummy variables, it is the model that incorporates community variables that works best. Overall, the likelihood of eating the recommended amount of 5 or more fruits and/or vegetables a day[21] increases with increasing age, income and education, and the likelihood is higher in those who are retired.

For men, the models based on both individual and community predictors (See Table 2) were superior to those using individual variables alone, based on the goodness-of-fit statistic.[19] Men who reside in rural counties are almost twice as likely to eat the recommended number of fruits and vegetables (odds ratio=1.92, 95% C.I.=1.14–3.27) than their urban counterparts. Black men were found to be more than twice as likely to consume the recommended amount of fruit and vegetables (odds ratio=2.22, 95% C.I.=1.34–3.70) when compared to white men. As the median

Table 1

Smoking in Men: Multivariate Logistic Regressions Showing Adjusted Differences Associated with Smoking Among Adult Male Kansans, According to Individual and Community Level Covariates

Variable	Odds Ratio	95% Confidence Interval	
		Lower	Upper
Age (years)			
18–24	0.345*	0.167	0.714
25–34	0.353*	0.183	0.684
35–44	0.209*	0.110	0.399
45–54	0.206*	0.108	0.394
55–64	0.360*	0.196	0.663
65 + #			
Race/ethnicity			
Non-Hispanic Black	1.147	0.669	1.967
Hispanic	1.348	0.760	2.392
Asian/Pacific Islander	1.781	0.477	6.654
American Indian	1.431	0.423	4.843
Non-Hispanic White #			
Marital status			
Never married	0.656*	0.484	0.888
Unmarried couple	0.609	0.306	1.210
Divorced/separated	0.496*	0.367	0.669
Widowed	0.378*	0.201	0.712
Married #			
Educational attainment (years)			
< 9	0.550	0.181	1.673
9–11	0.433*	0.189	0.991
12	0.569	0.322	1.005
13–15	0.696	0.470	1.032
16 + #			
Employment status			
Self-employed	1.534	1.000	2.353
Unemployed	0.883	0.388	2.013
Homemaker/student	2.721	0.969	7.641
Retired	1.937	0.565	6.632
Unable to work	2.825	0.503	15.860
Employed for wages #			

Table 1 *(continued)*

Smoking in Men: Multivariate Logistic Regressions Showing Adjusted Differences Associated with Smoking Among Adult Male Kansans, According to Individual and Community Level Covariates

Variable	Odds Ratio	95% Confidence Interval	
		Lower	Upper
Household income ($)			
< 10,000	0.871	0.210	3.614
10,000–19,999	1.031	0.300	3.542
20,000–34,999	0.861	0.370	2.002
35,000–49,999	1.076	0.697	1.662
50,000 + #			
Health care coverage			
Yes #			
No	1.520*	1.147	2.016
Population density (persons/sq.mi)			
Frontier	1.657	0.763	3.598
Densely-settled rural	1.398	0.824	2.371
Rural	1.134	0.806	1.597
Semi-urban	1.222	0.837	1.783
Urban #			
County level			
% unemployed	0.933	0.806	1.081
% w/ college degree	0.972	0.925	1.021
Median Household Income	0.990	0.942	1.041
Interaction work	1.000	0.999	1.001
Interaction education	1.009	0.997	1.020
Interaction income	0.979	0.931	1.029

Notes: * Indicates that the odds ratio is statistically significantly different from 1 ($p < 0.05$). For example, men who are under 65 years old are all more likely to smoke than men 65 years old or older. Men who do not have health insurance are more likely to smoke than men who have health insurance.

# Denotes the reference category.

household income in a county increased so did the likelihood of men eating the recommended number of fruits and vegetables (odds ratio=1.05, 95% C.I.=1.004–1.11). However, younger men, when compared to those who are 65 and older, were less likely to eat the recommended five or more fruits and vegetables daily. Divorced/separated men when compared to married men, as well as men whose annual household income is less than $35,000 when compared to men whose annual household income is $50,000 or more, were less likely to eat the recommended five or more fruits and vegetables daily.

Women who are homemakers, students, or retired are more likely to eat the recommended 5 or more fruits and vegetables a day than women who work for wages. Women who are under age 35 when compared to women who are 65 or older, and divorced/separated women when compared to married women, were less likely to eat the

Table 2

Nutrition in Men: Multivariate Logistic Regressions Showing Adjusted Differences Associated with Eating Five or More Fruits and Vegetables Daily Among Adult Male Kansans, According to Individual and Community Level Covariates

Variable	Odds Ratio	95% Confidence Interval	
		Lower	Upper
Age (years)			
18–24	0.308*	0.168	0.565
25–34	0.287*	0.173	0.477
35–44	0.336*	0.207	0.545
45–54	0.343*	0.208	0.565
55–65	0.369*	0.230	0.590
65 + #			
Race/ethnicity			
Non-Hispanic Black	2.221*	1.335	3.696
Hispanic	1.167	0.646	2.108
Asian/Pacific Islander	2.157	0.829	5.613
American Indian	0.729	0.197	2.693
Non-Hispanic White			
Marital status #			
Never married	1.129	0.823	1.550
Unmarried couple	1.129	0.516	2.471
Divorced/separated	0.697	0.482	1.007
Widowed	0.417*	0.223	0.777
Married #			
Educational attainment (years)			
<9	0.466	0.158	1.370
9–11	0.697	0.308	1.575
12	0.761	0.442	1.309
13–15	0.927	0.637	1.348
16 + #			
Employment status			
Self-employed	1.112	0.753	1.642
Unemployed	1.138	0.481	2.691
Homemaker/student	0.697	0.273	1.777
Retired	1.091	0.407	2.929
Unable to work	1.250	0.268	5.828
Employed for wages #			

Table 2 *(continued)*

Nutrition in Men: Multivariate Logistic Regressions Showing Adjusted Differences Associated with Eating Five or More Fruits and Vegetables Daily Among Adult Male Kansans, According to Individual and Community Level Covariates

Variable	Odds Ratio	95% Confidence Interval	
		Lower	Upper
Household income ($)			
<10,000	0.246*	0.064	0.942
10,000–19,999	0.254*	0.080	0.806
20,000–34,999	0.469	0.213	1.033
35,000–49,999	0.761	0.506	1.145
50,000 + =			
Health care coverage			
Yes #			
No	1.111	0.914	1.350
Population density (persons/sq.mi)			
Frontier	1.122	0.515	2.446
Densely-settled rural	1.925	1.142	3.247
Rural	1.292	0.900	1.854
Semi-urban	1.291	0.882	1.889
Urban #			
County level			
% unemployed	1.134	0.977	1.316
% w/ college degree	1.038	0.990	1.091
Median household income	1.053*	1.004	1.105
Interaction work	0.999	0.998	1.000
Interaction education	0.998	0.987	1.008
Interaction income	0.995	0.953	1.038

Note: * Indicates that the odds ratio is statistically significantly different from 1 ($p < 0.05$). For example younger men, when compared to those who are 65 and older, were less likely to eat the recommended five or more fruits and vegetables daily. Men who do not have health insurance are more likely to eat the recommended five or more fruits and vegetables daily than men who have health insurance.

# Denotes the reference category.

recommended 5 or more fruits and vegetables, as were women with less than a high school education compared to women with 16 or more years of education.

DISCUSSION

O UR models explain a relatively low proportion of the variances, typically between 4 and 16 percent, depending on the type of behavior and the model. This is not unexpected since we used cross-sectional data, which typically provide coefficients of determination (R^2) that are lower than those obtained from time series data. Further, changes in people's behavior occur over time whereas our data only provides information at one cross-sectional point in time. Even when the behavior is a direct response to social environmental changes, change in an individual's behavior, especially as regards long-ingrained habits, is rarely instantaneous, as some persons are faster and others slower adopters of new or changed behaviors. As the economy goes through cyclical changes and persons become unemployed and have less money to spend, they may be slow to diminish their consumption behavior, particularly when the good being consumed is addictive, as in the case of tobacco. Change in behavior may lag behind the time of occurrence of causative events. Our data would be insensitive to such lagged changes in behavior.

Our analysis attempted to determine the effect of community socioeconomic and demographic factors in addition to the effect of individual socioeconomic and demographic factors. Our community factors were measured at the level of the county. However, county-level data may not be the best measure of community influences. People may describe or think of their community in terms of the city or town they live in or, in a larger environment, in terms of their neighborhood, block, place of work, and so on. Therefore, the variables we used may not correspond to how individuals conceive of community and may not have captured the relative impor-

tance that community may have on an individual's behavior or indeed the relevant aspects of community that influence an individual's behavior.

The community variables we included were population density, income, education, and unemployment defined as persons per square mile, median household income, percent with a 4-year college degree, and percent unemployed respectively. One issue relates to the definitions we used. Whereas community education may indeed be of primordial importance in influencing a person's health behaviors, the aspect of it that we used in this study may not be the relevant aspect. Thus, in the case of education it may be that the percent of adults who have attained a high school diploma is more important than persons with a 4-year college degree for some behaviors. Another issue is that, whereas education is important, the specific aspect of education that is important may not be the one measured through formal years of education, but rather educational content matter (e.g., whether a high percentage of the population took a health class) or perhaps some administrative aspect of the educational system (e.g., availability of school-based extracurricular activities). Even when the relevant aspects of the variable are considered, it may be that the definition of the variable is not the most appropriate for that behavior. Thus, mean per capita income may be more appropriate than mean household income, which does not take into account the number of people within the household that must share the household income. Finally, it is possible that other community variables not considered here, such as prices and community sales tax rates on cigarettes that control availability, or the perception of appropriate social norms regarding the behavior, may be important community determinants of health behaviors. It would be useful if some future research could consider the effects of these additional factors.

That the models we developed were unequally satisfactory in statistical terms in explaining the behavior of the two genders is not surprising. Health behaviors involve the physical body in a very direct way. Biological differences as well as socially constructed gender roles contribute to differences in smoking,[18] nutrition and sedentariness.

In the case of smoking, community socioeconomic and demographic conditions are clearly important, especially for men. We believe that this may reflect the lengthy history of public control of tobacco. Smoking behavior has been subjected to public regulation for a very long time, first with the decades-old taxing of tobacco, the more recent regulation of public advertising for tobacco products (e.g., the ban of tobacco advertising on television), and more recently, the institution of smoke-free public spaces, and the stricter regulation of sales to minors. That community factors appear to influence women less than men may reflect the nature of anti-smoking programs that may be geared toward male smokers. Certainly trend data indicates that the rate of male smokers has decreased more than the rate of female smokers.[22]

In the case of nutrition, we found stronger community effects for men than for women, although we can only speculate as to their cause. One possibility may be that men eat out more than women because of employment outside the home. Food selection in ready-made meals bought outside the home may be influenced by availability of types of food on restaurant menus and communities with lower median income may have restaurants that offer a more limited variety of food items, with little or no fruit and vegetables available. Another element that may influence male food choices may be related to community food consumption norms for men, which in Kansas may correspond to the classic "meat and potatoes man." Such norms would lead restaurants to cater to the normative ideal of the "meat and potatoes man," as would possible perceived peer pressure from other male dining companions.

Women are more likely to eat at home where they have fuller control over the composition of meals. Women cook not only for themselves but also for their families, their children and spouses. In their concern to provide optimum conditions for their children, they are more likely to give attention to preparing nutritionally balanced meals for their children. Time pressures may induce women to eat the same food as their children. As women eat the same food they prepare for their children, they may be more likely to eat the recommended amount of fruits and vegetables, especially if they are concerned with modeling nutritious eating patterns for their children so that the children develop nutritious eating habits for a lifetime. Such food preparation and eating habits in women may persist even after the children are grown and may continue particularly in the later retirement years, which provide more time for time-consuming homebound activities such as food preparation or growing a home garden. These may also account for the greater likelihood of eating the recommended amount of fruit and vegetables among those who are unable to work. Furthermore, women may be concerned with personal issues surrounding their weight and body size and may be attempting to control their weight through diet.

Finally, there may also be biological and physiological differences in nutritional needs of men and women.

One difficulty in giving a full interpretation of patterns of nutrition in Kansans is that we only had data on fruits and vegetables, which form only a relatively small amount of the Kansan diet, and account for only a small proportion of eating behavior. Fruit and vegetables are typically eaten as part of meals and the effect of community socioeconomic and demographic variables may have influences first on the total food consumption and only indirectly and secondarily on the consumption of fruits and vegetables. At some future date we would like to examine the consumption of other food groups by Kansans.

We found little evidence of the effect of community socioeconomic and demographic factors on sedentary lifestyle. Because we had information on leisure time activity alone, the variable sedentary lifestyle did not fully measure the total amount of physical exertion that people have in their life. In particular, it did not include the effect of physical activity in the work setting. Thus, persons who are called upon to exert themselves physically on the job, as in lifting, carrying, climbing, walking or other activities common in certain industries such as construction, farm work, or warehouse and parcel delivery, where physical exertion is a normal expected part of the job duties, may not have the interest and energy to do physical exercise on their own time and may consider "resting" to be the appropriate leisure time behavior. Further research on this issue would need to consider not only the effect of work status but also of type of industry and industrial occupation, as they influence physical activity at work.

One drawback in this study is the lack of information on individual psychological variables, such as personal affect and mood, the perception of group norms, and perceived self-efficacy, as well as individual personality characteristics such as interests, attitudes, and opinions that may influence health behaviors. Future research would need to incorporate such factors to increase our knowledge of the mechanisms, both social and individual operating together, which account for health behaviors in the population.

In this paper we examined the effect of individual and community socioeconomic and demographic factors on smoking, nutrition, and sedentary lifestyle, which are some of the leading health behaviors linked to cardiovascular disease—the leading cause of death in Kansas. We found that individual socioeconomic and demographic variables were important in determining health behaviors in Kansas, and for smoking and nutrition we found that community socioeconomic and demographic variables were also important conditioning variables for health behaviors in men. With the increasing interest in the social determinants of health (viz the March,

1998 issue of the *American Journal of Public Health*), it becomes increasingly important to consider not only the effect of individual socioeconomic and demographic factors but also factors that are pervasive throughout the entire community. Although researchers in this field recognize the importance of community-based events and societal macro forces in influencing health and health behaviors,[13] most studies restrict themselves to the use of aggregate data alone.[21,22] In view of the increasing interest in considering both individual and societal level determinants of health and health behaviors, this is one of the first studies to have done so formally. We feel that this represents an important first step in examining this aspect of the society and health model and that it can contribute to a fuller understanding of the determinants of health behaviors and health in Kansas.

This study is one of the first attempts to understand the influence of specific community characteristics on health behaviors, behaviors heretofore considered by many to be primarily a matter of individual choice. We constructed statistical models to help understand the influence of individual person factors (already known to influence health behaviors) and community-level characteristics on smoking rates, sedentary lifestyle, and fruit and vegetable consumption, known factors for cardiovascular disease. We discovered that indeed even with limited measures of community context (population density, and the average level of education, income, and unemployment in each county) these community features did have an independent influence on tobacco smoking in both men and women in Kansas counties, in addition to the effect of individual person level characteristics. These findings, among the first to formally assess community context and health, suggest that both individual person level characteristics as well as community characteristics, acting independently and perhaps interactively, exert important influences on the adoption of health behaviors important to health outcomes.

NOTES

1. Dubos, R. J. (1965). *Man Adapting*. New Haven, CT: Yale University Press.

2. Cloninger, C. R., Sigvardsson, S., and Bohman, M. (1996). Type I and Type II Alcoholism: An Update. *Alcohol Health and Research World*, 20(1):18–23.

3. Anthenelli, R. M. and Schuckit, M. A. (1997). *Genetics*. In Lowinson, J. H., Ruiz, P., Millman, R. B. and Langrod, J. G. (Eds.) *Substance Abuse: A Comprehensive Textbook* 3rd ed, (pp.41–51). Baltimore, MD: Williams and Wilkins.

4. Howard, J. H., Rechnitzer, P. A., Cunningham, D. A., Wong, D. and Brown, H. A. (1990). Type A Behavior, Personality and Sympathetic Response. *Behavioral Medicine*, 16(4):149–60.

5. Howard, J. H., Rechnitzer, P. A., Cunningham, D. A., Wong, D. and Brown, H. A. (1991). Personality Type A Behavior, and the Effects of Beta-blockade. *Journal of Cardiovascular Pharmacology*, 18(2):267–77.

6. Bandura, A. (1986). *Social Foundations of Thought and Action: A Social Cognitive Theory*. Englewood Cliffs, NJ: Prentice-Hall.

7. Bandura, A. and Walters, R. H. (1963). *Social Learning and Personality Development*. New York: Holt, Rinehart and Winston.

8. Adrian, M., Dini, C., MacGregor, L. and Studute, G. (1995). Substance Use as a Measure of Social Integration for Women of Different Ethno-cultural Groups into Mainstream Culture in a Pluralist Society—The Example Canada. *International Journal of Addictions*, 30(6):669–734.

9. Fisher, J. D. and Misovich, S. J. (1990). *Social Influence and AIDS-Prevention Behaviors*. In Edwards, J., Tindale, R. S., and Poseva, E. J. (Eds.), *Social Influence Processes and Prevention* (pp. 39–70). New York: Plenum.

10. Winslow, R. W., Franzini, L. R. and Hwang, J. (1992). Perceived Peer Norms, Casual Sex, and AIDS Risk. *Journal of Applied Social Psychology*, 22:1809–1827.

11. Patrick, D. L. and Wickizer, T. M. (1995). Community and Health. In Amick, B. C., Levine, S., Tarlov, A. R. and Walsh, D. C. (Eds.), *Society and Health* (pp.46–73) New York: Oxford University Press.

12. Birch, S., Stoddart, G., and Beland, F. (1997). *Modeling the Community as a Determinant of Health*. Hamilton, Canada: McMaster University Centre for Health Economics and Policy Analysis Working Paper # 97–9, November 1997.

13. Brenner, M. H. (1995). Political Economy and Health. In Amick, B. C., Levine, S., Tarlov, A. R. and Walsh, D. C. (Eds.) *Society and Health*, pp 211–245. New York: Oxford University Press.

14. NCHS (1994).

15. Singh, G. K., Wilkinson, A. V., Song, F. F., Rose, T. P., Adrian, M., Fonner, E., and Tarlov, A. (1998). *Health and Social Factors in Kansas: A Data and Chartbook 1997–98*. Topeka, KS: Kansas Health Institute.

16. Perry, M. (1999). Local Behavioral Risk Data. *Kansas Health*, 2 (3):2–3.

17. Sokal, R. R. and Rohlf, F. J. (1969). *Biometry: The Principles and Practices of Statistics in Biological Research*. San Francisco, CA: W.H. Freeman & Co.

18. Walsh, D. C., Sorensen, G. and Leonard, L. (1995). Gender Health and Cigarette Smoking. In Amick, B. C., Levine, S., Tarlov, A. R., Walsh, D. C. (Eds.) *Society and Health*, pp. 131-171. New York: Oxford University Press.

19. Hosmer, D. W. and Lemeshow, S. (1989). *Applied Logistic Regression*. New York: John Wiley and Sons, Inc.

20. The President's Council on Physical Fitness and Sport (1996). *Patterns and Trends in Physical Activity*. Physical Activity and Health: a Report of the Surgeon General. Ch.5. National Center for Chronic Disease Prevention and Health Promotion. U.S. Dept. Health and Human Services.

21. Anon. (1996). Five-A-Day Power Play! *Chronic Disease Notes and Reports*, 9(1):16.

22. Adrian, M., Jull, P. and Williams, R. (1989). *Statistics on Alcohol and Drug Use in Canada and Other Countries*. Toronto: Addiction Research Foundation.

Ten

LABOR MARKETS AND HEALTH:
A FRAMEWORK AND SET OF APPLICATIONS

Benjamin C. Amick III and John N. Lavis

INTRODUCTION

W HY should firms consider health when designing organizational structures or formulating new human resource practices? Why should governments consider health when developing labor-market policies? In the next century, employee health will be a key factor underpinning the human capital of business, and thus in productivity and competitiveness.

THE BOTTOM LINE
IN THINKING ABOUT HEALTH

I T goes without saying that firms bear many costs associated with worker illness and injury and corresponding disability (Baldwin et al. 1996; Greenberg et al. 1993; Galizzi and Boden 1996; Personick 1997). Functional limitations associated with illness and injury or their treatment can affect worker performance (Berndt et al. 1997) and absenteeism (Amick and Wu 1998), and thus the productivity of the work unit. Illness and injury can also translate into higher health-

care benefit-plan costs in jurisdictions where experience rating of premia is permitted (e.g., the United States). There are also costs associated with worker disability (i.e., short- and long-term disability, STD and LTD) and the management of disability (Akabas et al. 1992). Both experience-rated workers' compensation premia and the costs of managing workers' compensation programs are directly linked to the number of work-related illnesses and injuries that a firm reports (Boden 1996). Moreover, workers who go on long-term disability must be replaced, and the firm's investment in the worker (e.g., training) is lost.

Diminished national competitive capacity represents a cost borne by society. Work-related illnesses and injuries alone cost the U.S. economy approximately $155 billion in 1992 (plus an additional $16 billion in administrative costs) (Leigh et al. 1997). A 1% productivity loss due to illness has been estimated to cost the U.S. economy $27 billion in 1990 (Berndt et al. 1997). Social Security disability benefit expenditures for

Dr. Amick is supported by grants from the Rockefeller Foundation, National Institute for Aging and the National Institute for Occupational Safety and Health

We would like to thank Ms. Jie Zhang and Dr. William H. Rogers for statistical and programming assistance. Judith Jacobs, Fabienne Peter, Dana Weinberg, Margaret Whitehead, Allard Dembe, Finn Diderichsen and Michael Handel provided valuable comments on an earlier version of this chapter. Ann Goodsell provided editorial guidance and Constance Kelley provided administrative support in the preparation of this manuscript.

people of working age are currently estimated at over \$36 billion annually. If we add to these figures the unmeasured costs to the families of injured workers, it is clear that society bears a very large burden because of worker illness and injury and the accompanying worker disability, part of which can be attributed to organizational and human resource decisions or to labor-market policies.

Turning this argument on its head to focus on producing health, rather than avoiding illness, injury, or disability, provides a new lens through which to view business practices and government policies. This chapter presents a framework for thinking about how business practices (specifically organizational and human-resource decisions) and government policies can influence labor-market experiences and their health consequences. One goal of our work is to provide evidence of the links between labor-market experiences and health to inform business practices and government policy. A second goal is to refocus labor market and health research on practice- and policy-relevant issues.

TOWARD A NEW FRAMEWORK

THIS section presents a general model of how society produces health, as well as a specific model of how labor markets produce health. Although it builds on current social epidemiological perspectives on the links between work and health (c.f. Karasek and Theorell 1996; Siegrist 1996; Lundberg 1996), the proposed framework, which we call the *labor market and health framework*, departs from recent health research that has combined work environment research with either social class research (c.f. Johnson and Hall 1995; Hallqvist 1998) or with family research (Walsh et al. 1995). The framework recontextualizes work as one of many labor-market experiences in a person's working career, thereby integrating disparate research, particularly unemployment studies and work environment studies.

The labor-market and health framework has three advantages. (1) It integrates experiences related to the availability of work and experiences related to the nature of work into the same model, focusing research on cumulative labor-market experiences. (2) It focuses research on the cumulative health effects of labor-market experiences, and on the reciprocal effects of health and these experiences. Combined, (1) and (2) establish a working-life-course perspective. (3) It recognizes employers and governments as institutional entities whose practices and policies directly affect labor-market experiences, thus making practice and policy interventions suitable subjects for health research. A distinctive feature of the labor-market and health framework is that the labor-market/health relationship is represented as a complex set of processes at several levels of analysis (the individual's work, the firm, and society).

Society and Health: A New Perspective

Study after study has found that a health disparity exists between those at the top of the social hierarchy and those lower down, regardless of whether the social-position indicator is related to education, income or occupation (Amick et al. 1995; Blane et al. 1996; Evans et al. 1994). To explain the relationship between social hierarchy and health, researchers have sought to relate the distribution of psychosocial, behavioral, and biological factors to the social hierarchy (Marmot et al. 1995; Marmot et al. 1997). Figure 1 depicts these factors as the mechanisms that link social hierarchy to health. The implicit assumption in this research has been that its results could pinpoint medical and public health interventions to reduce health disparities. Such research has tended to focus thinking "downstream" on individual-level factors (*Lancet* 1994)—leading to interventions focused on individual change— as opposed to "upstream" on societal-level factors leading to interventions focused on social change (Benzeval et al. 1995). As James House first observed, focusing on individual-level factors is like building a dam on a tributary of a raging river: the river will find its way to the flatlands regardless.

Diderichsen (1998) has proposed a new model assigning primacy to the social context. Context comes from the Latin and means "to weave together." The social context weaves together the social conditions of a society including processes of social stratification, institutional legitimization of behaviors and behavioral norms, cultural identification, and definition of self in daily life (Short 1986). Social context thus has a direct effect on social hierarchy, as well as an indirect effect on the relationship between hierarchy and health. For example, labor-market conditions are one aspect of the social context. Conditions such as competitive markets define the types of work available, sorting people into certain types of jobs on the basis of gender, race, education, and other factors (Kalleberg et al. 1997; Reskin and McBrier 1998; Tomaskovic-Devey 1993). Diderichsen (1998) further singled out policy as an important but understudied element of the society-and-health relationship in need of more research attention when social change is the ultimate goal.

The model depicted in Figure 1 compares two societies schematically to call attention to the importance of social action in a given society's labor market. Social action, which encompasses both the policies and actions of government (e.g., the Occupational Safety and Health Act) and employer practices (e.g., flexible work arrangements), can affect labor-market experiences and in turn health. These features of the new society-and-health framework are highlighted by dashed lines in Figure 1.

The advantages of this society-and-health framework are threefold. First, it acknowledges the consistently observed relationship between social hierarchy and health, in effect changing the question from what that relationship is to how gradients develop and persist within a society. Second, a societal focus allows for examination of the historical processes that produce and perpetuate such gradients. Third, introducing the concept of social action identifies key social-change levers capable of changing the underlying hierarchy.

Labor Markets and Health:
Building a New Research Framework

Figure 1 illustrates the relationship among context, labor-market experiences and health as essentially linearly connected, whereas Figure 2 allows greater complexity in the inter-relationships of these three phenomena. Figure 1 follows a general society-and-health-framework, while Figure 2 focuses on labor markets and health. We intend the labor market and health framework to generate new research directions that will illustrate new solutions for improving a society's health through changes in labor-market experiences or the social context in which those experiences occur.

The three dimensions of the cube are labor-market experiences, social context, and the health and productivity outcomes that follow from the experiences. Using a cube encourages the examination of the interaction between these experiences and the context in which they occur. The model suggests that how a person engages with the labor market over his or her working life (e.g., whether a person can find and keep a job, what type of work a person does, and in what type of environment) contributes to health and well-being. The context for these experiences operates at the individual level as well as at the business and societal levels. Linking health and productivity acknowledges that labor-market experiences are related to both, and that firms' bottom-line success is linked to health decisions and vice versa. The next three sections will examine each dimension in turn, with the first two sections using the generic terms health and productivity that will be more fully elaborated in the third section.

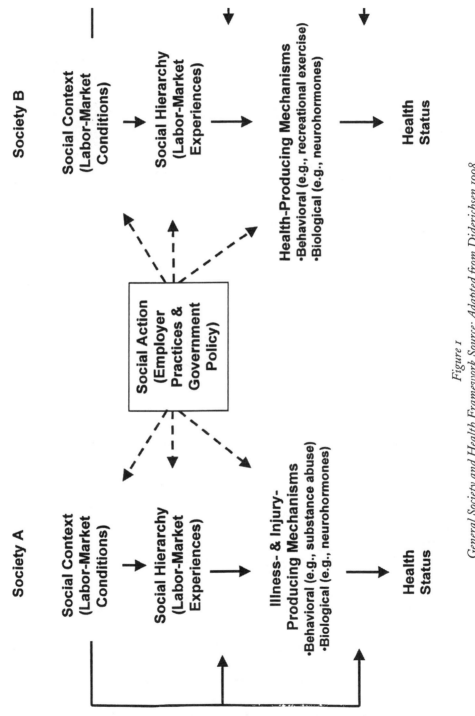

Figure 1

General Society and Health Framework Source: Adapted from Diderichsen 1998

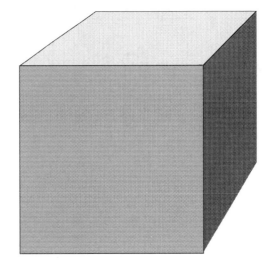

HEALTH
AND
PRODUCTIVITY

LABOR MARKET
EXPERIENCES
• Availability of Work
• Nature of Work

CONTEXTUAL
FACTORS
• Individual
• Firm
• Societal

Figure 2
General Framework for Understanding the Relationship Between Labor-Market Experiences and Health

LABOR-MARKET EXPERIENCES

Two sets of labor-market states—the availability of work and the nature of work—condition a person's labor-market experience (Lavis 1998a). Labor markets are subject to short-term or cyclical trends and long-term or structural trends. Thus, introducing a time dimension disaggregates labor-market states in ways that are important analytically for understanding health.

Table 1 lists six labor-market states related to the *availability of work*. Three are variants of "underwork"—discouraged worker, unemployed, underemployed—and a fourth represents fear of those states. The other two states are fully employed and overemployed/overworked.

Discouraged workers are those who are not working and have given up looking because of a lack of available work (World Bank 1995); underemployed workers are those who work less than full-time, not because they choose to but because more work is not available.

Examining these states by asking whether they are short-term or long-term, cyclical or structural, helps to ascertain which labor-market experiences have the most significant health consequences. Long-term unemployment is typically taken to mean unemployment lasting for longer than twelve months (ILO 1994). Cyclical unemployment results from business-cycle-related demand deficiency and is usually short-

Table 1

Labor-market experiences related to the availability of work

Labor-market experience	Short-term and/or cyclical	Long-term and/or structural
Discouraged workers	Lack of Work	Lack of skills
Unemployed	Temporary layoff	Permanent job loss
Underemployed	Forced work-sharing	Involuntary part-time employment
Fear of unemployment	Job or employment insecurity	Insecurity about employability
Fully employed		
Overemployed/overworked	Temporary increase in work hours	Permanent increase in work hours

Source: Lavis 1998a

term, whereas structural unemployment reflects a typically long-term mismatch between workers' skills (or location) and the available work. The health effects of short-term unemployment may be different from those of a long-term mismatch between skills and available work.

When we integrate a long-term/short-term time dimension with the six labor-market states, twelve unique labor-market experiences result. Examples of ten types appear in Table 1. For illustration, consider the two labor market experiences created when one labor-market state— fear of unemployment—is considered from both a short- and long-term perspective. Between the 1970s and the 1990s, job insecurity (measured on a six-point scale ranging from "secure" jobs to "insecure" jobs) increased from 3.5 to 4.5, or 1.5 standard deviations (Karasek et al. 1998). According to a survey of nonstandard work arrangements by the U.S. Department of Labor, over 8.5% of men and 9.8% of women work in jobs of uncertain or limited duration; these figures represent about 10.6 million jobs (Kalleberg et al. 1997). No longer do workers fear job loss only in periods of recession—fear of unemployment is constantly on the horizon as companies add and eliminate jobs. In a 1996 survey of U.S. companies by the American Management Association,

49% had eliminated jobs between June 1995 and June 1996, despite job growth of 68% (American Management Association, 1997). Old types of jobs, such as welders, are being eliminated and replaced by new types of jobs, such as telemarketers.

Incorporating a time dimension into Table I changes the focus from immediate job or employment insecurity to employability insecurity. A recent survey of firms in four metropolitan areas (Boston, Detroit, Los Angeles and Atlanta) found that "most employers require credentials like a high school diploma, specific experience, references, and/or previous training" (Holzer 1996, p. 127). Holzer concludes that these skill requirements reduce the hiring of blacks and Hispanics, and that because of the discriminatory attitudes of employers, blacks (especially males) are least likely to be hired. For these workers, the question is not whether they are secure in their current job (job security) or with another job in the firm (employment security); it is whether they have the skills, educational background, or skin color to be employable at all if they lose their job. Thus job or employment insecurity can become employability insecurity over time.

The evidence on the consequences for health

and disease of work availability has been reviewed by Lavis (1998b). The state of the evidence can be illustrated using research on unemployment and health. In studies from which results could be systematically extracted, unemployment is consistently associated with negative health outcomes. The absolute risk of a negative health consequence was consistently higher among unemployed than employed adults (Lavis 1998b), with the exception of smoking and alcohol consumption (which could be explained by their relatively high cost for unemployed individuals). Any one study has serious methodological limitations—the most significant being unexamined but possible baseline differences in health or other potential cofounders—but taken together the studies show a strong relationship between unemployment and health.

The *nature of work* encompasses the inherent characteristics of the job, its position within the firm and/or the position of the occupation within society, and the organizational characteristics of the firm (Table 2). The nature of a job can be described using a single characteristic, like work repetitiveness (Salvendy and Smith 1981), or multiple characteristics like the psychological demands of the job and the worker's decision latitude (Karasek and Theorell 1990). Job position within the firm has implications both for an individual's social status (e.g., laborer vs. doctor) and for the power or span of control that a person can exert at work. Job position within the firm and occupational position within society both correlate with a person's social and economic position. In the United Kingdom, for example, people are assigned to one of five occupational classes—professional, intermediate, skilled non-manual or manual, partly skilled manual, and unskilled manual—on the basis of their occupation (Whitehead 1990). The organizational characteristics of the firm define the specific work context and include: work organization, compensation systems, skills development programs, and workplace governance (Capelli et al. 1997; Kalleberg et al. 1996; O'Grady 1993).[1]

Table 2

Labor-market experiences related to the nature of work

Labor-market experiences	A single point in time (static perspective)	Over time (dynamic perspective)
Job characteristics		
Single characteristic	Repetitive work	Increasing job demands
Multiple characteristics	High demand, low control job	Cumulative job strain
Job position within the firm or society	Low employment grade	Lack of career mobility
Organizational characteristics of the firm		
Work organization	Involuntary self-employment	Contingent employment
System of remuneration	Lack of gain-sharing	Stagnant hourly wage
Skill upgrading/expansion	Lack of training	Deskilling
Workplace governance	Hierarchical or flat	Declining worker participation

Source: Lavis 1998a

Distinguishing labor-market experiences associated with the nature of work at a single point in time from such experiences over time enhances analytical leverage. Only by examining labor-market experience over time can working-life-course experiences be related to health through, for example, cumulative exposure models. The 14 labor-market experiences depicted in Table 2 result from integrating a time dimension with the seven states describing the nature of work. To illustrate, consider job position within a firm. A static analysis would identify a worker's employment grade at a given moment in time: the work and health experience of an unskilled manual laborer would clearly be different from that of a professional (c.f. Marmot et al. 1995; 1996; 1997). A dynamic analysis would identify a worker's career mobility or lack of it over time either within a firm or across firms as a factor potentially affecting health (Pavalko et al. 1993; Mare 1990).

The health consequences of the nature of work have been widely reviewed (c.f. Johnson and Hall 1995; Karasek and Theorell 1996; Kasl and Amick 1995; Lavis 1998b; Lundberg 1996; Siegrist 1996). The state of the evidence can be illustrated using one category of experience: job strain, defined as the combination of heavy psychological job demands with little opportunity to control those demands (Karasek and Theorell 1996). Examinations of job strain in terms of cardiovascular health outcomes have found the absolute risks of a positive coronary-heart-disease indicator or of mortality to be higher among individuals with low job-decision latitude, low job-decision latitude and low job support, or high job strain (i.e., high job demands and low job-decision latitude) (Lavis 1998b).

CONTEXTUAL FACTORS

The second dimension in Figure 2 is contextual factors, which can be subdivided into three levels: individual-level, firm-level and societal-level. The labor-market experiences addressed in

Tables 1 and 2 arise from conditions created by firm-level organizational and human-resource decisions and government-level public-policy decisions.[2] Contextual factors may profoundly alter the relationship between these labor-market experiences and health. Action could be targeted at these contextual factors, especially when the political climate makes it difficult to change labor-market experiences directly. Thus, in Table 3 examples of firm- and government-level responses are listed in the columns alongside the contextual factors.

Furthermore, the relationship between labor-market conditions and health can be affected by firm- and government-level responses that determine how labor-market experiences are differentially distributed within a society. For example, firm- and government-level actions create unique labor-market experiences for particular groups (e.g., women and blacks) that can have health consequences. Labor markets are social institutions, socially and culturally constructed, and as such embody the tendency of powerful interests to establish certain types of social arrangements. Fligstein and Byrkjeflot (1996) provide one illustration in a cross-national comparison of how societal values become embedded in labor markets:

> In the United States the dominant conception of the employment relation is that workers should be mobile factors of production and can be laid off whenever economic downturn occurs. Workers should treat the downturn as 'their' problem and they should thus move to where the jobs are. This contrasts with the view in Western Europe that firms should not lay workers off and that cutting hours is preferable. (Fligstein and Byrkjeflot 1996, p. 14).

Eight individual-level contextual factors listed in Table 3 characterize a person and his or her family/household. These traits can be subdivided into those that are relatively stable throughout working life (gender, race, and education) and those that change (age, health, family status, income, and availability of social support). These

Table 3

Contextual influences on the relationship between labor-market experiences and health

Contextual factors	Firm-level causes and/or responses (organizational and human resource practices)	Government-level causes and/or responses (public policy)
Individual-level factors		
Age	Statistical/institutional discrimination (hiring, promotion, pay and firing)	Equal Employment Opportunity ADAct, Equal Pay Act
Race		
Gender		
Health/disability status		
Family status (# and type of dependents)	Availability of flexible work arrangements	Child-care programs, Family and Medical Leave Act
Availability of support		
Educational status		
Income/wealth		
Firm-level factors		
Benefits	Benefits programs (compensation practices, health-care insurance, pension funds)	Minimum wage, Earned Income Tax Credit, tax law, OSHAct
	Skills-development programs	Labor laws, National Labor Relations Board rulings
	Human-centered management practices (provision of support)	
	Labor-management relations climate, safety culture	
Firm climate/culture	Corporate philanthropy	
Societal-level factors		
Labor-market conditions		Trade agreements
Financial conditions		Unemployment insurance generosity
		Workers compensation eligibility and generosity
		Other disability insurance (social security, private long-term disability)
		Health-insurance portability
Social-service conditions		Health-care system

characteristics relate to health by affecting labor-market experiences (e.g., type of employment and career mobility). For example, people of color are less likely to be employed in jobs requiring complex processing of information and more likely to be in jobs with more hazardous working conditions (Tomaskovic-Devey 1993). Individual factors can also affect the relationship between labor-market experiences and health: for example, the availability of social supports has been shown to cushion the impact of job loss on health (Gore 1978).

Firms and government can alter several of these individual-level contextual factors, and thus their health consequences. Firms can provide work arrangements that allow people (especially women) to manage work/family conflicts. Flexible work arrangements generate a greater sense of control and reduce the impact of unpaid work demands (i.e. family and child-care demands) on labor-market experiences (Galinsky and Bond 1996; Hall 1991; Christensen 1995; Spalter-Roth et al. 1997). Similarly, government-sponsored child-care programs support the increased participation of women in the labor market. The Family and Medical Leave Act of 1993 further supports workers with families if the employee takes an unpaid leave for family or medical reasons; employers must maintain the employee's existing level of health-care coverage, and must take the employee back at the same or an equivalent job. Governmental initiatives to prevent discrimination and ensure equal treatment for women, disabled and people of color, including Title VII of the Civil Rights Act of 1964, The Americans with Disabilities Act of 1990 (ADA) and the Equal Pay Act of 1963, have either directly or indirectly affected labor-market experiences and probably through these labor-market experiences, health. Employers are providing more accommodations after passage of the ADA (Burkhauser and Daly 1996), though it is still too early to assess the full impact of the law on employers' treatment of people with disabilities.[3] The consequences of these initiatives on

women's labor-market experiences have recently been documented: from 1970 to 1990, for instance, the disparity between the number of women in management jobs compared to men as a percentage of the U.S. labor force has dropped from 22% to 7% (Reskin and McBrier 1998).

Firm-level contextual factors can modify the relationship between labor market experiences and health (Soderfelt et al. 1997; Amick et al. 1997). What is unique about behavior in organizations is that the context of the organization somehow can shape behavior (Capelli and Scher 1991). Two key contextual factors at the level of the firm are its benefits programs and the climate or culture of the firm. Many U.S. workers are employed in non-standard work arrangements in which benefits are unavailable and not required by law; these are often workers of color, new immigrants, or minorities (Kalleberg et al. 1997). And many American workers discover that health-insurance contracts that deny coverage for pre-existing conditions can act as a powerful incentive to stay in a job even though work conditions may be worse than elsewhere. This predicament, known as "job-lock," is unknown to the citizens of countries with public health-insurance systems.

A firm's culture can have far-reaching effects, penetrating all aspects of the firm from the climate for job security, supervisor-employee relationships to the type and nature of outplacement programs for laid off workers (Schein 1992). A guaranteed job for life can eliminate insecurity about the availability of work. The Saturn automobile-production facility outside of Nashville, Tennessee, offers workers guaranteed job security (except in extreme circumstances) (Shaiken et al. 1997). Firms with a people-oriented culture—emphasizing trust, valuing human investments equally with productivity, and giving voice to workers—are more likely to value balancing work and family and to create skill-development programs through the implementation of internal labor markets or tuition-benefit programs (Christensen 1995). Such programs can mitigate the impact of job insecurity and reduce the amount of employability insecurity. The effects of firm climate or culture are also apparent in the management of work-related disability (Betcherman et al. 1994). Michigan firms with people-oriented cultures experienced less lost work time, fewer cases of work-related injury, and injuries of shorter duration than conventional firms (Hunt et al. 1993).

Laws and regulations governing firm-level contextual factors have implications for labor-market experiences and health. The Fair Labor Standards Act of 1938 established federal protections for maintenance of a minimum standard of living necessary for workers' health, efficiency, and general well-being (Amick 1987). Similarly, the Occupational Safety and Health Act of 1970 established the right to a safe and healthy workplace (Amick 1988). Enforcement of these and other laws by state and federal authorities can be a key factor in modifying the labor-market experiences of workers.

The societal-level context is a mix of labor-market conditions, the financial climate, and the range of social services available to the worker and his or her family. Labor-market conditions, such as the local unemployment rate, the occupational/job mix within a region, or the industries within a region can significantly modify whether a particular labor-market experience has a strong or weak impact on health. Trade agreements (e.g., NAFTA) are one important labor-market condition that can directly affect the availability and nature of work. The financial climate of the parent company profoundly affects the opportunity for the development of business-supported community service programs or the likelihood of a merger and thus the type and availability of jobs. In bad financial times companies may merge and sell off some of their businesses. In good financial times companies may invest in local communities. The financial climate of the state or country can define the types of jobs in the local job market. The types and

availability of unemployment, workers' compensation, and health insurance, to name but a few, can significantly moderate the negative impact of certain labor-market experiences. Finally, social services provided by the government can affect employability (through training programs) and the type of health care available to workers and their families.

Both firms and government can change the societal-level context for labor-market experience. Firm's responses at this level typically consist of financial contributions to social-service programs and corporate philanthropy to offset costs that would otherwise fall on the broader society. An example of the latter is the decision by the president of Massachusetts-based Malden Mills, a manufacturing plant that was partially destroyed by fire, to pay salaries and benefits to all employees until the mill reopened. Pertinent government actions include the establishment of social-service programs, trade agreements, and the promotion of new industries through labor market policy. One example of a social-service program is the Health Insurance Portability and Accountability Act of 1996. This act guarantees the portability of health insurance for employees and their families in case of job loss or job change, mitigating one aspect of the potentially deleterious health consequences of unemployment. Furthermore, it provides workers with a mechanism for reducing the time in potentially hazardous work conditions due to "job lock" (O'Brien and Barker 1997).

THE HEALTH AND PRODUCTIVITY IMPLICATIONS
OF LABOR-MARKET EXPERIENCES
The third dimension of the model is the possible health and productivity consequences of labor-market experiences and their social context (Figure 2). Our typology of consequences draws on Evans and Stoddart's framework for analyzing the determinants of health (Evans and Stoddart 1990). Their framework has three components: environments and endowment (that is, the social

and physical environment, and individuals' genetic endowments), individual responses, and outcomes. Our labor market and health framework illustrates one aspect of the social environment, the centerpiece of the Evans and Stoddart framework.[4] The other two components of their framework—individual responses and outcomes—provide a useful organizing perspective on the possible health and productivity consequences of labor-market experiences (Figure 3).

An individual's response to labor-market experiences can include both behavioral and biological elements, and can be health-enhancing or health-damaging. Behavioral responses range: from some forms of consumption (e.g., smoking, drinking, drug use) to help-seeking (e.g., seeking social support, visiting a health-care provider, contacting a union representative), from some forms of avoidance (e.g., repeatedly missing work) to taking preventive action (e.g., use of protective eye wear or hearing-protection devices in the workplace, use of a seatbelt in a delivery van). These behaviors reflect in part the coping strategies that individuals use to respond to their social environment. Biological responses, including neuroendocrine, immunologic, and physiologic responses (Lundberg 1996), are presumably less amenable to direct intervention than is behavior (Sorensen and Himmelstein 1992).

Outcomes, the final component of Evans and Stoddart's framework, include health outcomes and a broader but related outcome, well-being. Disease and disability, one class of health outcomes, is reserved for professionally designated medical conditions, such as carpal-tunnel syndrome (CTS), a compression of the median nerve in the wrist diagnosed through patient history, physical exam, and nerve-conduction studies (Szabo and Madison 1995). A second category of health outcomes, mental and physical health and function, represents an individual's assessment of his or her own health. Again consider CTS: a functional limitation would be defined

through patient responses to questions about daily activities like opening a jar, holding a book, or answering a phone (Levine et al. 1993). Mental-health problems often accompany musculoskeletal injuries (Kasl and Amick 1995). Symptoms of depression, for instance, could result from the pain associated with the nerve compression or from the inability to engage in valued social roles.

Mental and physical health and function are in turn distinguished from a higher order concept, well-being, defined as an individual's interpretation of his or her own general happiness. Health is a component of well being, but some individuals may be willing to sacrifice gains in health status for something else, like higher income, that translates more directly into improved well-being. Different individuals with CTS, for example, may well define its implications for their well-being differently.

Productivity outcomes are critical to the tradeoffs that employers make in choosing between different policies that affect labor-market experiences. Productivity and other economic outcomes drive business decision-making. Such economic outcomes encompass absenteeism (which may or may not be health-related), worker performance, health-care benefit-plan costs, worker-replacement costs, workers' compensation premia (if experience-rated), and (private) disability plan costs.

Productivity—the effectiveness of productive effort—is the outcome to which improvements in health may contribute; it is often also the desired outcome against which improvements in health must compete. If one alternative available to an employer leads to improvement in both health status and productivity, the case is easily made for adopting it. If these outcomes diverge, the case is much less clear. As yet, unfortunately, few studies on the links between labor-market experiences and health have measured both health and productivity consequences concurrently. One study of the relationship between

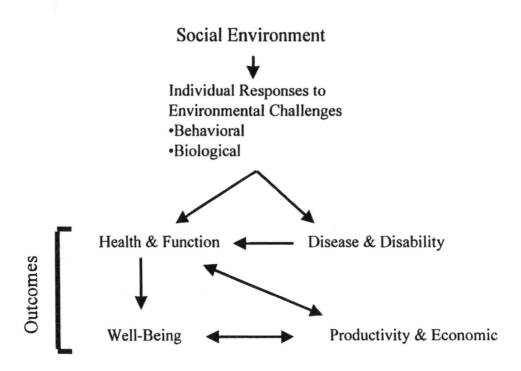

Figure 3
The Relationship Between Health and Productivity (modified from Evans and Stoddard 1990)

work-role performance and carpal tunnel syndrome, reported in Figure 4, found that the relationship between health and productivity depends on the health measures chosen. Limitation in work activities related to managing a schedule, not severity of CTS symptoms or limitations in household activities, predicts lost productivity. For every 25% increase in the difficulty of performing work-scheduling activities[5] due to CTS, 2.7 additional workweeks are lost (Amick and Wu 1998). The costs in lost productivity of this 25% increase (assuming a mean weekly wage of $605, including all overtime) is about $1573. Surprisingly, lost work weeks were not related to the degree of CTS symptoms severity.

THE LABOR MARKET AND HEALTH FRAMEWORK: A CONCEPTUAL ILLUSTRATION

AN important criterion for assessing the utility of our proposed framework is that it leads to different ways of asking questions. The illustration that we provide in this section highlights several key elements of the framework: the temporal dimension, the interconnectedness of health and productivity, and the reciprocal relationships between health and labor-market experiences. Curiously, little research has examined reciprocal relationships between health and labor-market experiences (c.f. Ostlin

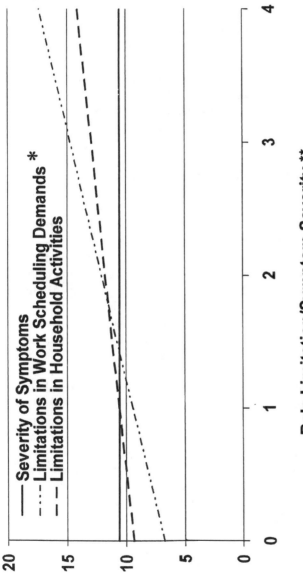

Figure 4

The Relationship Between Carpal Tunnel Syndrome Symptom Severity and Role Limitations and Lost Work Weeks

1989). In occupational epidemiology this relationship is treated as merely methodological bias—the healthy-survivor effect or health selection bias (Arrighi and Hertz-Picciotto 1994). The healthy-survivor effect is an observation about the consequences of sampling an employed population; unhealthy workers having left work, the working population appears healthier and has lower risks of disease than expected. The labor market and health framework presented in Tables 1–3 suggests that, in fact, multiple contextual factors determine a person's labor-market experiences and that health is only one such factor. Functionally limiting injuries don't typically end careers; but they often change work-life courses.

Instead of conceptualizing these issues as bias, a perspective developed within psychosocial epidemiology argues for studying the effects of health on social mobility in its own right. Mobility is a possible alternative explanation for the observed relationship between socioeconomic gradients and health (Bartley and Lewis 1997): the healthy members of society may climb up the social gradient while those less healthy drop down. This perspective posits that health affects a person's position in society, but it does not integrate work-life-course experiences in work and other life-course experiences into the explanation. This unidimensional view fails to identify key factors that can redirect or change work-life courses.

Another perspective, drawn from labor economics, considers the role of health in departures from the workforce. Health status predicts exits from the workforce, whereas benefits, age, and duration of disability affect the likelihood of return to work (Arrow 1996; Burkhauser and Daly 1996; Galizzi and Boden 1996). While debate continues about these reciprocal relationships, studies have not yet examined the interactive or synergistic effects of health on labor-market experiences or labor-market experiences on health. Without addressing this complex dynamic, the effects of labor-market experiences on health are likely to vary depending on the working-life-course status of study participants. The virtual disappearance of lifelong employment with a single employer necessitates a more dynamic perspective that recognizes the push-and-pull between working-life-course experiences and health trajectories.

Few studies have examined working-life-course experiences. Research on white-collar workers whose job sequences appear haphazard and incoherent—such as a progression from lawyer to undertaker to teacher—finds that such careers place a person at greater risk of mortality (Pavalko et al. 1993). By contrast, careers characterized by increasing status and diminishing physical demands over time—such as from laborer to service worker—enjoy lower risk of death (Mare 1990). Sometimes, no change in career trajectory can be hazardous: workers in laboring occupations at the beginning and end of their careers rather than professional/technical occupations had an 80% greater mortality risk (Mare 1990). These findings suggest that career dynamics influence mortality.[6]

If health is indeed influencing career dynamics, a more complex model of working life is clearly required. As a first approximation, Figure 5 presents two illustrations of the complex relationship between health and working life. Productivity, the other main socially-valued work outcome in the labor market and health framework, is also considered. In case 1, illness amplification, the person starts his or her career in reasonably good health and early labor-market experiences (related to the availability or nature of work) bring about change for the worse. Diminished health may cause the person to perform less well, transfer to a new job, or exit the labor force. Productivity is likely to suffer. Future costs to society in the form of disability or other types of income support are likely.

Case 2, health amplification and sustained performance, illustrates a different trajectory.

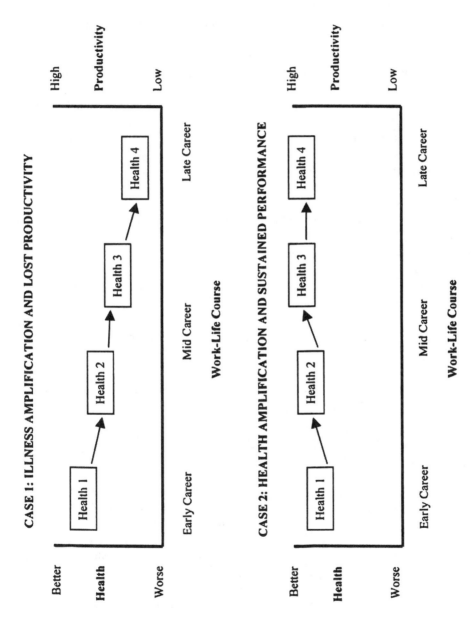

Figure 5
The Relationships Between Work–Life Course and Health,
Including Hypothesized Productivity Consequences

Here, work is a positive influence on a person's health, promoting increased productivity. Other research has shown the impact of positive work experiences on activities outside of work, such as political participation (Gardell 1971; Elden 1981) and parent-child dynamics (Menaghan and Parcel 1991). From an employer's perspective, an experienced worker, with accumulated tacit knowledge, who can share such knowledge with other workers is a valuable asset. In tight labor markets and in competitive industries where workforce flexibility is a competitive advantage, health could be a core element of the added value that an experienced employee contributes to the firm.

These examples are presented as scenarios because so little data exist on the interplay of health and career trajectories. These scenarios do, however, illustrate the potential usefulness of the labor market and health framework. To test the framework will require the development of new data sources to answer more complex questions.

THE LABOR MARKET AND HEALTH FRAMEWORK: EMPIRICAL ILLUSTRATIONS FROM A NEWLY ESTABLISHED DATA LABORATORY

T O answer questions posed within the labor market and health framework, we have begun building a new data laboratory. Funding from the National Institute of Aging and the National Institute for Occupational Safety and Health has allowed us to enrich the Panel Study of Income Dynamics (PSID) dataset to create a national data laboratory (Amick et al. 1998). The PSID is an ongoing longitudinal study of a representative sample of U.S. men, women and children and of the family units in which they reside (Hill 1992). Using the PSID to study labor markets and health has several advantages. First, because it is representative of the U.S. labor market, its findings are generalizable to the U.S. population as a whole (Hill 1992; Fitzgerald et al.

1998). Second, annual collection of information on labor-market experiences allows for both short-term (static) and long-term (dynamic) dimensions to be characterized. This survey design also minimizes problems of recall bias (Mathiowetz 1992; 1994). Third, annual collection of health information allows for the reciprocal effects of labor-market experiences and health to be estimated, while again minimizing recall bias. Fourth, the PSID is a public resource, with most data available through an internet site (html:/www.isr.umich.edu/soc/psid). Finally, because the survey oversampled poor households in 1968 (the baseline year), working women (2,243 or 51% of all women in the sample) and working blacks (1,664 or 70% of blacks in the sample) are well represented in the sample in the early years.

The Availability of Work, Social Context, and Health

The labor market and health framework posits that it is not only loss of a job that is bad for health: the duration of unemployment can be harmful as well. The health outcome used in this analysis is age at death or censoring (Korn et al. 1997). It is hypothesized that being unemployed increases the risk of death, and that the longer the duration of an unemployment spell the greater the risk of early death (Lavis 1998c). A cohort of 2,868 male household heads was followed over 25 years. Unemployment was measured as a time-varying predictor of death in a Cox proportional hazard model. All models include measures of race, marital status, household income, family size, education, and employment grade. Compared to those who were working, unemployed men had a 3.23 greater likelihood of death (hazard rate 3.23, with 95% confidence limits of 1.6–6.5). Duration of the unemployment experience was associated with a 3 percentage point increase in risk of death with each extra week of unemployment (1.03; 1.00–1.05) (Lavis

1998c). Because the 95% confidence limits include 1.00, the added risk must be interpreted with caution.

Contextual factors, as suggested in Table 3, may modify this relationship. Specifically, labor-market conditions could create a social context in which unemployment is the norm; in such circumstances unemployed individuals may enjoy more support and community cohesion than they would in areas where the local unemployment rate is low. Unemployed men in areas with low unemployment rates tended to die earlier than either employed men or unemployed men in areas with high unemployment rates (3.5; 0.78–15.7) (Lavis 1998c). These data are suggestive of a contextual effect, and illustrate the importance of attending to the context of labor-market experiences. But the small sample size and resulting small number of deaths make it difficult to state definitively that social support should be targeted to men in areas with low local unemployment rates.

The Nature of Work, Social Context and Health

One hypothesis generated by the framework defined in Table 2 is that there are health consequences associated with long-term exposure to job conditions. As a first approximation of the health consequences of cumulative exposure to work conditions, an individual's work-life course was summarized as the percentage of the person's working life spent in one of four quartiles (ranging from low to high) for each of the nine work conditions (see Appendix A).[7] Each measure of the nature of work along with gender, race, baseline health status and mean income over working life is entered as a predictor of death in Cox proportional hazard models (Korn et al. 1997). For all three measures of job control (job decision latitude, skill discretion, decision authority), there is a significant linear trend (p < 0.001); job control protects workers from death (see Table 4). Neither psychological nor physical job de-

mands had consistent effects, nor did the expected linear trend appear; perhaps because of confounding by health selection or social position (Hallqvist 1998; Johnson and Hall 1995), or the imprecision of these imputed measurements given the potential for intra-occupational variability (Johnson and Stewart 1993). These cumulative or work-life-course exposure models show the importance of time dimension in the labor market and health framework.

As suggested in Table 3, gender is an important contextual element: men and women may be hired and fired differently, and women have greater unpaid work responsibilities (c.f. Johnson and Hall 1995; Walsh et al. 1995). Table 5 presents Table 4 results stratified by gender. There are two important findings.[8] First, whereas for men both skill discretion and decision authority are significant (as well as job decision latitude), women are protected only when they work in jobs with high decision authority most of their working lives. Since women are more likely to interrupt work for childbearing, caregiving, and household responsibilities (Moen 1985; Frankenhaueser et al. 1991), it is plausible that decision authority indicates the importance of control over work hours through flexible work arrangements, position in the firm, or family-sensitive benefits (Christensen 1995). Second, a supportive supervisor is protective for men, but does not have an effect on women's health. Women may in fact find interaction with supervisors burdensome rather than supportive because of either social conflict specific to the workplace or societal norms that cast women as the caretakers of social relationships— both potential sources of stress rather than support. Alternatively, a supervisor could see flexible arrangements as counter to productivity, for which the supervisor is held accountable, and thus the supervisor may be unsympathetic. These gender-stratified results confirm the differential labor market experiences of men and women and their health consequences, and the necessity of treating gender as an important contextual factor in the labor market and health framework.

Table 4

Risk of Death by Amount of Working Life in Psychosocial Work Environment Exposure Groups[1]

Work Condition[2]	1[4]	Quartiles of Exposure[3]			Test of Trend
		2	3	4	
Job Demands					
Psychological	1.0	1.07 (.61, 1.73)	1.61 (.99, 2.63)	0.89 (.59, 1.35)	χ^2=4.36 (p=.2250)
Physical	1.0	1.39 (.92, 2.10)	1.67 (1.13, 2.46)	1.13 (.76, 168)	χ^2=7.87 (p=.0489)
Job Control					
Job Decision Latitude	1.0	.76 (.52, 1.12)	.57 (.40, .82)	.52 (.37, .73)	χ^2=18.83 (p=.0003)
Skill Descretion[5]	1.0	1.00 (.68, 1.48)	.54 (.37, .80)	.58 (.41, .84)	χ^2=20.85 (p=.0001)
Decision Authority[5]	1.0	.72 (.42, .92)	.56 (.39, .82)	.50 (.34, .71)	χ^2=18.55 (p=.0004)
Social Support					
Coworker Support	1.0	1.02 (.03, 1.63)	.82 (.52, 1.29)	.72 (.48, 1.08)	χ^2=3.68 (p=.2981)
Supervisor Support	1.0	.79 (.50, 1.24)	.61 (.40, .94)	.86 (.58, 1.29)	χ^2=5.55 (p=.1358)

1 All models adjust for race, gender, income and health status. There were 793 deaths in a split-half random sample of 4,280 people.
2 All exposures were imputed using the JCSS job exposure matrix (Schwartz, et al 1988).
3 For comparability, each measure is standardized and then divided into quartiles; 1 is the bottom quartile of the distribution and 4, conceptually, is the top quartile. For psychological and physical job demand, the higher the more hazardous to health; for the remaining measures, the lower the more hazardous to health. Then the fraction of working life a person has spent in each category is calculated. The interpretation of a coefficient is the risk of death if a person spent 100% of working life in that particular quartile compared to that of 100% in the lowest quartile.
4 Reference category.
5 A subscale of the job decision latitude index.

Reciprocal Relationships Between Labor Market Experiences and Health

An underlying, yet complex, pathway implicit in the labor market and health framework is that labor-market experiences influence an individual's health which contributes over time to an individual's employability. We illustrate these paths with two analyses of the PSID.

ANALYSIS I

To examine the reciprocal relationships between skill use and health, we first examine how skill underutilization—having at least 1 more year of education than is required for one's job—is related to early death. Second, we examine how becoming work disabled predicts changes in skill use. Because women and blacks may experience

Table 5

Gender Differences in Risk of Death by Amount of Working Life in Psychosocial Work Environment Exposure Group[1]

Work Condition[2]	1[4]	Quartiles of Exposure[3]			Test of Trend
		2	3	4	
Job Demands					
Psychological					
Men	1.0	1.20 (.65, 2.2)	1.79 (1.0, 3.22)	.92 (.58, 1.48)	χ^2=4.64 (p=.1988)
Women	1.0	.73 (.29, 1.84)	1.33 (.54, 3.26)	.83 (.33, 2.04)	χ^2=1.04 (p=.7920)
Physical					
Men	1.0	1.49 (.93, 2.40)	1.74 (1.11, 2.74)	1.22 (.78, 1.91)	χ^2=6.56 (p=.0873)
Women	1.0	1.07 (.46, 2.52)	1.47 (.72, 3.02)	.83 (.33, 2.09)	χ^2= 2.50 (p=.4750)
Job Control					
Job Decision Latitude					
Men	1.0	.63 (.39, 1.00)	.52 (.36, .78)	.50 (.34, .74)	χ^2=.10.95 (p=.0007)
Women	1.0	1.18 (.60, 2.31)	.79 (.36, 1.74)	.45 (.20, 1.04)	χ^2=5.66 (p=.1296)
Skill Discretion[5]					
Men	1.0	.94 (.57, 1.56)	.49 (.32, .78)	.57 (.38, .87)	χ^2=10.95 (p=.0007)
Women	1.0	1.00 (.57, 2.12)	.81 (.34, 1.94)	.50 (.19, 1.34)	χ^2=5.66 (p=.1296)
Decision Authority[5]					
Men	1.0	.43 (.41, .99)	.48 (.31, .73)	.54 (.36, .82)	χ^2=15.16 (p=.0016)
Women	1.0	.57 (.24, 1.33)	.89 (.49, 1.99)	.31 (.14, .68)	χ^2=8.63 (p=.0346)
Social Support					
Coworker Support					
Men	1.0	.94 (.55, 1.59)	.69 (.41, 1.15)	.75 (.48, 1.16)	χ^2=3.30 (p=.3475)
Women	1.0	1.47 (.54, 4.04)	1.73 (.69, 4.32)	.46 (.6, 1.26)	χ^2=0.78 (p=.8535)

1 All models adjust for race, gender, income, and health status. There were 520 deaths among 2,158 men and 273 deaths among 2,122 women.
2 All exposures were imputed using the JCSS job exposure matrix (Schwartz et al. 1988).
3 For comparability, each measure is standardized and then divided into quartiles; 1 is the bottom quartile of the distribution and 4, conceptually, is the top quartile. For psychological and physical job demand, the higher the more hazardous to health; for the remaining measures, the lower the more hazardous to health. Then the fraction of working life a person has spent in each category is calculated. The interpretation of a coefficient is the risk of death if a person spent 100% of working life in that particular quartile compared to that of 100% in the lowest quartile.
4 Reference category.
5 A subscale of the job decision latitude index.

Appendix A:

Work environment measures used in the job-characteristics scoring system

Work condition	Meaning	High score interpretation	Low score interpretation
Psychological job demands	The pace and degree of difficulty of the work within the time required to do the work, contingent on other demands being placed on the worker	A job whose pace is fast and work is hard	A job free of conflicting demands, where there are no excessive demands and enough time to get the work done
Job decision latitude (combination of skill discretion and decision authority)	Opportunity for the worker to decide when and how to proceed and what skills to use, to develop new skills and to participate in decisions affecting oneself	A job with opportunities to grow and to do a variety of tasks	A repetitive job with little say over how or what to do
Skill discretion	Opportunity for the worker to develop and use a variety of skills in non-repetitive work	A job that offers the opportunity to be creative, develop and learn new skills and do a variety of tasks	A repetitive job
Decision authority	Oppportunity to decide what, when, and how to do work and to participate in decisions affecting oneself	A job that offers ample say in what to do and freedom to choose how to do the job	A job with no say how to work or what tasks to do
Coworker support	The degree to which coworkers are friendly, helpful, personally interested in the worker and competent	Friendly, helpful coworkers, personally interested in the worker and quite competent	Incompetent, unfriendly, unhelpful coworkers not personally interested in the worker
Supervisor support	The degree to which the supervisor shows concern and is attentive to the worker, fosters teamwork and helps get work done	A supervisor who shows concern, is attentive to the worker, helps get work done and fosters teamwork	Inattentive, unhelpful supervisor who shows no concern for the worker, and doesn't foster teamwork
Job insecurity	Likelihood of being laid off and lack of steady work	High likelihood of being laid off	Good job security and steady work
Skill underutilization	Use of only a fraction of the worker's skills	High disparity between worker skills and job requirements	Low disparity between worker skills and job requirements
Physical demands	The amount of physical effort the job requires	Job requires regular physical exertion	Job does not require regular physical exertion

Source: Schwartz et al. 1988

greater discrimination in hiring, firing, and promotion (see Table 3), and thus be more subject to skill underutilization, we examined separate logistic regression models for sex and race; adjusting for health status and log-income. The results are further stratified by age (<45, >=45).

As Figure 6 shows, non-black males are the only group with high skill underutilization to have an elevated risk of mortality (odds ratio [OR] 1.84); the effect is most pronounced among those at mid-career or late in their careers (OR 2.21). This may indicate a health consequence of downsizing (e.g., job loss) for older non-black males, especially mid-level managers with a college education who find it difficult to gain employment in similar jobs that exercise their skills in the new service economy. It may be that blacks and women only experience stress early in their working lives and become inured to it over time, but this phenomenon is difficult to identify due to the small number of deaths in the early years of work for these groups. Conversely, non-black males who experience unexpected skill underutilization at mid-career may find it a significantly stressful experience with negative health consequences. Alternatively, skill underutilization could be traceable to a change in jobs in response to a health problem; a job that requires less skill may enable a person to continue working with a disabling health condition.

To examine the effect of health on skill utilization, we created two new measures of change in skill utilization states. One measures whether a change has occurred from a good state—a good match between a person's education and the education required by the job—to a bad state—at least one year more education than the job requires. The second measure is the reverse—a change from bad to good. The results, shown in Figures 7a and 7b, suggest the effect of disability on changes in skills is pervasive, not just among non-black males. For non-black men, there is a significant risk (OR 2.33) of disability preceding a transition from a good skills

match to skill underutilization, yet the risk is greater for black men (OR 2.89) (Figure 7a). Interestingly, for non-black males under 45, disability is likely to predict a transition from skill underutilization to a good skills match (OR 2.03); the same is true for young black women (OR 2.08) and older non-black women (OR 1.6) (Figure 7b). Disability management may be an important firm-level response not only for preventing poor skill use, but for encouraging better skill use. Overall, these findings suggest complex dynamics between labor-market experiences and health states as we argued earlier and illustrated hypothetically in Figure 5.

ANALYSIS 2

To examine the more complex dynamics, as suggested by Figure 5, a new statistical model was developed exploring the reciprocal relationships between the substantive complexity of jobs and self-rated health (1 excellent to 5 poor); each measured every year from 1984 onward in the PSID. Substantive complexity, imputed using the Dictionary of Occupational Titles (Cain and Treiman 1981), measures the complexity of a job in terms of its skill requirement or content. The higher a job's complexity, the more education and training it requires and the more it calls for complex data processing, people-management skills, and work with technically advanced machines. Using longitudinal psychometric modeling[9] (c.f. Arminger et al 1995), the dynamic relationship between substantive complexity and health is described. With adjustment for age, sex, race, marital status, and year of measurement, predictive models are used to simulate how substantive complexity and self-reported health change over time (Figure 8). The statistical simulation assigns people to one of four states at age 35: good health and high substantive complexity, good health and low substantive complexity, poor health and high substantive complexity, and poor health and low substantive complexity,[10] and follows them to age 60. These results are both preliminary and designed to show an

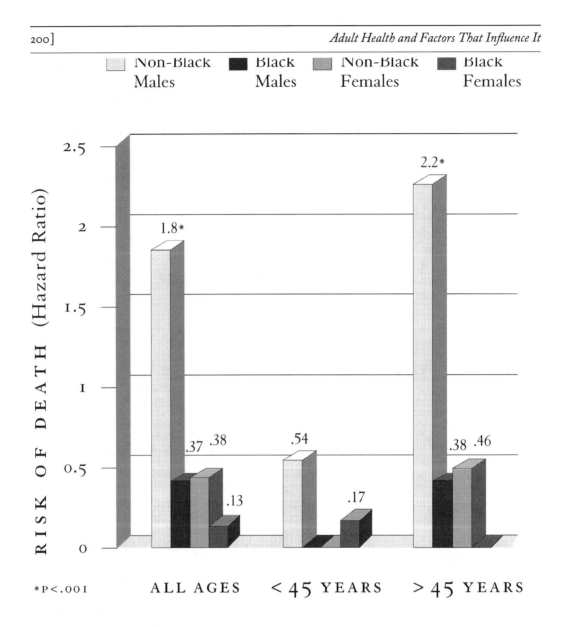

Note: Age-stratified results are not shown for groups in which no deaths occurred.

Figure 6
Risk of Mortality for Workers with High Skill Underutilization by Gender, Race, and Age, 1968–1992

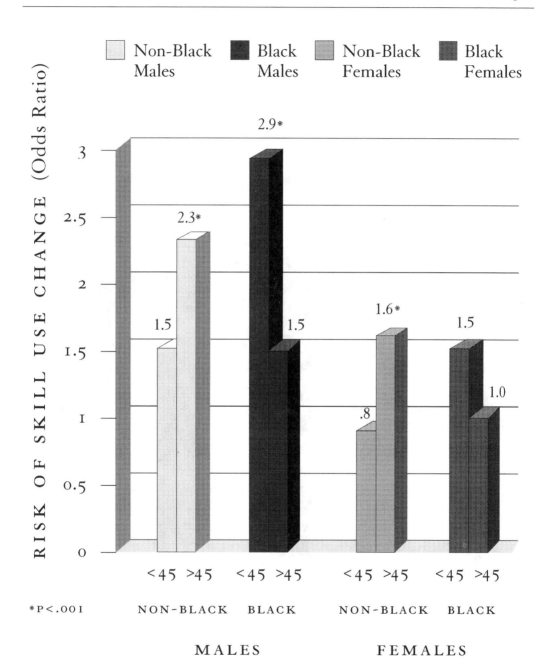

Figure 7a
*Risk of Changing from Good Skill Utilization to Skill Underutilization for Persons with
a New Work-Related Disability, by Gender, Race, and Age, 1968–1992*

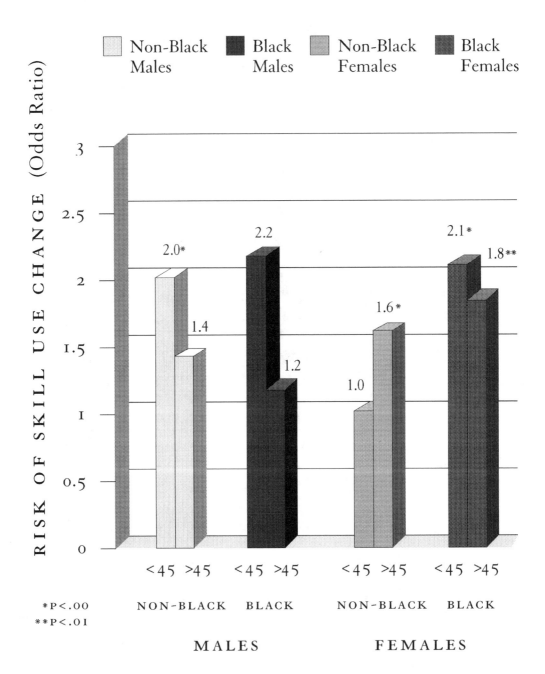

Figure 7b
Risk of Changing from Skill Underutilization to Good Skill Utilization for Persons with
a Work-Related Disability, by Gender, Race, and Age, 1968–1992

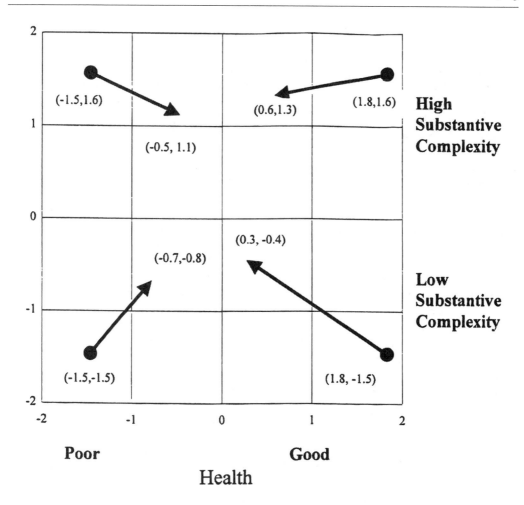

Note: The large circle • indicates age 35 in 1980 and the end of the arrow → indicates a predicted location for a person age 60 in 2005. The lines represent work and health trajectories over the 25 year working life course. The coordinates show health (x) and substantive complexity (y).

Figure 8
Dynamic Relationships Between Substantive Complexity of Work and Self-Reported Health Status
(original source data The Panel Study of Income Dynamics)

approach to modeling complex dynamic relationships. Not unexpectedly, people in good health working in a job with high substantive complexity at age 35 experience declining health but not a significant change in substantive com-

plexity (upper right quadrant). This trajectory describes an underlying aging process: health typically declines with age. Contrast this with people in good health working in a job with low substantive complexity (lower left quadrant).

Here people have a significant drop in health. So, when people in good health are working in jobs with different levels of complexity their health trajectory differs. It could be hypothesized that jobs with limited job content (as represented by substantive complexity) accelerate the aging-related health decline. A cursory examination of Figure 8 would lead one to believe that the effect being illustrated is "regression to the mean," but if this was the case we would expect all four arrows to look very similar in terms of their slope. However, for those starting in high substantive complexity jobs the rate of change is less compared to those starting in low substantive complexity jobs. These findings are preliminary and intended to demonstrate the importance of understanding the complex interplay between work and health in the context of a person's life course. Typical regression modeling may not allow researchers to capture the complex interplay we have illustrated here using longitudinal psychometric models. More work is needed to disentangle the role of work in retarding the aging process and possibly promoting a healthy working life course.

CONCLUSION

THIS chapter has proposed a labor-market and health framework to help build an understanding of how firms and government can promote labor-market experiences that in turn promote health and productivity. This framework is linked to a broader society-and-health framework that encourages research on the labor-market conditions (that is, the social context) that influence the relationship between labor-market experiences and health, and on the actions on the part of firms and government (that is, the social action) necessary to promote change. Our approach treats employers and government as active contributors to labor-market-related health gains or losses.

This chapter also provided empirical support for many of the relationships described in the

framework using a newly established data lab. First, unemployed men were found to have a higher risk of death than employed men. As well, social context (i.e. labor market conditions—the unemployment rate) was found to modify the relationship. Second, working in a job with little control increases the risk of death, but small changes in control over a person's working life course can reduce the mortality risk. Third, gender differences in the effect of job control show the importance of the social context. While for men small changes in job control can make a difference, for women it is only substantial amounts of decision authority over the working life. Fourth, health is not only an outcome of working, but often is determinant of a person's transition from a job with a reasonable skill–education match to one where the there is a poor match (skill underutilization). Taken together, these findings provide some insights into the usefulness of the labor markets and health framework.

This framework suggests that a key goal of research is to define the competitive advantage to firms of sustaining worker health, illustrated hypothetically in Figure 5 and supported by the exploratory finding that jobs with high substantive complexity are associated with less of a health decline over the life course. A key challenge is to promote a shift on the part of firms from viewing workers as costs to viewing workers as investments. Interestingly, a systematic study of companies that "downsized" from 1980 to 1994 (Cascio et al. 1997) found no relationship between downsizing and corporate profitability (as measured by return on investment). Conventional wisdom to the contrary, companies that increased their payrolls tended to produce higher returns for their stockholders than companies that cut their payrolls (Cascio et al. 1997). This finding highlights the importance of a human-investment strategy—a strategy that improves the abilities as well as the health of workers.

A new human-investment strategy requires research on labor-market experiences over time, and on the role of employers and government in shaping these experiences. One approach might be to foster collaborative research arrangements (Cummings et al. 1985). The world of work is dynamic; decision-makers in the marketplace need new information in a short time frame. Researchers, by contrast, need long time horizons to understand the processes that contribute to health and disease. Multiple stakeholders must thus be involved to produce knowledge that is useful to everyone concerned. Since the goal is to improve health, in part, through change in firm's behavior, mutual commitments between researchers and firms must be long-term. The involvement of multiple stakeholders will increase the likelihood that each understands the relevance of both the research and its potential application; a long-term commitment makes the investment of time worthwhile.

A second research need is for measures of short-term changes in health that can be linked to productivity, either directly or indirectly through effects on performance. Evidence must be presented in ways that firms and employees can understand tradeoffs they are making (Levine 1995). Measures of role functioning appear to be the most likely candidates because of their importance to the work role and sensitivity to health status.

Research must focus on the dynamics of social change and how the change processes can influence labor-market experiences. A recent case study of a participatory ergonomics program at the NUMMI (New United Motor Manufacturing Inc.) car assembly facility in California after OSHA citations for insufficient attention to hazardous ergonomic conditions illustrates the complexity of these dynamics. "When management reliance on employee involvement is complemented by strong employee voice and strong regulators," the authors concluded, "managers may find it in their interest to improve safety as a means of maintaining high employee commitment and thereby improving business performance" (Adler et al. 1997, p. 416). Government is a key player, especially in the short

term. As the above quote suggests, policies that encourage certain firm behaviors can improve both business performance and health. Unfortunately, research has not yet focused on these important change levers, focussing instead on individual psychosocial processes. Our labor market and health framework suggests that labor market and industrial policies are important determinants of worker health through their effects on business practices and firm behavior.

Policy development takes time. What can government and businesses do now? The data we have presented support three key actions.

1. First, keep people participating in the labor market so they are active members of society as well as more healthy.
2. Second, enhance decision authority in all jobs. Approaches range from job redesign, self-managing teams, and flexible work arrangements to employee ownership and changing organizational culture. There is no single best solution; what works in one industry may not be suited to another. State agencies can provide technical assistance or workshops and disseminate successful approaches.
3. Third, build a labor market characterized by high-skill jobs which will promote long-term maintenance of health, reduce the costs of managing illness and disability, and improve productivity.

NOTES

1. It could be argued that labor-market experiences are an individual-level experience and that these characteristics of the organization should be assigned to the labor-market context as firm-contextual factors. Often these conditions are conceptualized at the work unit or organizational level but measured as individual-level phenomena.

2. Other social institutions affect the labor market as well, especially educational institutions, which determine the type of skills that a person brings to the labor market and socialize people to expect certain types of work. The judicial system also affects labor market. Currently, a number of court cases are examining employment-at-will doctrines and the discretionary authority of firms to fire employees whenever they want. Trade unions and other forms of worker representation also have an important effect.

3. This also shows how cost can be affected. If effective, the ADA should reduce the societal costs of injury by reducing Social Security Disability Insurance awards for people of

working age. The ADA will do so less by speeding up exits from the disability rolls than by decreasing the likelihood that someone with a disability will experience job loss.

4. Many of the contextual factors will also help in addressing problems in the physical environment. The interconnectedness of the physical and social conditions of work deserves greater attention. This ecology of work exposure is another element to be integrated into the current framework.

5. The work scheduling activities measured include: sticking to a routine, working without taking frequent rest or breaks, working the required number of hours, and getting to work on time. The scale measures the difficulty meeting these demands given Corpel Tunnel Syndrome.

6. It is important to note that this research has focused on white men. Clearly, generalizing to women from men's career experiences may not be appropriate. Women's careers are characterized by interruptions and longer periods of absence from the labor force (Moen 1985). Consequently, women have less tenure in their jobs, and are less likely to get promoted or to receive new assignments (Baron et al. 1986).

7. For example, a person who had spent 100% of his or her working life in jobs with large amounts of decision latitude would have a value of 1 (for 100%) for 4, the top quartile, and 0 for each of the other three possible categories, quartiles 1, 2 and 3. Most people, however, spend their working lives in a series of jobs with varying levels of job decision latitude. Thus, they may not have received a 1 for a single category but have a series of values summing to 1 across the four categories.

8. The results should be seen as suggestive. When gender is interacted with the cumulative work exposures in unstratified models, no significant interactions are identified. This formal statistical test merely indicates the power problems inherent in this analysis and should not detract from the four categories.

9. These models have been developed at The Health Institute of New England Medical Center by Dr. William Rogers.

10. The four states were defined by cross-classifying substantive complexity and health at their 0 value. Both variables were standardized with a mean of 0 and a standard deviation of 1. So 1 on either the health or substantive complexity scale represents the 68 percentile above the mean of health or substantive complexity and 2 the 97.5 percentile.

REFERENCES

Adler, P. S., Goldoftas, B. and Levine, D. I. Ergonomics, employee involvement, and the Toyota production system: A case study of NUMMI's 1993 model introduction. *Industrial and Labor Relations Review* 50(3):416–437, 1997.

Akabas, S. H., Gates, L. B. and Galvin, D. E. *Disability Management: A Complete system to reduce costs, increase productivity, meet employee needs, and ensure legal compliance.* New York: AMACON, 1992.

American Management Association. *Corporate Downsizing, Job Elimination and Job Creation: Summary of Key Findings.* Chicago, IL: AMA, November, 1997.

Amick, III, B. C. The politics of the quality of worklife in automated offices in the USA. *Behavior and Information Technology* 6(4), 1987.

Amick, B. C. Health and safety in the automated office: National policy, organizational initiatives and individual choices. *Office: Technology and People* 3:341–360, 1988.

Amick, III, B. C., Levine, S., Tarlov, A. R. and Walsh, D. C. *Society and Health.* New York: Oxford University Press, 1995.

Amick, B. C., Wu, V., Mangione, T. and Levine, S. Putting the Organization Back into the social epidemiology of work. Paper presented at the *1997 American Sociological Association Meetings*, Toronto, Canada, August 9, 1997.

Amick, III, B. C. and Wu, V. Work, Household and Leisure Time Limitation in Work-Related Carpal Tunnel Syndrome. *Paper presented at the Workers' Compensation Research Group Meeting*, Cambridge, MA, 1998.

Amick, III, B. C., McDonough, P., House, J., Duncan, G., Williams, D. and Rogers, W. Cumulative exposure to psychosocial work organization and mortality: Preliminary evidence for the US 1968–1992. *Am J Public Health* (submitted), 1998.

Arminger, G., Clogg, C. C. and Sobel, M. E. (eds.). *Handbook of Statistical Modeling for the Social and Behavioral Sciences.* New York: Plenum Press, 1995.

Arrighi, H. M., and Hertz-Picciotto, I. The evolving concept of the healthy worker survivor effect. *Epidemiology* 4:189–196, 1994.

Arrow, J. O. Estimating the influence of health as a risk factor on employment: A survival analysis of employment durations for workers surveyed in the German socioeconomic panel (1984–1990). *Soc Sci Med*, 1996.

Baldwin, M. L., Johnson, W. G. and Butler, R. J. The error of using returns-to-work to measure the outcomes of health care. *Am J Ind Med* 29:632–641, 1996.

Baron, J. N., Davis-Blake, A. and Bielby W. T. The structure of opportunity: How promotion ladders vary within and among organizations. *Administrative Science Quarterly* 31:248–273, 1986.

Bartley, M. and Lewis, I. Does health-selective mobility account for socioeconomic differences in health? Evidence from England and Wales, 1971 to 1991. *J Health Soc Behav* 38(4):376–386, 1997.

Benzeval, M., Judge, K. and Whitehead, M. *Tackling Inequalities in Health: An Agenda for Action.* London: Kings Fund Publishing, 1995.

Berndt, E. R., Finkelstein, S. N., Greenberg, P. E., Keith, A. and Bailit, H. Illness and productivity: objective workplace evidence. Working Paper #42–97. *Program on the Pharmaceutical Industry.* Cambridge, MA: Sloan School of Management, MIT, 1997.

Betcherman, G., McMullen, K., Leckie, N. and Caron, C. *The Canadian Workplace in Transition: Final Report of the Human Resources Management Project.* Kingston, Ontario: IRC Press, 1994.

Blane, D., Brunner, E. and Wilkinson, R. *Health and Social Organization: Towards a Health Policy for the 21st Century.* London: Routledge, 1996.

Boden, L. I. Workers' compensation in the United States: High costs, low benefits. *Ann Rev Public Health* 16:189–218, 1996.

Burkhauser, R. V. and Daly, M. C. Employment and economic well-being following the onset of a disability. In: Mashaw, J. L., Reno, V., Burkhauser, R. V. and Berkowitz, M. (eds). *Disability, Work and Cash Benefits.* Kalamazoo, MI: W. E. Upjohn Institute for Employment Research, 1996.

Cain, P. S. and Treiman, D. J. The D.O.T. as a source of occupational data. *Am Soc Rev* 56:253–278, 1981.

Cappelli, P., Bassi, L., Katz, H., Knoke, D., Osterman, P. and Useem, M. *Change at Work.* New York: Oxford University Press, 1997.

Cappelli, P. and Sherer, P. D. The missing role of context in OB: The need for a meso-level approach. *Res Org Behav* 13:55–110, 1991.

Cascio, W. F., Young, C. E. and Morris, J. R. Financial consequences of employment-change decisions in major U. S. corporations. *Academy of Management Journal* 40(5):1175–1189, 1997.

Christensen, K. *Contingent Work Arrangements in Family-Sensitive Corporations.* Boston, MA: Center on Work & Family, 1995.

Cummings, T. G., Mohrman, S. A., Mohrman, A. M. and Ledford, G. E. Organization design for the future: A collaborative research approach. In: Lawler, III, E. E., Mohrman, Jr., A. M., Mohrman, S. A., Ledford, Jr., G. E., Cummings, T. G. and Associates (eds.). *Doing Research That Is Useful for Theory and Practice.* San Francisco, CA: Jossey-Bass Publishers, pp. 275–323, 1985.

Diderichsen, F. The future work on formulating national health targets and strategies. In: The National Public Health Commission. Towards a Healthy Sweden: The first step towards national health targets, Chapter 8, p. 199. *SOU* 30: Stockholm, 1998.

Elden, J. M. Political efficacy at work: The connection between more autonomous forms of workplace organization and a more participatory politics. *The American Political Science Review* 75:43–58, 1981.

Evans, R. G. and Stoddart, G. L. Producing health, consuming health care. *Soc Sci Med* 31:1347–63, 1990.

Evans, R. G., Barer, M. L. and Marmor T. R. (eds.). *Why Are Some People Healthy and Others Not?* New York:Aldine De Gruyter, 1994.

Fitzgerald, J., Gottschalk, P. and Moffitt, R. An analysis of sample attrition in Panel data: The Michigan Panel Study of Income Dynamics. Technical Working Paper #220. Cambridge, MA: National Bureau of Economic Research, February, 1998.

Fligstein, N. and Byrkjeflot, H. The logic of employment systems. In: Baron, J. N., Grusky, D. B. and Treiman, D. J. (eds.). *Social Differentiation and Social Inequality: Essays in Honor of John Pock.* Boulder, CO: Westview Press, p. 14, 1996.

Frankenhaeuser, M., Lundberg, U. and Chesney, M. (eds.). *Women, Work, and Health: Stress and Opportunities.* New York: Plenum Press, 1991.

Galinsky, E. and Bond, J. T. The experiences of mothers and fathers in the US labor force. In: Costello, C. and Krimgold, B. B. (eds.). *The American Woman 1996–1997: Where We Stand.* New York: W. W. Norton & Company, 1996.

Galizzi, M. and Boden, L. I. *What Are the Most Important Factors Shaping Return to Work: Evidence from Wisconsin.* Cambridge, MA: Workers Compensation Research Institute, 1996.

Gardell, B. Alienation and mental health in the modern industrial environment. In: Levi, L. (ed.). *Society, Stress and Disease,* Vol. 1. The Psychosocial Environment and Psychosomatic Diseases. London: Oxford University Press, pp. 148–180, 1971.

Gore, S. The effect of social support in moderating the health consequences of unemployment. *Journal of Health and Social Behavior* 19:157–165, 1978.

Greenberg, P. E., Stiglin, L. E., Finkelstein, S. N. and Berndt, E. R. The economic burden of depression in 1990. *Clin Psychiatry* 54:11, November 1993.

Hall, E. Gender, work control, and stress: A theoretical discussion and empirical test. In Johnson, J. V. and Johansson, G. (eds.), *The Psychosocial Work Environment: Work Organization, Democratization and Health*. Amityville, NY: Baywood Publishing, pp. 89–108, 1991.

Hallqvist, J. *Socioeconomic Differences in Myocardial Infarction Risk: Epidemiological Analyses of Causes and Mechanisms*. Department of Public Health Sciences, Karolinska Institute, Sundbybreg, Sweden, 1998.

Hill, M. *The Panel Study of Income Dynamics*. Beverly Hills, CA: Sage, 1992.

Holzer, H. J. *What Employers Want: Job Prospects for Less-Educated Workers*. New York: Russell Sage Foundation, 1996.

Hunt, H. A., Habeck, R. V., VanTol, B. and Scully, S. M. *Disability Prevention Among Michigan Employers*. Final report submitted to the Michigan Department of Labor (Upjohn Institute Technical Report No. 93–004). Kalamazoo, MI: W. E. Upjohn Institute for Employment Research, 1993.

ILO. *World Labor Report 1994*. Geneva: International Labor Office, 1994.

Johnson, J. V. and Hall, E. M. Class, work and health. In: Amick, B. C., Levine, S., Tarlov, A. R. and Walsh, D. C. (eds.). *Society and Health*. New York: Oxford University Press, pp. 247–271, 1995.

Johnson, J. V. and Stewart, W. F. Measuring work organization exposure over the life course with a job-exposure matrix. *Scand J Work Environ Health* 19:21–28, 1993.

Kalleberg, A. L., Knoke, D., Marsden, P. V. and Spaeth, J. L. *Organizations in America: Analyzing Their Structures and Human Resource Practices*. Thousand Oaks, CA: Sage Publications, 1996.

Kalleberg, A. L., Rasell, E., Hudson, K., Webster, D., Reskin, B. F., Cassirer, N. and Applebaum, E. *Nonstandard Work, Substandard Jobs: Flexible Work Arrangements in the U.S.* Washington, DC: Economic Policy Institute, 1997.

Karasek, R. and Theorell, T. *Healthy Work: Stress, Productivity, and the Reconstruction of Working Life*. New York: Basic Books, 1990.

Karasek, R. A. and Theorell, T. Current issues relating to psychosocial job strain and cardiovascular disease research. *J Occup Health Psychol* 1(1):9–26, 1996.

Karasek, R., Brisson, C., Amick, B., Bongers, P., Houtman, I. and Kawakami, N. The Job Content Questionnaire (JCQ): An instrument for internationally comparative assessments of psychosocial job characteristics. *J Occup Health Psychol* (submitted February, 1998).

Kasl, S. V. and Amick, III, B. C. Work stress. In: MacDonald, J. C. (ed.). *The Epidemiology of Work Related Diseases*. BMJ Press, 1995.

Kasl, S. V. and Amick, III, B. C. Cumulative Trauma Disorder Research: Methodological Issues and Illustrative Findings From the Perspective of Psychosocial Epidemiology. In: Moon, S. and Sauter, S. (eds.) *Factors and Musculoskeletal Disorders in Office Work*. New York: Taylor and Francis, 1996.

Korn, E. L., Graubard, B. I. and Mudthune, D. Time-to-event analysis of longitudinal follow-up of a survey: Choice of the Time-scale. *Am J Epidemiol* 145:72–80, 1997.

Lancet, Editorial, 343:88–95, 1994.

Lavis, J. N. *The Links Between Labor-Market Experiences and Health: Towards a Research Framework*. Working Paper 62. Toronto, ON: Institute for Work & Health, 1998a.

Lavis, J. N. Labour-market experiences and health: A systematic review of cohort studies. In: Hurley, J., et al. *Health Policy in the Era of Population Health: An Exploration of Changing Roles*. Report submitted to Health Canada through the National Health Research and Development Program (NHRDP), February 1998b.

Lavis, J. N. Unemployment and Mortality: A Longitudinal Study in the United States, 1968–92. Working Paper 63. Toronto, ON: Institute for Work & Health, 1998c.

Leigh, J. P., Markowitz, S. B., Fahs, M., Shin, C. and Landrigan, P. J. Occupational injury and illness in the United States: Estimates of costs, morbidity, and mortality. *Arch Intern Med* 157:1557–1568, 1997.

Levine, D., Simmons, B. P., Koris, M. J., Daltroy, L. H., Hohl, G. G., Fossel, A. H. and Katz, J. N. Development and validation of symptom severity and functional status scales for carpal tunnel syndrome. *J Bone Joint Surg* 75A:1585–1592, 1993.

Levine, D. I. *Reinventing the Workplace: How Business and Employees Can Both Win.* Washington, DC: Brookings Institution, 1995.

Lundberg, U. Paid and unpaid employment: A review of health effects. *J Occup Health Psychol* 1(1):36–48, 1996.

Mare, R. D. Socio-economic careers and differential mortality among older men in the U.S. In: Vallin, J., D'Souza, S. and Palloni, A. (eds.). *Measurement and Analysis of Mortality—New Approaches.* Oxford: Clarendon Press, pp. 362–387, 1990.

Marmot, M. and Feeney, A. Work and health: Implications for individuals and society. In: Blane, D., Brunner, E. and Wilkinson, R. (eds.). *Health and Social Organization: Towards a Health Policy for the 21st Century.* London: Routledge, pp. 235–25, 1996.

Marmot, M., Bobak, M. and Smith, G. D. Explanations for social inequalities in health. In: Amick, B. C., Levine, S., Tarlov, A. R., and Walsh, D. C. (eds.). *Society and Health.* New York: Oxford University Press, pp. 172–210, 1995.

Marmot, M. G., Bosma, H., Hemingway, H., Brunner, E. and Stansfield, S. Contribution of job control and other risk factors to social variations in coronary heart disease incidence. *Lancet* 350:235–239, 1997.

Mathiowetz, N. A. Errors in reports of occupation. *Public Opinion Quarterly* 56:352–355, 1992.

Mathiowetz, N. A. Autobiographical memory and the validity of survey data: Implications for the design of the Panel Study of Income Dynamics. *PSID Working Paper* (March), 1994.

Menaghan, E. and Parcel, T. Determining children's home environments: The impact of maternal characteristics and current occupational and family experience. *J Marriage Fam* 53:417–431, 1991.

Moen, P. Continuities and discontinuities in women's labor force activity. In: Elder, G. H. (ed.). *Life Course Dynamics.* Ithaca, NY: Cornell University, pp. 113–155, 1985.

O'Brien, K. P. and Barker, R. B. HIPAA's nondiscrimination rule: Agencies see green light for regulating health plan design. *Benefits Law Journal* 10(2), Summer 1997.

O'Grady, J. *Direct and Indirect Evidence on the Extent of Changes in Work Organization in Canada.* Unpublished mimeo, prepared for the Secretariat, Premier's Council on Economic Renewal, Toronto, ON, 1993.

Östlin, P. *Occupational Career and Health: Methodological Considerations on the Healthy Worker Effect.* Uppsala University, Department of Social Medicine, University Hospital, Uppsala, Sweden, 1989.

Pavalko, E., Elder, G. H. and Clipp, E. C. Work lives and longevity: Insights from a life course perspective. *J Health Soc Behav*, 34(4):363–380, December 1993.

Personick, M. Types of work associated with lengthy absences from work. *Compensation and Working Conditions* Fall: 51–54, 1997.

Reskin, B. and McBrier, D. Organizational determinants of the sexual division of managerial labor. Paper presented at *Work Organizations* Seminar, Cambridge, MA, March 1998.

Salvendy, G. and Smith, M. J. (eds.). *Machine Pacing and Occupational Stress.* London: Taylor & Francis Ltd., 1981.

Schein, E. *Organizational Culture and Leadership*, second edition. San Francisco, CA: Jossey Bass Publishers, 1992.

Schwartz, J. E., Pieper C. F. and Karasek, R. A. A procedure for linking psychosocial job characteristics data into health surveys. *Am J Public Health* 78:904–909, 1988.

Short, Jr., J. F. *The Social Fabric: Dimensions and Issues.* Newbury Park, CA: Sage Publications, 1986.

Shaiken, H., Lopez, S. and Mankita, I. Two routes to team production: Saturn and Chrysler compared. *Industrial Relations* 36(1):17–45, 1997.

Siegrist, J. Adverse health effects of high-effort/low-reward conditions. *J Occup Health Psychol* 1(1):27–41, 1996.

Söderfeldt, B., Söderfeldt, M., Jones, K., O'Camp, P., Muntaner, C., Ohlson, C. G. and Warg, L. E. Does organization matter? A multilevel analysis of the demand-control model applied to human services. *Soc Sci Med* 44(4):527–534, 1997.

Sorenson, G. and Himmelstein, J. Worksite intervention. In: Ockene, I. S. and Ockene, J. K. (eds.). *Prevention of Coronary Heart Disease.* Boston, MA: Little, Brown and Company, 1992.

Spalter-Roth, R. M., Kalleberg, A. L., Rasell, E., Cassirer, N., Reskin, B. F., Hudson, K., Webster, D., Applebaum, E. and Dooley, B. L. *Managing Work and Family: Nonstandard Work Arrangements Among Managers and Professionals.* Washington, DC: Economic Policy Institute and Women's Research and Education Institute, 1997.

Szabo, R. M. and Madison, M. Carpal Tunnel Syndrome as a work-related disorder. In: Gordon, S. L., Blair, S. J. and Fine, L. J. (eds.). *Repetitive Motion Disorders of the Upper Extremity.* Rosemont, IL: American Academy of Orthopaedic Surgeons, pp. 421–434, 1995.

Tomaskovic-Devey, D. *Gender and Racial Inequality at Work: The Sources and Consequences of Job Segregation.* Ithaca, NY: ILR Press, 1993.

Walsh, D. C., Sorensen, G. and Leonard, L. Gender, health, and cigarette smoking. In: Amick, B. C., Levine, S., Tarlov, A. R. and Walsh, D. C. (eds.). *Society and Health.* New York: Oxford University Press, pp. 131–171, 1995.

Whitehead, M. The health divide. In: Townsend, P., Davidson, N. and Whitehead, M. *Inequalities in Health.* London: Penguin, 1990.

World Bank. *World Development Report 1995: Workers in an Integrating World.* New York: Oxford University Press, p. 28, 1995.

❦

Eleven

SOCIAL RELATIONS, HIERARCHY, AND HEALTH

Richard G. Wilkinson

This paper argues that the most important influence on health in modern societies is the nature of the social environment which is, in turn, powerfully determined by the extent of economic inequality in society.

INTRODUCTION

WHAT the accumulated body of research on health inequalities tells us is, above all, that social and economic factors are much the most powerful determinants of population health. That is not because medical care is ineffective; rather it is because the small improvements which medical care makes to survival rates once a person has some life-threatening disease are completely overshadowed by what may be the two to five fold differences in the rates at which richer and poorer people get these diseases. This is particularly clear in countries where the vast majority of the population have access to the same medical care system.

DIFFERENCES WITHIN AND BETWEEN SOCIETIES

TO say that health is determined by socioeconomic factors is little more than to say that people's health is affected by the kind of life they lead. We know that individuals who are better-off, who are better educated, or live and work in better conditions tend to be healthier. Figure 1 shows the remarkably steep and regular gradients in self-reported health among Kansans classified by years of education and by household income. But although the data is impressive and these gradients have been replicated hundreds of times, it does not necessarily mean that if everyone was twice as well educated or twice as rich, that the health of the whole society would improve as much as this data might seem to suggest.

One of the most important issues in gaining an understanding of population health has gone almost unnoticed for many years because research has concentrated on studies of individuals—albeit sometimes very large numbers of individuals. It is possible that much of the advantage of a better education to the individual is that it slots you into a higher status position in societies by giving you access to higher status jobs. Similarly, it might be that richer people are healthier than poorer people not just because their physical circumstances are healthier, but perhaps also because they have a superior social status. If social status does make a significant contribution to why richer or better educated individuals are healthier, then higher standards across society as a whole may not produce all the expected benefits. In a world that suggests that

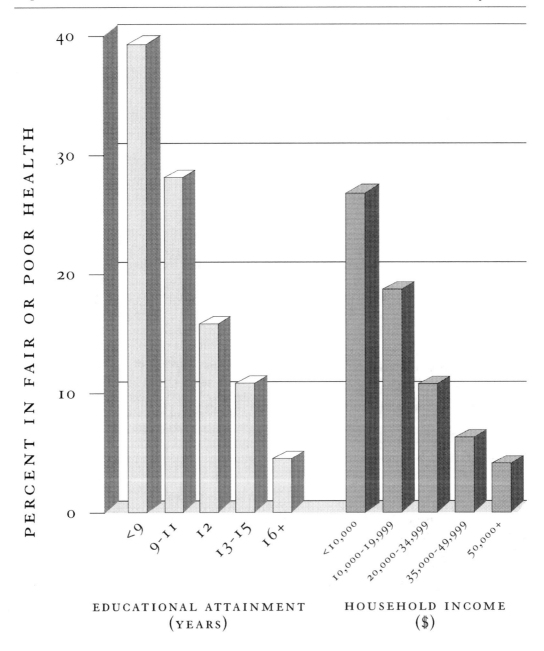

Source: Derived from 1993-1995 Kansas Behavioral Risk Factor Surveillance System Data Files.

Figure 1
Self-Assessed Health Status by Education and Household Income, Kansas, 1993–1995

standards of material consumption are what life is about, it may seem to stretch plausibility to question whether the most important part of the association between socioeconomic circumstances and health springs from the direct effects of the material environment itself. However, a closer look at the data shows that we do need to question it.

Let us look at the contrast in the relationship between income and health at different levels of analysis. Figure 2 shows that there is very little relationship between median state income and age-adjusted mortality rates for each state. In 1990 the correlation was -0.26. Cross-sectional and time series data for countries belonging to the Organization for Economic Cooperation and Development (OECD)—the rich market democracies—show an equally weak relationship. One U.S. state or developed country may be twice as rich as another and yet not enjoy lower mortality rates. Nor can the idea of a close relationship between living standards and mortality be saved by suggesting that it is hidden behind the effects of differences in income distribution. Rather than revealing a closer underlying connection, the effect of controlling the relationship shown in Figure 2 for income distribution is to entirely remove what little suggestion of a relationship there was. The correlation drops from -.026 to 0.06.[1]

The reason for this lack of relationship becomes clear when we look at the international relationship between Gross National Product per capita (GNPpc) and mortality among both rich and poor countries. The curve rises steeply among the poorer countries, but flattens out to become almost horizontal among the rich developed countries. Beyond a threshold level of material standards, additional consumption seems to make less difference to mortality rates.[2][3]

However, when we look at health or mortality data grouped by income levels within countries we see the kind of regular gradient shown for Kansans in Figure 1. Another example comes from men screened for the Multiple Risk Factor Intervention Trial (MRFIT). Their mortality rates are shown in Figure 3 grouped according to the median income of the zip code areas in which they lived.[4] Death rates are almost perfectly rank ordered across all 14 categories of income.

Why is the relationship between income and mortality so extraordinarily different within societies from what it is between societies and states? It is a difference that cannot be simply shrugged off or ignored. The suggestion that the relationship among OECD countries is somehow obscured by differences in national culture, by the healthy Mediterranean diet, or whatever, is belied first by the fact that you do not find a close relationship even when looking at changes in mortality and in GNPpc over a 23-year period (that is comparing each country with itself as it gets richer),[5] and second, by the fact that there is no clear relationship among the U.S. states although cultural differences are smaller and people shop at many of the same chain stores.

The only way of making sense of the contrasting picture coming from data within and between societies (or states), is to say that it is not absolute, but relative, income which is related to health. Where income has implications for social position or social status—as it does within societies—then it is related to measures of health. Where it has little or no implication for social status—the differences between societies for example—then it is not closely related to health.

The effect of this comes close to saying it is social position itself which influences health. But before going into that, let us first look at another similar but opposite pattern. Although the median incomes of the 50 U.S. states are not closely related to state mortality rates, the scale of income *inequality* (the gap between rich and poor) within each state is.[16] International comparisons show that the same is true of whole countries.[3] But if we move from these large areas to the opposite end of the scale, to small areas such as census tracts, we see the opposite picture. Median incomes for zip code areas are very closely related

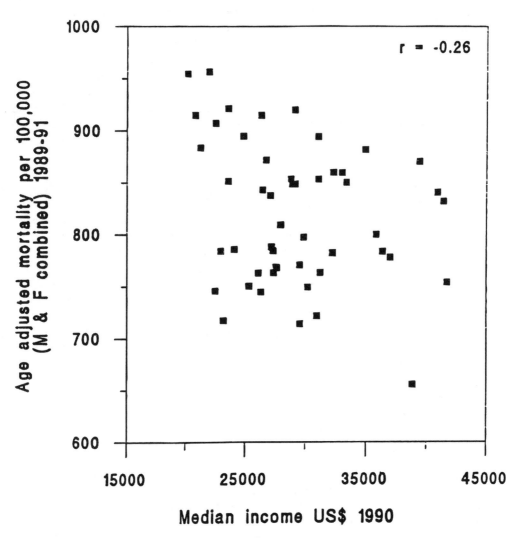

Figure 2
Age-Adjusted Mortality per 100,000 (M & F Combined) 1989–91
in Relation to Median Income in 1990 Among the 50 U.S. States

to mortality (as in Figure 3), but there is only a very weak relationship with income inequality within each area.[7][8] In large areas average income does not matter but income distribution does, whereas in small areas the situation is reversed. At the intermediate level, for instance among counties within the USA, there is some relationship with both income distribution and with average income.[9][8]

It is perhaps worth mentioning at this point that the picture of stronger relationships between health and inequality in larger than in smaller

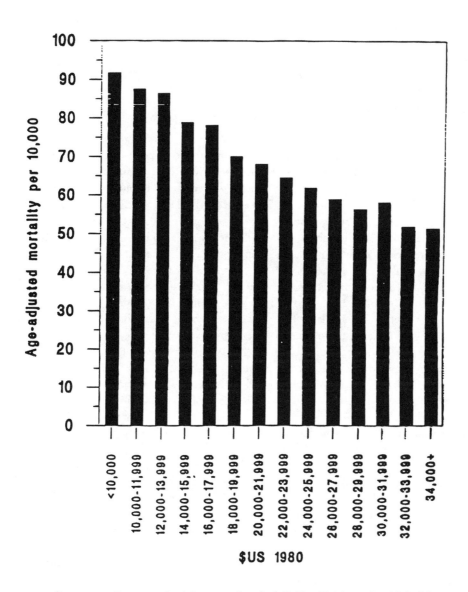

$US 1980

Source: Davey Smith et al., A.J.P.H. 1996; 86: 486-96

Figure 3
Age–Adjusted Mortality Rates by Median Family Income of Zip Code Areas: 300,000 White Men

areas has also been observed in studies of homicide and violent crime. A meta-analysis shows that they are reliably related to income inequality and that the relationships are stronger when the units of analysis are larger than when they are smaller.[10]

Once more, the most plausible interpretation of these patterns seems to be in terms of the health effects of social position and the scale of status differences. Income inequality is almost certainly related to health primarily because it serves as an indicator of the scale of the problem of relative deprivation or low social status in a society.[11 3] When we get down to the smallest areas, the patterns reverse because—at the extreme—we are getting closer to socially homogenous one class neighborhoods. In those areas people do not have bad health because of the inequality between them and their neighbors, but because they are all relatively deprived in relation to the wider society. Harlem has bad health not because of inequality within Harlem, but because the people of Harlem are so disadvantaged in relation to the wider society.[12] This tells us that what does the damage is less a matter of face to face inequality with neighbors, than something closer to the inferiority and low social status that come from a person's identity in terms of their class position in the wider society.

Although it might seem a major departure from the conventional wisdom to think that the relationship between people's socioeconomic circumstances and their health may be less a matter of the direct health impact of the material environment than of something closer to social status itself, it is hard to imagine how the data we have discussed could provide clearer support to that position. Such a view also makes it easier to understand why much of the data on socioeconomic circumstances and health does not show a sharp distinction between the poor, who do often have to contend with difficult material circumstances, and the rest of the population who rarely do. It tends instead to show a continuous health gradient across the whole society. We need a theory able to explain why there should be threefold differences in death rates for instance between senior and junior white collar workers in Government offices in London—almost all of whom would have called themselves "middle class."[13]

PSYCHOSOCIAL PATHWAYS AND SOCIAL STATUS

INCREASINGLY the evidence suggests that some of the most powerful influences on health in modern societies are psychosocial risk factors. If the socioeconomic gradient in health is less a matter of the absolute standard of living than it is of relative income and social status, then psychosocial pathways would seem to provide the most plausible links. Epidemiology has demonstrated the importance of a number of psychosocial risk factors including social integration,[14 15] being able to control one's work,[16 17] bereavement,[18] hopelessness,[19] anger,[20 21] life events,[22 23] as well as job and housing insecurity.[24 25]

My very limited understanding of the biology through which psychosocial factors affect physical health suggests that they do so because they are sources of chronic anxiety. As such, they trigger the stress response that prepares the body for muscular exertion. But as well as mobilizing energy for the muscles, resources are reduced for a wide range of other bodily functions which are not essential when facing a brief emergency. These include tissue maintenance and repair, digestion, immunity, growth, and reproductive functions.[26] If the emergency—escaping from an imminent physical threat—is short and everything can go back to normal as soon as you are safe, then there are no serious consequences. But when the anxiety lasts for weeks, months, or years, there is a wide range of possible health consequences. In addition, there are mechanisms through which exposure to chronic stress leads to a vicious circle ratcheting up the basal level of stress hormones such as cortisol. Higher levels of cortisol then damage the neurones in the hippocampus which are the sensors for the regulatory mechanism controlling cortisol levels, thus causing the whole system to move up a point on the ratchet.[27]

The wide range of health problems for which risks are increased by chronic anxiety means that the results may look much like more rapid aging.[26] Indeed, this kind of mechanism, if it is biologically sound,[28] [29] seems to provide something close to the general vulnerability factor which several people have suggested was implied by the very wide range of causes of death that show a socioeconomic gradient.[30] [31] It also enables us to understand how three different kinds of contribution to this general vulnerability come together. For some years there has been a tendency for research workers to emphasize either the lifelong effects of the environment in early childhood, or the health effects of people's cumulative experience of deprivation throughout life, or the more immediate importance of current circumstances. But now we know that stress responses can be set differently throughout life by the effects of the early emotional environment;[32] [33] [34] we also know that the effects of chronic anxiety are cumulative as they ratchet up basal cortisol levels; and lastly, we know that living with stress in the current environment is also important. Thus the biological effects of chronic anxiety are a candidate for unifying what once seemed very different approaches to understanding the social gradient in health.

Although it is still too early for much research specifically on the role of cortisol in the socioeconomic health gradient in human populations, there is beginning to be evidence suggesting a major contribution. Kristenson[35] found that both the class gradients in health in Lithuania and Sweden as well as the differences between the two countries were related to higher basal cortisol levels and to an attenuated cortisol response to stress—both of which are known to be indicative of chronic anxiety. This seemed to be one of the most important pathways underlying the differences in coronary deaths and atherosclerosis found within and between the two countries. Other studies have also found an association between atherosclerosis and raised basal cortisol levels.[36] Arnetz et al[37] reported that HDL cholesterol and basal cortisol increased in people threatened with job loss and unemployment. A case-control study of breast cancer patients found that higher basal levels of cortisol and attenuated cortisol responses to stress were associated with breast cancer.[38] Several studies have reported that rising basal cortisol levels are related to cognitive impairment among the elderly.[39] [40]

The most likely explanation of the main psychosocial factors which epidemiological research has identified as risks for poor health and premature death is that they are all sources of chronic anxiety. For example, a sense of being in control of things suggests that there is nothing in your immediate situation—or on the horizon—that seems too big a threat to manage. Insecurity, on the other hand, whether about jobs, housing, or income, represents almost the opposite of control: you feel insecure because something disastrous may happen which you can do very little about. "Life events" research is similarly concerned with major events that pose worrying problems and may be important sources of anxiety. On the other hand, you would expect social support to reduce anxiety.

The Kansas data can be used to illustrate the component of general susceptibility in the socioeconomic gradient in health. Correlations between socioeconomic factors and all causes of death combined tend to be stronger than the correlations between those factors and any specific causes of death. Using data provided by the Kansas Health Institute, the variables picked out in a multiple regression as predictors of the age-adjusted all-causes death rates for the 105 Kansas counties were firearm injuries (here used as a so-cial indicator), the teenage pregnancy rate, and unemployment. These variables, acting as prox-ies effects of relative poverty on the social envi-ronment, produce a multiple r-square suggesting that they account together for about 44 percent of the variance in all causes of death among Kan-sas counties. But they are linked with the all-causes mortality rate not because they have an overwhelming influence on one or two particu-larly important causes of death. Instead, they are strongly linked to it because they have a minor influence on many different causes of death. Singh was kind enough to supply me with age-adjusted death rates from a number of specific causes of death among Kansas counties to illus-trate this. Table 1 shows that firearms injuries, teenage pregnancies, and unemployment are re-lated strongly to all causes of death because of the cumulative effects of weaker relationships with separate causes of death (i.e. the correlations in the first column are stronger than those in other columns). This is a very typical finding.

It can also be seen that the cause-specific death rates are pointing to the same source of increased health risk. The bottom row of Table 1 shows correlations between each cause of death and the predicted value of the all-causes death rate given by the regression which picked out firearms in-juries, teenage pregnancies, and unemployment. From that row it can be seen that it is not only the correlation with the all-causes death rates which

is highest against the predicted value. Almost all the cause-specific death rates show correlations as high or higher in the bottom row as in the other rows. (The most notable exception is for injuries, where the correlation with firearms in-juries is higher simply because firearm injuries are a large component of all deaths due to inju-ries.) Although other explanations for these pat-terns could be suggested, they are consistent with the existence of a common component of mor-tality in each cause that arises from the same so-cial environment as is identified by the mix of the three independent variables related to all-cause mortality.

The same process of widespread but minor in-fluences on many different causes of death ex-plains why, in the international data, each country can have a major socioeconomic gradient in health despite the contributions to the gradi-ent coming from quite different causes of death. Death rates from each specific cause of death are influenced by other more powerful factors that differ substantially from one country to another. But whatever a country's dominant causes of death, they are likely to contribute to a marked social gradient in the all-causes death rate.

To some, psychosocial pathways will seem less suitable for explaining the ill-health of the least well-off than they are for explaining the social gradient in health among better off people—such as the office workers in the Whitehall

Table 1

Correlations Between Social Indicators and Death Rates: 105 Counties in Kansas

Social indicator:-	All-causes	Infections	Respiratory	Cancers	Cardiovascular	Diabetes	Injury
Firearms injuries	0.44	0.17	0.27	0.20	0.20	0.13	0.36
Teenage pregnancies	0.52	0.36	0.38	0.29	0.34	0.24	0.10
Unemployment	0.54	0.34	0.23	0.39	0.42	0.15	0.15
Predicted all-causes dth rt.	0.68	0.39	0.38	0.41	0.44	0.22	0.28

Data provided by G. Singh.

Studies. But insecurity over jobs and housing, and worrying about debts or about whether you have enough money for food are potent sources of anxiety. Because material problems are inevitably a crucial source of stress, it will always be difficult to distinguish the pathways clearly. However, Sapolsky tells an indicative story about the bodies of paupers on which medical students in London used to learn anatomy. For a century or so up to the 1920s they worked almost exclusively on the bodies of paupers and became used to seeing what we now know were unusually large adrenal glands.[41] They assumed these were the normal size until they started to see much smaller adrenal glands from bodies donated by middle-class people for medical education and research. Sapolsky says the small size of these adrenals was initially put down to a disease— "idiopathic adrenal atrophy"—invented for the purpose. Only when it was realized that the paupers had enlarged adrenals because poverty is chronically stressful was this disorder transformed "into an embarrassing footnote." The result of absolute poverty is not therefore only its direct physical effects: the poor also suffer intense psychosocial effects.

One of the clearer signs of the role of anxiety in the causation of the ill-health associated with socioeconomic circumstances comes from the work on unemployment and health. When people started to do factory closure studies (partly as a way of finding out whether the unemployed were unhealthy because of their unemployment or whether they had become unemployed partly because of their poor health) they found that health began to worsen not simply when people became unemployed, but often months or even years before, when they first knew that there were going to be redundancies and so started to worry about losing their jobs.[24 42 43 44] This has led to the literature on the effect of job insecurity on health.

If stress is so closely related to the difficulties of material life it may seem to make little differ-

ence whether the pathways are psychosocial or not. But it does make a difference. First, to know that the health impact of unemployment has a large psychosocial component (as the research on job insecurity demonstrates) changes the way we understand the experience of unemployment. It shows that it is not normally a carefree state chosen by a happy-go-lucky minority who happen to expose themselves to some physical and behavioral health risks while enjoying their leisure. The psychosocial links to poor health (including raised suicide rates) show that the subjective reality is very different and much less likely to be a state which people would choose voluntarily. So the psychosocial links provide an important indicator of the experience of socioeconomic differences which modern societies need to understand. Second, to know that some of the health effects of material circumstances result from the way the anxiety they cause makes people more vulnerable to a wide range of diseases, is knowledge which is generalizable to numerous other situations that cause chronic anxiety in a way which a knowledge of disease-specific biochemical pathways is not. The psychosocial links empower people to think about the health implications of social and economic life themselves rather than being dependent on scientific expertise. Third, the psychosocial links with health are also the links that account for a wide range of other social problems. They make it clear why so many social problems are rooted in relative deprivation and so make it more likely that policy makers will avoid underestimating the benefits accruing to a new policy initiative. Lastly, the involvement of psychosocial pathways shows us how directly and profoundly human subjectivity is affected by social structure.

Material problems are not the only sources of anxiety related to socioeconomic status. Work on the physiological effects of social status among non-human primates shows that even when the diet and environment are held constant and social status is manipulated, lower social status can still be expected to have major health consequences. Shively has shown that among macaques in captivity lower social status is directly linked to increased atherosclerosis, central obesity, and higher cortisol levels. She says that her results "suggest that the stress of social subordination causes hypothalamic-pituitary-adrenal and ovarian disfunction."[45] Sapolsky, studying baboons in the wild, has also demonstrated strong links between lower social status and raised basal cortisol levels and lower cortisol responses to stress.[46]

If subordinate social status still has physiological effects among non-human primates even when social status is experimentally manipulated and diet and environment are held constant, it is hard to avoid the conclusion that low social status may itself be directly stressful. Monkeys do not after all suffer job insecurity or worry about paying the rent. Among humans the lack of a relationship between health and median state income—discussed above—points in the same direction. If health were related to material living standards themselves—whether through psychosocial or direct physical pathways—then there would surely be a relationship between median state income and health. These very different kinds of evidence both point to the centrality of social status itself as a cause of the socioeconomic gradient in health in human societies.

However, we should not assume that this is necessarily separate from the very much greater burden of financial and material problems faced by people on lower incomes. Worrying about debt, insecure jobs, housing, paying for children's clothes with the right brand labels or whatever, must be potent sources of chronic anxiety. If this is a source of ill health, as epidemiological studies suggest it is, how can this be consistent with the data showing that U.S. states or developed countries with higher absolute living standards show little or no tendency to have better health? The most likely way in which this apparent inconsistency could have arisen is for

the extent of worries about debts, insecurity, housing etc. to be a function not of absolute living standards but of income inequality. If the pressure to consume and the likelihood of people's resources getting overstretched was related to maintaining their self-respect and social position relative to rising societal standards of consumption, then it would lead to the scale of what appear to be poverty related problems in society being a function of income inequality rather than of inadequate economic growth.

A number of considerations point in this direction. First is the modern emphasis on defining poverty in relative rather than absolute terms.[47] The European Union defines poverty as the proportion of the population living on less than half the average income. Strong evidence of the empirical justification for using relative standards is provided by surveys of public opinion that show that an ever increasing range of goods is now regarded as necessities.[48] [49] Between 1973 and 1996 the proportion of Americans who regarded air conditioning as a necessity doubled from 26 to 51 percent, while those who regarded a second car as a necessity increased from 20 to 37 percent.[50] The importance of maintaining one's social position is demonstrated by studies that show the health effects and psychological trauma of downward mobility.[51] [52] [45] [53] Another indication that the apparent difficulties of material life are driven by social status rather than by the desire to attain some absolute level of living comes from the economic literature that suggests that saving is related to relative income.[54] During the last decade or so, while income differences have widened rapidly, the so-called aspirational incomes—which people imagine would satisfy all their material desires—shot up, while savings decreased and debt increased.[50] An economist who has produced a sustained argument that consumption and expenditure are motivated primarily by social status pressures rather than by a desire for any absolute level of material consumption is Frank.[55] In her book *The Overspent*

American, Schor[50] also argues that consumption is a competitive process fueled by insecurities about status. As she says, "We live with high levels of psychological denial about the connection between our buying habits and the social statements they make" (p. 19).

But rather than seeing the health gradient only as a consequence of the various material difficulties that may—in one society or another—happen to be the cultural concomitants of low social status, we need to think more about the direct (as opposed to the indirect effects) of low social status itself. Social status has always been so inseparable from material differences because it is, most fundamentally, a ranking of access to resources. What links human status hierarchies to social ranking in animals is that they are about what Gilbert[56] called "resource holding power." This is the common component behind all the different class schemas—whether we use the Erikson-Goldthorpe classification, the Cambridge scale, the British Registrar General's or—for that matter—the class divisions between freeman and slave, patrician and plebeian, lord and serf, guildmaster and journeyman, bourgeois and proletarian, which Marx saw as the driving force of history. In all of them, the hierarchy of access to resources is inevitably bound to the hierarchy of power which is needed to protect it.

So deeply rooted in us is this status hierarchy that we have different cardiovascular responses according to whether we are interviewed by a person of higher or lower social status than ourselves.[57] As every television sitcom writer knows, we quake before our superiors and look askance at those below us. But at the same time, the social hierarchy is read as a hierarchy of ability, as a ranking from the most able to the most inadequate, as if from the brightest to the stupidest. Indeed, in Sennett and Cobb's[58] study of U.S. auto workers, the message that comes across most clearly is that we infer ability—our own as well as that of others—from social position. Numerous psychological experiments make the same point. Status becomes synonymous with

social distance and important parts of our culture and aesthetic choices seem to be used as vehicles through which to express social distinctions.[59] Even without a caste system, social status permeates almost every aspect of life.

VIOLENCE AND SOCIAL RELATIONS

IN the Kansas Health Institute data book, the correlation between homicide and the age-adjusted death rate among the 50 U.S. states is -0.85. At a different level, Wilson and Daley showed that among some 77 neighborhoods in the Chicago area there was a 0.9 correlation between homicide and all other causes of death (excluding homicide). The implication is that the social milieu that produces high homicide rates is also the social milieu that produces high death rates from other causes. At first this may seem nothing more than a reflection of a relationship between deprivation and crime. But in an analysis of relationships among the U.S. states between income distribution, mortality, and different kinds of crime, Kawachi, Kennedy and I found that both mortality from all other causes and income distribution were specifically related to homicide and *violent* crime: there was no relationship at the state level between *property* crime and either mortality or income distribution.[60]

The association between homicide and other causes of death seems to be telling us something about the nature of the relationship between income distribution and mortality. We found that controlling for homicide rates entirely removed the close correlation between income distribution and mortality from all other causes (i.e. all-causes excluding homicide).[60] The relationship between mortality and income distribution has a number of characteristics in common with the relationship between homicide and income inequality. Both relationships have been shown at several different levels within the USA and internationally.[10 3] In addition, both show a tendency toward stronger relationships to be reported where income distribution is measured across larger areas. The implication seems to be that the relationship between income inequality and homicide is much like the relationship between income distribution and other causes of death. If we could identify the environmental component of homicide which is related to income inequality, it is likely that it would have much in common with the component of mortality which is related to income inequality.

When looking at literature on the causes of violence, we were struck by the repeated observation that it is often an attempt to defend one's dignity from insult triggered by people feeling that they had not been respected. Gilligan was a prison psychiatrist for 25 years before becoming director of the Center for the Study of Violence at the Harvard School of Public Health. He says:

> ". . . the prison inmates I work with have told me repeatedly, when I asked them why they had assaulted someone, that it was because 'he disrespected me' or 'he disrespected my visit' (meaning 'visitor'). The word 'disrespect' is central in the vocabulary, moral value system, and psychodynamics of these chronically violent men that they have abbreviated it into the slang term, 'he dis'ed me'."[61]

A few pages further on Gilligan continues:

> "I have yet to see a serious act of violence that was not provoked by the experience of feeling shamed and humiliated, disrespected and ridiculed, and that did not represent the attempt to prevent or undo this 'loss of face'—no matter how severe the punishment, even if it includes death." (p.110)[61]

This is not a view that applies only to prison violence or merely reflects the vantage point of the psychiatrist. McCall,[62] who was brought up in considerable poverty in Virginia and was himself imprisoned for violence before becoming a journalist, says in his autobiography:

> "For as long as I can remember, black folks have had a serious thing about respect. I guess it's because white people disrespected them so blatantly for so long that blacks viciously protected what little morsels of self-respect they thought they had left. Some

of the most brutal battles I saw in the streets stemmed from seemingly petty stuff . . . But the underlying issue was always respect. You could ask a guy, "Damn, man, why did you bust that dude in the head with a pipe?"
>
> And he might say, "The motherfucka disrespected me!"
>
> That was explanation enough. It wasn't even necessary to explain how the guy had disrespected him. It was universally understood that if a dude got disrespected, he had to do what he had to do.
>
> It's still that way today. Young dudes nowadays call it "dissin'."
>
> They'll kill a nigger for dissin' them. Won't touch a white person, but they'll kill a brother in a heartbeat over a perceived slight. This irony was that white folks constantly disrespected us in ways seen and unseen, and we tolerated it. Most blacks understood that the repercussions were more severe for retaliating against whites than for doing each other in. It was as if black folks were saying, "I can't do much to keep whites from dissin' me, but I damn sure can keep black folks from doing it."[62]

This description of street violence from someone who had experienced it firsthand is almost identical to Gilligan's. But Gilligan also emphasizes the importance of an underlying sense of shame which makes respect such an important and sensitive issue. He says:

> "Behind the mark of 'cool' or self-assurance that many violent men clamp onto their faces—with a desperation born of the certain knowledge that they would 'lose face' if they ever let it slip—is a person who feels vulnerable not just to 'loss of face' but to the total loss of honor, prestige, respect, and status—the disintegration of identity, especially their adult, masculine, heterosexual identity; their selfhood, personhood, rationality, and sanity."[61]

In this context, it would be obtuse to avoid the conclusion that the most plausible reason for the relationship between income inequality and homicide is that wider income differences exacerbate problems of respect. By making the status differences bigger, and excluding more people from the traditional economic and social sources of status, sensitivity to these issues is inevitably heightened.

The evidence that greater income inequality leads to increased violence, but not to increased property crime, suggests that what is hardest to bear about low relative income is less the material deprivation itself but its social meaning, the lack of a sense of being valued and respected and the shame or stigma which attach to low social status. We are perhaps inherently sensitive to this social dimension of inequality. Indeed, it has been suggested that depression and violence have served evolutionary as two different responses to low social status.[56][63] Depression, it has been suggested, is a form of submission and reflects acceptance of defeat, whereas violence has often served as a contestation of social status. Interestingly, both are linked to low serotonin[64][65][63] which in turn is linked to low social status in a number of species.[66][67][63] (Without an explanation that suggests that in a pre-human existence the submissive/subordinate behavior associated with depression may at least have had the survival value of avoiding further conflict with superiors, it is difficult to see why we should all be so vulnerable to such an extraordinarily incapacitating frame of mind. Apart from the serotonin link, the work on learned helplessness and depression is probably the most obvious indication of a possible link with acceptance of defeat.)

From the health point of view, homicide perhaps serves as a signal of the anxiety and stressfulness of low social status and how these problems are exacerbated by wider income differences. The same anxieties that come from feeling put down, ashamed, not respected or valued, and that feed into what we should perhaps see as a kind of defensive violence, also feed into the chronic anxiety that seems to operate as a general health vulnerability factor. It is not that social status matters more to the poor than the rich: it is simply that getting it is more problematic for the poor. Indeed, Adam Smith[68] saw the desire for what he called "regard" as one of the great driving forces in everyone's economic activity. He asked:

"What is the end of avarice and ambition, of the pursuit of wealth, of power and pre-eminence? Is it to supply the necessities of nature? The wage's of the meanest labourer can supply them . . . what are the advantages which we would propose to gain by that great purpose of human life which we call bettering our condition? To be observed, to be attended to, to be taken notice of with sympathy, complacency, and approbation, are all the advantages which we can propose to derive from it." (Book i, ch. ii.i)

Another piece of this social status and health jigsaw comes from the work on social relations (or social integration) and health. What is puzzling about this work is not only that almost any measure of social relations seems to be related to health, but also that many of these relationships are so strong. Thus Cohen et al.[14] showed that when people are given nasal drops containing cold viruses, those with friends in few areas of life are over four times as likely to develop colds as people with friends in many areas of life. In a review of epidemiological studies of social integration, House et al.[69] reported that death rates were two, three, and four times as high among those who were less highly integrated in their communities than those who were more socially integrated. In a more recent review, Berkman reported that studies had shown survival rates after myocardial infarction were sometimes almost halved among people who were socially isolated. In terms of relative risk, these differences are very large: in terms of population attributable risk, they are likely to be among the most important risk factors known. But the question I want to ask is what is it about our psychosocial make up which accounts for these powerful associations between health and social relationships?

Among our pre-human ancestors friendship has always been very important in relation to hierarchy. Frequently one's safety depended on ones ability to make alliances. Similarly, position in the social hierarchy and success in improving or defending one's social position were dependent on alliances. Non-human primates spend a vast amount of time grooming each other in order to make these alliances. As Jolly[70] said, grooming constitutes "the social cement of primates from lemur to chimpanzee." Given that other members of one's own species can compete with us for everything (food, shelter, jobs, clothing, sexual partners), but can also be the greatest source of comfort, help, love, and support, people's ability to keep social relationships sweet has always been a crucial determinant even of their material welfare. Small wonder then that touch—grooming—remains emotionally soothing and comforting for us and a powerful indicator of a sympathetic bond. So much so that even having a pet seems to have a beneficial effect on cardiovascular function.[71] The close relationship between these alliances and position in the social hierarchy can be judged from the fact that among some non-human primates position in the social hierarchy does not correlate well with size or strength but seems to have more to do with an animal's social skills.[72]

At this point it might be worth mentioning the work of Erdal and Whiten[73] on the egalitarianism of primitive hunting and gathering societies. Surveying the literature from over 100 anthropological accounts of some 24 recent hunter and gatherer societies spread over four continents, they were led to the conclusion that these societies were characterized by:

> "Egalitarianism, cooperation and sharing on a scale unprecedented in primate evolution . . . They share food, not simply with kin or even just with those who reciprocate, but according to need even when food is scarce . . . There is no dominance hierarchy among hunter-gatherers. No individual has priority of access to food which . . . is shared. In spite of the marginal female preference for the more successful hunters as lovers, access to sexual partners is not a right which correlates with rank. In fact rank is simply not discernible among hunter-gatherers. This is a cross cultural universal, which rings out unmistakably from the ethnographic literature, sometimes in the strongest terms." (pp. 140–144)

I mention this now not primarily to show that our human ancestors avoided the social and psychic costs of inequality—though that is important, but because it is suggested that they did so on the basis of a kind of alliance which Erdal and Whiten call a "counter dominance strategy." Rather than reflecting an outbreak of selflessness, Erdal and Whiten[74] say that the sharing was what they characterize as "vigilant" sharing, with people watching to see fair play and to ensure that they were not disadvantaged. They suggest that a counter-dominance strategy functioned as an alliance of everyone against anyone who tried to gain a superior position.

Alliances are then in some sense a protection from hierarchy, creating islands of equality cutting across the divisive dominance hierarchy. They are areas of mutuality that contrast with the dominance hierarchy based on power and self-interest. Friendship is about mutuality and provides a haven running counter to the hierarchical relations with their marked absence of mutuality. Friendship is safety, security, and mutual support, whereas hierarchy is competitive, oppositional, dog eat dog. This is surely why social relations are seen as offsetting the effects of stress. We evolved, after all, in a situation where the most important resources were not hoards of private goods or wealth, but friendship and relations of mutuality.

The opposition between these two can be seen in some work on social cohesion and inequality. In his work on the strength of civic life in Italy, Putnam[75] says: "Political leaders in the civic regions are more enthusiastic supporters of political equality than their counterparts in less civic regions" (p. 102). "Citizens in the more civic regions, like their leaders, have a pervasive distaste for hierarchical authority patterns" (p. 104). He concludes by saying, "Equality is an essential feature of the civic community" (p. 105).

These observations are based partly on empirical measures of the strength of people's involvement in local community life, and partly on interviews with people and politicians in each region. Throughout he is talking more of an egalitarian social ethos than of income inequality itself. However, in a footnote (p. 224 note 52) he does say that there is a correlation of 0.81 between greater income inequality in each of the Italian regions and a lower score on his index of the strength of people's involvement in community life.

Kawachi and Kennedy[76] found that a measure they called "social trust" (the proportion of people in each state who agreed that "most people would try to take advantage of you if they got the chance") was very closely correlated with income distribution (r = 0.7) and mortality (r = 0.8) across the states. On the basis of a path analysis they suggested that the relationship between income inequality and mortality went through social trust—which should perhaps be interpreted as an indicator of how hostile or hospitable people experience their social environment as being.

Another example of the relationship between the amount of inequality and the nature of the social environment is derived from Williams et al.[77] Following work on hostility as a risk factor for cardiovascular disease, they commissioned Gallup to administer the Minnesota Hostility Scale to ten samples of 200 people, one in each of ten U.S. cities chosen as cities with a wide spread of different mortality rates. They found a close correlation between the average hostility scores in each city and its mortality rate. Surprised that there were such important differences in each city's hostility scores, I checked and found them also to be closely related to income distribution (income distribution data was kindly supplied by John Lynch—personal communication).

We have then four indications that there is a strong connection between the extent of inequality and the nature of the social environment in different places. First is the relationship between income inequality and homicide which has been reported within the U.S. as well as internationally; second are Putnam's[75] observations from his study of civic community in Italy; third is Kawachi et al.'s[76] data on social trust and mortality; and fourth is the relationship between Williams et al.'s[77] hostility scores, mortality and income distribution in ten U.S. cities.

In addition to this statistical data, I have discussed a number of examples of societies that were unusually egalitarian and unusually healthy.[3] They included the Italian American town of Roseto in Pennsylvania,[78] Britain during the First and Second World Wars, Japan, and Eastern Europe during the 1970s and '80s. Each example showed remarkably clear evidence that trends in health were related to trends in social cohesion and inequality.

The combined weight of this evidence makes it clear that wider income differences are inimical to good social relations. The most plausible guess is that, as inequality increases, the agonistic relations of hierarchy grow stronger at the expense of the mutuality of friendship. In Putnam's terms, vertical links (such as patron/client dependencies) come to predominate over the more sociable horizontal links.

In the light of the evidence of less good social relations in societies with bigger income inequalities, the work on social integration and health seems to provide the necessary stepping stone allowing us to cross from income distribution to health. However, I am not convinced that these measures of social relations at the societal level, that is to say of social cohesion, are doing all the work simply on that level. The studies of the links between social relations and health show that the relationship between them works perfectly well at the individual level. Rather than having to live in more cohesive societies, they show that if any *individual* has more friends, better social support, or is more involved with local associations, he or she will have better health. So social cohesion may not be involved in the causation of health or illness as a societal variable, but simply as a summary of individual social integration. But if the health causation need not work at the societal level, then we have to assume that it is involved in the reasons why the average person in more egalitarian communities (whether they are whole countries, U.S. states, or cities) has more friends or is more socially integrated—or, if we stick closer to the evidence we have, why they are more trusting of others, less hostile and less likely to be violent— than people in less egalitarian communities.

There seems little reason to believe that these social relations variables—which are merely those that happen to have been measured in relation to income distribution—are themselves doing all the work in relation to health. They probably derive much of their statistical power from acting as proxies for a range of related social variables. It is likely that different measures of the quality of social relations move together with similar patterns of variability—and this is probably true whether the units of observation are individuals or communities. Homicide should probably not be regarded simply as a bizarre form of behavior unrelated to anything else. The fact that violent crime and hostility measures are also related to income inequality means that there is a shift in the whole tenor of relationships toward the more aggressive, conflictual end of the spectrum and there is no reason to think that it is limited to life on the streets. The chances are that if we had the data we would find that domestic conflict also occurred more frequently, and close confiding relationships less frequently, in less egalitarian places. At the individual level, there are well established links both between the psychosocial stresses of living in relative poverty and the increased likelihood of domestic conflict, and between the experience of domestic conflict in childhood and later violence.[79]

Rose showed that the reason why more people were at high risk from different risk factors (such as blood pressure, cholesterol levels, alcohol intake) in one society rather than another, was not that the distribution of that risk factor had a longer tail of high risk in that society, but that the whole society's distribution of risk was shifted upward. In other words, the proportion at high risk in a society is a function of the average risk in that society: more people are hypertensive, obese, or have drinking problems in a society because the average blood pressure, body mass index, or alcohol intake is higher. Perhaps we should think in terms of a distribution of the character of social interaction in a society, moving from highly supportive to highly aggressive, and interpreting measures such as homicide or violent crime simply as the extreme end of these distributions of risk telling us where the whole pattern of social interaction in a society is centered—whether nearer the more supportive or aggressive end of the spectrum.

GENDER

BUT perhaps we can perhaps go farther than that and identify what might be called a *"culture of inequality."* Although all the major categories of causes of death (such as respiratory diseases, infections, cardiovascular diseases, cancers etc.) tend to be more common in less egalitarian countries, the closest relationships in terms of the percentage increases are found in causes like homicide, accidents, alcohol related deaths, and infections.[1][80] These seem indicative of effects on the social fabric and are added to the picture of social causation in the link between income distribution and mortality. But accidents, alcohol, and violence also suggest that the mortality impact might be greatest among young men, particularly single young men. As a result, one might expect the mortality differential both between men and women and between married and single people to be greater in less egalitarian places. There is evidence supporting both these expectations. Look first at Eastern Europe in the 1970s and 1980s when mortality rates ceased to fall or started to rise (long before 1989). These adverse trends can most plausibly be laid at the door of the growth of inequality and the loss of social cohesion in those societies.[81] Particularly prominent are the rises in mortality from deaths related to alcohol and violence. But what is most interesting is that the rise in mortality seems to have been largely confined to single men and women and was particularly marked among single men.[82 83]

Another pointer to how these things fit together comes from Kawachi et al.[84] Compiling indices of women's economic and political status among the 50 states of the USA, they found that improved status was significantly associated with lower mortality rates for women. However, they also found that there were closer relationships between improved status of women and lower male mortality. In short, improvements in women's status were more closely related to lower male than female mortality. (The position of women has long been recognized as a powerful correlate of mortality in developing countries.[85] Kawachi et al. refer to evidence provided by Yllo[86] indicating that rates of severe marital violence against women were highest in the states where gender inequality was greatest. A plausible explanation of these connections is that the more aggressive culture associated with wider income differences is also a more macho culture in which women are subordinated and their political and economic status suffers. It has already been shown that where income inequality is greater among men, women suffer a larger economic disadvantage.[87] Improvements in women's status depend on more sociable conditions (where violence less often prevails) which are associated with greater equality. Male mortality then shows bigger improvements than female mortality because the more aggressive, macho culture of inequality affects male death rates even more than female.

An important problem which has not yet been mentioned centers on the fact that widening income differences appear to do more damage to social cohesion among the poor than they do to any notional cohesion between rich and poor. Except during riots and revolutions, the increased violence is not between rich and poor so much as among the poor themselves. This is part of a fairly general tendency to try to gain or main-

tain status by putting down those who may be considered weaker. The phenomenon of scapegoating racial and other minorities in times of high unemployment is only too familiar. In general, processes of discrimination and intolerance thrive when people are denied access to other forms of social and economic status. We have already touched on two examples: one was the tendency to greater oppression of women where there is greater inequality among men, and the second was the violence directed at other blacks rather than whites which McCall mentioned in the quote above (p. 216). The links between a male sense of inferiority, a macho culture, and repression of women are clearly expressed in this quote from Anzaldua,[88] who comes from the Hispanic Chicano culture where the machismo developed its current meaning. She says:

> "For men like my father, being 'macho' meant being strong enough to protect and support my mother and us, yet being able to show love. Today's macho has doubts about his ability to feed and protect his family. His 'machismo' is an adaptation to oppression and poverty and low self-esteem. It is the result of hierarchical male dominance. The Anglo, feeling inadequate and inferior and powerless, displaces or transfers these feelings to the Chicano by shaming him. In the Gringo world, the Chicano suffers from excessive humility and self-effacement, shame of self and self-deprecation.

> "The loss of a sense of dignity and respect in the macho breeds a false machismo which leads him to put down women and even to brutalize them. Coexisting with his sexist behavior is a love of the mother which takes precedence over that of all others. Devoted son, macho pig. To wash down the shame of his acts, of his very being, and to handle the brute in the mirror, he takes to the bottle, the snort, the needle and the fist."[88]

The tendency to assert status over inferiors when threatened with a loss of status is widely recognized among primatologists. When an animal loses a battle for rank with another there is often a tendency to show what can easily be dismissed simply as "displaced" aggression. But in fact, the aggression is systematically turned on subordinate animals as if to reassert, or prevent further loss of, status. Volker Sommer (personal communication 1997) explained:

> "the phenomenon is termed *"radfahrer-reaktion"* in German, (bicycling-reaction), because the animal shows its back to the top (of the social hierarchy) while kicking towards the bottom. It is very common in non-human primates: after having received aggression from a higher ranking individual, they will redirect aggression towards lower ranking ones."

This does not necessarily mean the behavior has a genetic component in humans: it could instead reflect a common situational logic. But either way, it is a dangerous effect that seems to be rooted in status insecurity which we would do well to recognize. McCall described people who "viciously protected what little morsels of self-respect they thought they had left," Anzaldua and Gilligan talked about violent responses to shame. We can see this pattern not only in the situations of individual violence already mentioned and in the rise of extreme right-wing nationalist movements of racial intolerance during periods of high unemployment, but also in things like school bullying, where the perpetrators are likely to be insecure children who have been put down or exposed to violence at home or elsewhere. As well as the actual violence which may come from this source, we are all familiar with a wide range of social behavior rooted in insecurity—criticisms intended to put people down, scoring off people or attempts to demonstrate some cheap superiority, and so on. Essentially, they are forms of behavior which more confident and secure people should find it easier to avoid.

Childhood Socialization

AT this point we arrive at what seems to be the boundary between a more sociological analysis, centered on social structure, and a more psychological analysis that seems to be based on personality characteristics. There is of course a

remarkable contrast between the sociological and psychological literature in the treatment of social status. Social stratification and social class are the backbone of sociology—the literature is full of them. In contrast, social status seems almost absent from the psychological literature. On the other hand, the psychological literature is full of material on the importance of emotional experience in early childhood. But despite the apparent contrast between them, in a very important sense both these literatures are about fears of inadequacy, security, and insecurity. The emotional insecurity that comes from not having experienced love and appreciation as a child feeds directly into the insecurities about social status and whether one is respected and valued as an adult. It is a truism to talk about the psychological parallels between the experience of being a child in the family and an adult in society; or between the way we experience the authority of parents and the authority of those in positions of power over us in society. But although there are psychological echoes from one to the other, it would be a mistake to suggest that we cannot experience them independently. There are reasons for thinking that a large part of what often appear to be personality characteristics is in fact dependent on the social situation.[89] Nevertheless, insecurities from childhood are likely to exacerbate the insecurities which go with low social status in society. If, as suggested earlier, the social hierarchy presents itself to us as if it were a hierarchy of human adequacy, from the most superior to the most inferior human being, both sources of insecurity will seem to call into question our personal adequacy and confidence.

The extent to which these two sources of security or insecurity lead to vicious or virtuous spirals can be seen from an analysis of data from the cohort of Britons born in 1958 whose growth, development, education and careers have been followed through since birth. It has long been known that taller people are more likely to move up the social ladder and tend to be healthier. The common assumption was that this was somehow because they were better physical specimens and that perhaps there is a psychological tendency to look up to taller people and give them the benefit of the doubt at interview. However Montgomery et al.[90] found that upward social mobility was actually much more closely related to height at age seven than to adult height. The implication of this is that the success of tall people is nothing to do with their physical presence as adults, but is related to something in early childhood that affects both their growth and their later social mobility. In trying to identify what this factor was, it became clear that there are a number of psychosocial correlates of slow growth,[91] and some evidence from a natural experiment that psychosocial factors play a causal role in slow growth.[92] Most recently, Montgomery et al.[93] showed that slow growth in childhood was strongly associated with family conflict and that the association could plausibly be explained in terms of the influence of stress on the growth hormone. If height was a reflection of emotional trauma in childhood, then it is likely that the less good social mobility of these children in adulthood was a reflection of their social and emotional development—in other words tall people are more likely to be upwardly mobile because they are also more likely to be in good emotional shape.

As well as the psychological literature showing the life-long importance of early social environment, there is a growing body of experimental evidence from other mammalian species showing that the early environment has effects on stress responses throughout life. Neonatal handling of rats has been shown to lead to lower endocrine responses to stress, lower basal cortisol levels, and less stress-related impairment of cognitive functioning.[94][32] Similar effects have been shown to follow from the amount of maternal licking and grooming neonatal rats get: indeed, a study concludes that maternal behavior serves to "program" hypothalamic-pituitary-adrenal responses to stress in the offspring.[33] Similar changes in stress responses have been found

among monkeys brought up without parental attention.[95] Among humans it has also been shown that there are important differences in cognitive functioning (suggestive of differences in basal cortisol levels) attributable to differences in childhood circumstances.[96][39][97]

If we were to draw a kind of flow diagram, the socialization of children in the family would form a kind of subsystem increasing vulnerability to the main effects of economic inequality in society. As the inequality increases, the socialization of children is pervaded more and more by the aggressive culture of inequality. Instead of the family forming what Lasch[98] called a "haven in a heartless world," an island of mutuality providing some protection from the antagonisms of inequality in the wider society, those antagonisms increasingly leak into it. Family life in conditions of relative poverty becomes increasingly strained, the incidence of domestic conflict rises, and a higher proportion of children grow up with varying amounts of insecurity and emotional damage, predisposing them to educational failure and violence.[79]

At one level there is the feedback from the harshness of the adult environment to childrearing practices. If life on the streets is tough and children get bullied at school, then parents have to bring up their children tougher—if they grow up too soft in a tough culture, they will be picked on. But the social skills and behavior appropriate to surviving on the streets in the poor inner city areas are not the most appropriate for getting on in the job market. Although the resulting higher basal cortisol levels and stress responses would perhaps have had survival value in a harsher social environment, too often family life is rendered dysfunctional: the associations between relative poverty and increased domestic conflict show how the effects of a more stressful environment for parents shorten fuses and increase the amount of conflict in childrearing.

On top of this are the problems of the legitimacy of the social institutions in societies that exclude a significant proportion of the population from the jobs, incomes, status and respect available to others. As income differences widen, political participation diminishes.[76] Although most of the conflict is among the poor themselves, the antagonism toward mainstream society is expressed in the counterculture. If you cannot join it, you can perhaps maintain some self-respect and avoid some of the humiliation of being excluded by expressing your rejection of its values.

Both countercultural values and higher basal cortisol levels embedded from childhood are strongly related to health in later life. Not only is domestic conflict in early childhood predictive of health in adulthood,[99] [100] but in the 1958 cohort study it was found that teachers' assessment of children's behavior was the best single predictor of health in early adulthood—a finding that neatly expresses the role of social stress and conflict in health.[101]

POLICY

ONE of the most important reasons for recognizing the psychosocial nature of the link between relative deprivation and health is that there is then no difficulty in understanding why relative poverty, low social status, and inequality carry such a wide range of social costs. We have already seen that violence is closely related to inequality and it is well established that the repercussions of inequality on family life and childhood experience also feed into crime[102] [103] and a wide range of other problems, including educational failure.[3] Unless the psychosocial connections are recognized, the way ill health and other social problems arise from relative deprivation will remain mysterious and the likelihood of the necessary policy initiatives will become more remote.

In terms of policy, there are two points to be made. The first concerns the need to change our understanding of the quality of life so that we recognize that improvements in the quality of the social environment are now more important than increased levels of material consumption. The second is to bear in mind that the evidence suggests somewhere between one-third and two-thirds of the variations in death rates, in homicide and in measures of social cohesion seem to be accounted for by differences in income distribution alone. The social environment is built on economic foundations, and its most powerful known determinant seems to be income inequality. While that must be the prime objective, there are almost certainly other things that also make a difference. If the key issues are inequality, low social status, and people feeling belittled, inferior and excluded, then perhaps we should do a social audit of schools, workplaces, and other institutions to try to minimize practices that divide people, put people down, which emphasize marks of distinction and hierarchy by raising some at the expense of others. Instead we need to improve the cohesiveness of our institutions and strengthen the ways in which they give people a sense of belonging and of being valued.

The view I have rejected—of health being influenced primarily by the direct material effects of relative deprivation—reflects what seems to me to be an insufficiently social view of humanity. In societies less dominated by the values of the market and consumerism we might start out from a more social view of ourselves and be better able to understand the impact of social structure itself.

The impact of hierarchy and social fragmentation is perhaps what lies behind the age rise in blood pressure found in all but the earliest forms of society. Reviewing data from some 84 societies Waldron et al.[104] and more recently Eyer[105] have suggested that the more monetized and developed an economy is, the greater the age rise in blood pressure. They found no age rise among hunting and gathering societies or among pastoralists. The age rise in blood pressure begins among agriculturalists and increases with economic development. Given the possibility that both the age rise in blood pressure and in cortisol may reflect some common causes, this is particularly interesting. Although Waldron et al. controlled for salt intake, their data do not allow us to do more than guess at causes. However, Timio et al.[106] suggest that the key factor is social relations. Over 20 years follow-up, they found no age rise in blood pressure among Italian nuns belonging to a closed order—despite the fact that they were eating a diet much like that eaten by a control group of local women whose blood pressure continued to rise. Timio et al. concluded: "Increased blood pressure in women over 20 years may be avoided by living in a stress-free monastic environment characterised by silence, meditation, and isolation from society."

The secondary part played by absolute material standards is strikingly demonstrated by the fact that in 1990 China's life expectancy was as high as the USA's had been only 20 years earlier in 1970. Yet the large majority of the Chinese still lived in what would seem to us pretty squalid conditions, often overcrowded and eating adequate, but very basic food. With a real Gross Domestic Product per capita of less than one-tenth of that of the U.S., only one in five households had a refrigerator and only just over a quarter had a washing machine.[107] Most had neither. How many were without hot water, proper drainage or flush lavatories is not clear, but it must have been a large proportion. It would be wise therefore to see the material standards within the U.S. as related to health in relative rather than absolute terms. That also makes clear why, in that famous paper by McCord,[12] we find death rates in Harlem in New York to be higher at most ages than they are in rural Bangladesh.

NOTES

1. Kaplan GA, Pamuk, E, Lynch, JW, Cohen, RD and Balfour, JL. Inequality in income and mortality in the United States: analysis of mortality and potential pathways. *British Medical Journal* 1996; 312: 999–1003.

2. Wilkinson, RG. The epidemiological transition: from material scarcity to social disadvantage? *Daedalus* (Journal of the American Academy of Arts and Sciences) 1994; 123(4): 61–77.

3. Wilkinson, RG. *Unhealthy Societies: the afflictions of inequality*. Routledge, London 1996a.

4. Davey Smith, G, Neaton, JD and Stamler, J. Socioeconomic differentials in mortality risk among men screened for the Multiple Risk Factor Intervention Trial I. White Men. *American Journal of Public Health*, 1996; 86: 486–96.

5. Wilkinson, RG. (1997a) Health inequalities: relative or absolute material standards? *British Medical Journal*; 314: 591–5.

6. Kennedy, BP, Kawachi, I and Prothrow-Stith, D. Income distribution and mortality: cross sectional ecological study of the Robin Hood index in the United States. *British Medical Journal* 1996; 312: 1004–7. See also: Kennedy, BP, Kawachi, I and Prothrow-Stith, D. Important correction. Income distribution and mortality: cross sectional ecological study of the Robin Hood index in the United States. *British Medical Journal* 1996; 312: 1194.

7. Wilkinson, RG. (1997b) Income, inequality and social cohesion. *American Journal of Public Health*; 87: 104–6.

8. Soobader, M-j and LeClere, FB. (Forthcoming.) Aggregation and the measurement of income inequality: effects on morbidity. *Social Science and Medicine* (special issue for Sol Levine) 1998?.

9. Fiscella, K and Franks, P. Poverty or income inequality as predictors of mortality: longitudinal cohort study. *British Medical Journal* 1997; 314: 1724–8.

10. Hsieh, CC and Pugh, MD. Poverty, income inequality, and violent crime: a meta-analysis of recent aggregate data studies. *Criminal Justice Review* 1993; 18: 182–202.

11. Kennedy, BP, Kawachi, I, Glass, R and Prothrow-Stith, D. Income distribution, socioeconomic status, and self-rated health: a US multi-level analysis.

12. McCord, C and Freeman, HP. Excess mortality in Harlem. *New England Journal of Medicine* 1990; 322: 173–7.

13. Marmot, MG, Rose, G, Shipley, M and Hamilton, PJS. Employment grade and coronary heart disease in British civil servants. *Journal of Epidemiology and Community Health* 1978; 32: 244–9.

14. Cohen, S, Doyle, WJ, Skoner, DP, Rabin, BS and Gwaltney, JM. Social ties and susceptibility to the common cold. *Journal of the American Medical Association* 1997; 277: 1940–44.

15. Berkman, LF. The role of social relations in health promotion. *Psychosomatic Research* 1995; 57: 245–54.

16. Karasek, R and Theorell, T. *Healthy work: stress, productivity and the reconstruction of working life.* New York: Basic Books, 1990.

17. Marmot, MG, Bosma, H, Hemingway, H, Brunner, E and Stansfield, S. Contribution of job control and other risk factors to social variations in coronary heart disease. *Lancet* 1997; 350: 235–40.

18. Helsing, KJ and Szklo, M. Mortality after bereavement. *American Journal of Epidemiology* 1981; 114: 41–52.

19. Everson, S, Kaplan, G, Goldberg, DE, Salonen, R and Salonen, JT. Hopelessness and 4-year progression of carotid atheroscerosis. *Arteriosclerosis, Thrombosis, and Vascular Biology* 1997; 17(8): 1490–5.

20. Salonen, JT, Julkunen, J, Salonen, R and Kaplan, A. Cynical distrust and anger control associated with accelerated progression of carotid atherosclerosis. *Circulation* 1991; 83: 722.

21. Williams, BB, Haney, TL, Lee, KL, Blumenthal, JA and Whalen, RE. Type A behaviour, hostility, and coronary atherosclerosis. *Psychosomatic Medicine* 1980; 42(6): 539–549.

22. Chen, CC, David, AS, Nunnerley, H, Michell, M, Dawson, JL and Berry, H et al. Adverse life events and breast cancer: case-control study. *British Medical Journal* 1995; 1527–9.

23. Rosengren, A, Orth-Gomer, K, Wedel, H and Wilhelmsen, L. Stressful life events, social support, and mortality in men born in 1933. *British Medical Journal.* 1993; 307: 1102–5.

24. Ferrie, JE, Shipley, MJ, Marmot, MG, Stansfield, S and Davey Smith, G. Health effects of anticipation of job change and non-employment: longitudinal data from the Whitehall II study. *British Medical Journal* 1995; 311: 1264–9.

25. Nettleton, S and Burrows, R. Insecure home ownership and health. In: *The Sociology of Health and Inequalities*: a Sociology of Health and Illness Monograph 1998.

26. Sapolsky, RM. *Why zebras don't get ulcers. A guide to stress, stress-related disease and coping.* New York: WH Freeman, 1994.

27. Uno, H, Tarara, R, Else, JG, Suleman, MA and Sapolsky, RM. Hippocampal damage associated with prolonged fatal stress in primates. *Journal of Neuroscience* 1989; 9: 1705–11.

28. Stratakis, CA and Chrousos, GP. Neuroendocrinology and pathophysiology of the stress system. In: *Stress: Basic Mechanisms and Clinical Implications*, edited by Chrousos, GP et al. The New York Academy of Sciences 1995; Vol 771: Annals of the New York Academy of Sciences.

29. Lovallo, WR. *Stress and health: biological and psychological interactions.* Sage, London 1997.

30. Marmot, MG, Shipley, MJ and Rose, G. Inequalities in death — specific explanations of a general pattern. *Lancet* 1984; 1(8384): 1003–6.

31. Cassel, J. The contribution of social environment to host resistance. *American Journal of Epidemiology* 1976; 104: 107–23.

32. Meaney, MJ, Aitken, DH, van Berkel, C, Bhatnagar, S and Sapolsky, RM. Effect of neonatal handling on age-related impairments associated with the hippocampus. *Science* 1988; 239: 766–8.

33. Liu, D, Diorio, J, Tannenbaum, B, Caldji, C, Francis, D, Freedman, A, Sharma, S, Pearson, D, Plotsky, PM and Meaney, MJ. Maternal care, hippocampal glucocorticoid receptors, and hypothalamic-pituitary-adrenal responses to stress. *Science* 1997; 277: 1659–1662.

34. Smythe, JW, Rowe, WB and Meaney, MJ. Neonatal handling alters serotonin (5-HT) turnover and 5-HT2. *Developmental Brain Research* 1994; 80: 183–189.

35. Kristenson, M. *Possible causes for the differences in coronary heart disease mortality between Lithuania and Sweden: The LiVicordia Study.* Linkoping University Medical Disserations No 547, Linkoping University 1998.

36. Troxler, RG, Sprague, EA, Albanese, RA, Fuchs, R and Thompson, AJ. The association of elevated plasma cortisol and early atherosclerosis as demonstrated by coronary angiography. *Atherosclerosis* 1977; 26: 151–62.

37. Arnetz, BB, Brenner, S, Hjelm, R, Levi, L and Petterson, I. *Stress reactions in relation to threat of job loss and actual unemployment: physiological, psychological and economic effects of job loss and unemployment.* Stress Research Report No 206, Karolinska Institute, Stockholm. 1988.

38. van der Pompe, G, Antoni, MH and Heijnen, CB. Elevated basal cortisol levels and attenuated cortisol responses to a behavioral challenge in women with metastatic breast cancer. *Psychoneuroendocrinology* 1996; 21(4): 361–74.

39. Lupien, S, Lecours, AR, Lussier, I, Schwartz, G, Nair, NPV and Meaney, MJ. Basal cortisol-levels and cognitive deficits in human aging. *Journal of Neuroscience* 1994; 14: 2893–2903.

40. Seeman, TE, McEwen, BS, Singer, BH, Albert, MS and Rowe, JW. Increase in urinary cortisol excretion and

memory declines: MacArthur studies of successful aging. *Journal of Clinical Endocrinology and Metabolism*, 1997; 82(8): 2458–2465.

41. Sapolsky, RM. Poverty's remains. *The Sciences* (NY) 1991; 31: 8–10.

42. Mattiasson, I, Lindgarde, F, Nilsson, JA and Theorell, T. Threat of unemployment and cardiovascular risk factors: longitudinal study of quality of sleep and serum cholesterol concentrations in men threatened with redundancy. *British Medical Journal* 1990; 301: 461-6.

43. Beale, N and Nethercott, S. Job-loss and family morbidity: a study of factory closure. *Journal of the Royal College of General Practitioners* 1988; 35: 510–14.

44. Cobb, S and Kasl, SC. *Termination: the consequences of job loss.* Cincinnati: Department of Health, Education and Welfare—US National Institutes for Occupational Safety and Health, publication no. 77-224, US National Institutes for Occupational Safety and Health. 1977.

45. Shively, CA, Laird, KL and Anton, RF. The behavior and physiology of social stress and depression in female cynomolgus monkeys. *Biological Psychiatry* 1997; 41: 871–82.

46. Sapolsky, RM. Endocrinology alfresco: psychoendocrine studies of wild baboons. *Recent Progress in Hormone Research* 1993; 48: 437–68.

47. Townsend, P. *Poverty in the United Kingdom.* Penguin, Harmondsworth. 1979.

48. Mack, J and Lansley, S. *Poor Britain.* Allen and Unwin 1985.

49. Hallerod, B. Deprivation and poverty—a comparative analysis of Sweden and Great Britain. *Acta-Sociologica* 1996; 39,2: 141–168.

50. Schor, J. *The overspent american: when buying becomes you.* Basic Books 1998.

51. McDonough, P, Duncan, GJ, Williams, D and House, J. Income dynamics and adult mortality in the U.S. 1972-89. *American Journal of Public Health* 87; 1997.

52. Siegrist, J. Threat to Social Status and Cardiovascular Risk. *Psychotherapy and Psychosomatics* 1984; 42: 90–96.

53. Newman, KS. *Falling from grace: the experience of downward mobility in the American middle class.* Free Press, N.Y. 1988.

54. Duesenberry, KS. The relative income hypothesis (1962).

55. Frank, RH. *Choosing the right pond: human behavior and the quest for status.* Oxford University Press. 1985.

56. Gilbert, P. *Depression: The Evolution of Powerlessness.* Erlbaum, Hove 1992.

57. Long, JM, Lynch, JJ, Machiran, NM, Thomas, SA and Malinow, K. The effect of status on blood pressure during verbal communication. *Journal of Behavioral Medicine* 1982; 5: 165–71.

58. Sennett, R and Cobb, J. *The Hidden Injuries of Class.* Knopf, N.Y. 1973.

59. Bourdieu, P. *Distinction: a social critique of the judgement of taste.* Routledge, London 1984.

60. Wilkinson, RG, Kawachi, I and Kennedy, B. Mortality, the social environment, crime and violence. *Sociology of Health and Illness.* Special edition edited by M. Bartley. 1998.

61. Gilligan, J. *Violence: Our Deadly Epidemic and Its Causes.* G.P. Putnam 1996.

62. McCall, N. *Makes me wanna holler. A young black man in America.* Random House, New York. 1994.

63. James, O. *Britain on the Couch: a treatment for the low serotonin society.* Random House, London 1997.

64. Moller, SE. Serotonin, carbohydrates, and atypical depression. *Pharmacology and Toxicology* 1992; 71: 61–71.

65. Higley, JD, King, ST, Hasert, MF, Champoux, M, Suomi, SJ and Linnoila, M. Stability of interindividual differences in serotonin function and its relationship to severe aggression and competent social behavior in rhesus macaque females. *Neuropsychopharmacology* 1996; 14(1): 67–76.

66. Raleigh, MJ, McGuire, MT, Brammer, GL and Yuwiler, A. Social and environmental influences on blood serotonin concentrations in monkeys. *Archives of General Psychiatry* 1984; 41: 405–10.

67. Raleigh, MJ et al. Serotenergic mechanisms promote dominance acquisition in adult male vervet monkeys. *Brain Research* 1991; 559: 181–90.

68. Smith, A. *The theory of the moral sentiments.* Liberty Classics, Indianapolis 1982.

69. House, JS, Landis, KR and Umberson, D. Social relationships and health. *Science.* 1988; 241: 540–5.

70. Jolly, A. *The evolution of primate behavior.* (2nd edition) Macmillan, NY 1985.

71. Walster, D. The role of the human/companion animal bond in the mental health of the elderly. Scottish Health Education Unit. Edinburgh, 1979.

72. Byrne, R. *The thinking ape: Evolutionary origins of intelligence*. Oxford University Press, Oxford 1995.

73. Erdal, D and Whiten, A. Egalitarianism and Machiavellian intelligence in human evolution. In: *Modelling the early human mind*. Edited by Mellars, P. and Gibson, K. McDonald Institute Monographs 1996; 139–160

74. Erdal, D and Whiten, A. On human egalitarianism: an evolutionary product of Machiavellian status escalation? *Current Anthropology* 1994; 35(2): 176–83

75. Putnam, RD, Leonardi, R and Nanetti, RY. *Making democracy work: civic traditions in modern Italy*. Princeton U.P. 1993.

76. Kawachi, I, Kennedy, BP, Lochner, K and Prothrow-Stith, D. Social capital, income inequality and mortality. *American Journal of Public Health* 1997; 87: 1491–8

77. Williams, RB, Feaganes, J and Barefoot, JC. Hostility and death rates in 10 US cities. *Psychosomatic Medicine* 1995; 57(1): 94.

78. Bruhn, JG and Wolf, S. *The Roseto Story*. Norman: University of Oklahoma Press 1979.

79. James, O. *Juvenile violence in a winner-loser culture*. Free Association Books 1995.

80. McIsaac, SJ and Wilkinson, RG. Income distribution and cause-specific mortality. *European Journal of Public Health* 1997; 7: 45–53.

81. Wilkinson, RG. Health and civic society in Eastern Europe before 1989. In: *The East-West life expectancy gap in Europe*. Edited by C. Hertzman, S. Kelly and M. Bobak. Kluwer, Dordrecht 1996b.

82. Watson, P. Explaining rising mortality among men in Eastern Europe. *Social Science and Medicine* 1995; 41: 923–34.

83. Hajdu, P, McKee, M and Bojan, F. Changes in premature mortality differentials by marital status in Hungary and England and Wales. *European Journal of Public Health* 1995; 5: 529–64.

84. Kawachi, I, Kennedy, BP, Gupta, V and Prothrow-Stith, D. Women's status and the health of women: a view from the States. Forthcoming.

85. Caldwell, JC. Routes to low mortality in poor countries. *Population and Development Review* 1986; 12: 171–220.

86. Yllo, K. Sexual equality and violence against wives in American states. *Journal of Comparative Family Studies* 1983; XIV(1): 67–86.

87. Blau, FD and Kahn, LM. The gender earnings gap — learning from international comparisons. *American Economic Review* 1992; 82: 533–8.

88. Anzaldua, G. *Borderlands*. Aunt Lute Books, San Francisco 1987.

89. Mischel, W. Introduction to personality: a new look (4th edition) Holt, N.Y. 1986.

90. Montgomery, SM, Bartley, MJ, Cook, DG and Wadsworth, MEJ. Health and social precursors of unemployment in young men. *Journal of Epidemiology and Community Health* 1996.

91. Power, C and Manor, O. Asthma, enuresis, and chronic illness — long term impact on height. *Archives of Diseases in Childhood* 1995; 73(4): 298–304.

92. Widdowson, EM. Mental contentment and physical growth. *Lancet* 1951; June 16: 1316–18.

93. Montgomery, SM, Bartley, MJ and Wilkinson, RG. Family conflict and slow growth. *Archives of the Diseases of Childhood* 1997; 77: 326–30.

94. Rostene, W, Sarrieau, A, Nicot, A, Scarceriaux, V and Betancur, C. Steroid effects on brain functions — an example of the action of glucocorticoids on central dopaminergic and neurotensinergic systems. *Journal of Psychiatry and Neuroscience* 1995; 20: 349–356.

95. Suomi, SJ. Early stress and adult emotional reactivity in rhesus monkeys. In: *The childhood environment and adult disease*. Edited by Ciba Foundation. John Wiley & Sons 1991; 171–86.

96. Meaney, MJ, ODonnell, D, Rowe, W, Tannenbaum, B and Steverman, A. Individual-differences in hypothalamic-pituitary-adrenal activity in later life and hippocampal aging. *Experimental Gerontology* 1995; 30: 229–251.

97. Hayakawa, K, Shimizu, T, Ohba, Y and Tomioka, S. Risk factors for cognitive aging in adult twins. *Acta Genet Med Gemellol* 1992; 41: 187–195.

98. Lasch, C. *Haven in a heartless world: the family besieged*. Basic Books 1977.

99. Lundberg, O. The impact of childhood living conditions on illness and mortality in adulthood. *Social Science and Medicine* 1993; 36: 1047–52.

100. Wadsworth, MEJ. Early stress and associations with adult health, behaviour and parenting. In: *Stress and disability in childhood*, edited by Butler, NR and Corner, BD. Wright, Bristol 1984.

101. Power, C, Manor, O and Fox, J. *Health and class: the early years*. Chapman and Hall 1991.

102. McCord, J. Early stress and future personality. In: *Stress and disability in childhood*. Edited by Butler, NR and Corner, BD. Wright, Bristol 1984.

103. Rutter, M and Giller, H. *Juvenile Delinquency: trends and perspectives*. Penguin Books 1983.

104. Waldron, I, Nowotarski, M, Freimer, M, Henry, JP, et al.Cross-cultural variation in blood pressure: a quantitative analysis of the relationships of blood pressure to cultural characteristics, salt consumption and body weight. *Social Science and Medicine* 1982; 16: 419–30.

105. Eyer, J. Capitalism, health, and illness. In: *Issues in the political economy of health care*. Edited by J.B. McKinlay. Tavistock, N.Y. 1984.

106. Timio, M, Verdecchia, P, Venanzi, S, Gentili, S, Ronconi, M, Francucci, B, Montanari, M and Bichisao, E. Age and blood pressure changes: a 20-year follow-up study in nuns in a secluded order. *Hypertension* 1988; 12: 457–61.

107. *China Statistical Yearbook 1997*. State Statistical Bureau of the People's Republic of China. Beijing 1997.

Twelve

RACE AND HEALTH IN KANSAS: DATA, ISSUES, AND DIRECTIONS

David R. Williams

T HE first census of the United States, conducted in 1790, paid attention to major subdivisions within the United States population. In compliance with Paragraph 3, Section II, Article 1, of the United States Constitution, this census enumerated whites, black slaves as three-fifths of a person, and only those Indians who paid taxes.[1] Numerous changes have been made to these officially recognized racial categories over time. The Thirteenth Amendment to the Constitution abandoned the three-fifths rule, and Congress voted in 1924 to grant U.S. citizenship to all American Indians.[2] As non-white immigrants entered the United States the racial taxonomy was revised to include them.[2] Chinese was added as a new racial group in the 1870 Census, Japanese in the 1890 Census, and Filipino, Hindu, and Korean in the 1920 Census. Mexicans were classified as a separate race in the 1930 Census, reclassified as white in the 1940 Census, and designated as the "Spanish surname" population in the southwestern states in the 1960 Census.

The United States continues to evaluate a broad range of societal outcomes, including health, on the basis of these racial groups. Current guidelines require federal agencies to report statistics for four racial groups (American Indian and Alaska Native, Asian and Pacific Islander, black, and white) and one ethnic category (Hispanic origin).[3] Table 1 reveals that although almost 9 out of every 10 persons in Kansas are white, all of the major racial/ethnic categories are represented in the population of Kansas.[4] In Kansas, there are over 140,000 blacks, 22,000 American Indians, 32,000 Asians, and almost 100,000 Hispanics.

RACE/ETHNICITY AND HEALTH

T HESE racial categories importantly predict variations in health status. Table 2 presents black/white ratios for the leading causes of death in the U.S. and Kansas for 1994.[5] A ratio greater than 1.0 reflects a higher rate of mortality for blacks compared to whites. The national mortality data reveal that African Americans (or blacks) have an overall death rate that is more than one-and-a-half times higher than that of whites. The magnitude of the racial difference in death rates varies by the specific cause of death, but a pattern of elevated death rates for blacks compared to whites exists for almost all the leading causes of death in the United States. Table 2

Table 1

Racial Composition of the State of Kansas, 1990

Race and Ethnicity	Percent[1]	Numbers
Non-Hispanic White	88.4	2,190,524
Non-Hispanic Black	5.7	140,761
Hispanic Origin of Any Race	3.8	93,670
Asian or Pacific Islander	1.3	31,750
American Indian, Eskimo, or Aleut	0.9	21,965
Other Race	2.0	48,797

Source: reference 4.
[1]The numbers do not add to 100 percent because Hispanics can be of any race.

also reveals that the black/white ratios for the leading causes of death in Kansas are very similar to those for the overall United States population. In nationally reported data, all of the other racial groups have an overall death rate that is lower than that of whites.

However, these overall data mask important patterns of variations for subgroups of these populations and for specific health conditions. The Indian Health Service, for example, indicates that age-adjusted mortality rates for American Indians in its service area are higher than the national average for several causes of death.[6] These include tuberculosis (520% higher), alcoholism (433% higher), diabetes (188% higher), accidents (166% higher), homicides (71% higher), suicides (54% higher), and pneumonia and influenza (44% higher). Moreover, even within a specific state, considerable tribal variation is evident. Similarly, while Hispanics have lower death rates for heart disease and cancer than do non-Hispanics, they have higher mortality rates than non-Hispanic whites for tuberculosis, septicemia, chronic liver disease and cirrhosis, diabetes, and homicide.[7,8] Hispanics also have elevated rates for several infectious diseases. Subgroups of the Asian and Pacific Is-

lander population also have elevated mortality rates for some health conditions.[9] For example, the Native Hawaiian population has the highest death rates due to heart disease of any racial group in the United States.[10]

Table 3 presents infant mortality rates for the United States and the state of Kansas.[11] Whites, Hispanics, and Asians in Kansas have infant death rates that are higher than the national infant death rates for their group. In contrast, black and American Indian babies born in Kansas are less likely to die before their first birthday than their counterparts nationally. At the same time, these racial categories importantly capture variations in infant mortality. Whites have the lowest death rate of any racial group in Kansas, with the rate for blacks being almost twice as high as that of whites. In contrast to the national level, where Asians have the lowest rate of infant mortality, Asians in Kansas have the second highest infant mortality rate.

TRENDS OVER TIME

THESE racial disparities in health are not new. Black/white differences in health in the United States have been monitored for a long

Table 2

Black/White Ratios for Leading Causes of Death in Kansas and the United States, 1994

Cause of Death	Black/White Ratio	
	Kansas	U.S.
All Causes	1.6	1.6
Heart Disease	1.5	1.5
Cancer	1.3	1.4
Stroke	1.7	1.9
Pulmonary Diseases	0.8	0.8
Unintentional Injuries	1.3	1.3
Pneumonia and Influenza	1.2	1.4
Diabetes	2.3	2.4
Infectious Diseases	2.6	3.7
HIV/AIDS	2.4	4.4
Atherosclerosis	0.8	1.3
Suicide	0.5	0.6
Kidney Disease	3.0	2.7
Homicide and Legal Intervention	12.1	6.6
Liver Disease and Cirrhosis	2.7	1.4

Source: reference 5.

Table 3

Infant Mortality per 1,000 Live Births in Kansas and the United States, 1989–1991

Race/Ethnicity	Kansas	U.S.
Non-Hispanic White	7.8	7.3
Non-Hispanic Black	15.4	17.2
Hispanic	8.7	7.6
Asian	9.7	6.6
American Indian	8.2	12.6

Source: reference 11.

time, and the earliest health data reveal striking black/white disparities in health. Some evidence suggests that these disparities in health have been widening in recent decades. Table 4 presents infant mortality rates for blacks and whites between 1950 and 1990.[12] It indicates that death rates for both racial groups declined over this 40-year period. In 1950, 27 out of every 1,000 white infants born in the United States died before their first birthday, compared to 44 out of every 1,000 black infants. The infant mortality rate for blacks was 1.6 times higher than that of whites. Although the death rates for both racial groups are considerably lower in 1990, a black infant born in 1990 is 2.2 times more likely to die before his first birthday than a white infant. Thus, over the last 40 years infant death rates for whites have declined more rapidly than those for blacks, leading to a widening of the differential between them.

The report of the Secretary's Task Force on Black and Minority Health indicated that there were 80,000 excess deaths for minority populations in the United States in 1980.[13] That is, 80,000 minority individuals died that year who would not have if the mortality experience of minority populations was the same as that of the white population. Sixty-thousand of these excess deaths were for the African-American popula-tion. A recent update of this report indicates that the annual number of excess deaths for the African-American population increased from 60,000 in 1980 to 66,000 in 1991.[14] This report also reveals that the black/white gap in life expectancy widened between 1980 and 1991 for both males and females. The data on life expectancy indicates that at least part of the growing black/white disparities in health is driven by the absolute deterioration of the health status of the black population for some health indicators. National life expectancy data reveal that for the five years following 1984 there was a decline in life expectancy at birth for the black population from the 1984 level.[15] By 1990, life expectancy for African Americans began to increase again, so that by 1992 the level was slightly higher than that of 1984. In contrast, over the same time period there was a progressive annual increase in life expectancy for whites, so that the black/white gap in life expectancy in 1992 (6.9 years) was wider than it was in 1984 (5.8 years). Research reveals that a slower rate of decline among blacks than whites for heart disease is the chief contributor to the widening racial gap in life expectancy, while HIV infection, homicide, diabetes, and pneumonia are major causes of decreasing life expectancy for blacks.[16]

Table 4

Infant Mortality Rates (per 1,000 Live Births) for Whites and Blacks in the United States, 1950–1990

Year	White	Black	Black/White Ratio
1950	26.8	43.9	1.6
1960	22.9	44.3	1.9
1970	17.8	32.6	1.8
1980	11.0	21.4	1.9
1990	7.7	17.0	2.2

Source: reference 12.

WHAT IS RACE?

HEALTH researchers and practitioners routinely use race in an uncritical manner. Discussions on racial variations in health have historically been dominated by a genetic model that views race as primarily reflecting biological homogeneity and racial differences in health as largely genetically determined. Understanding and addressing the role of race in health require a clear understanding of what race is and the identification of the specific risk factors and resources linked to race that may be responsible for variations in health status. There is growing recognition in the public health field that the prevailing conceptualization of race is flawed. It predated modern scientific theories of genetics and carefully executed genetic studies.

Although widely shared in our society, the belief that races are human populations that differ from each other primarily in terms of genetics is not supported by the existing scientific data.[17-19] There is more genetic variation within races than between them, and racial categories do not capture biological distinctiveness. Regardless of geographic origin or race, all human beings are identical for about 75 percent of known genetic factors.[20] In addition, some 95 percent of human genetic variation exists within racial groups. Thus, our current racial categories are more alike than different in terms of biological characteristics and genetics, and there is no specific scientific criteria to unambiguously classify the human population into discrete biological categories with rigid boundaries. The fact that we know what race we belong to tells us more about our society than about our genetic background.[21] Racial taxonomies are arbitrary, and race is more of a social category than a biological one.[22,23]

RACE AND SES

ALTHOUGH the current racial categories do not tell us much about underlying biological risks for diseases, they do capture an important part of the inequality and injustice in American society.[24] There are important power and status differences between groups. This can readily be illustrated by looking at differences in socioeconomic status (SES) across racial groups. Table 5 presents selected socioeconomic profiles of the population of Kansas by race.[25]

Blacks, Hispanics, and American Indians have lower rates of high school and college completion than whites. Rates of high school graduation are especially low for Hispanics. The API population is overrepresented at both ends of the educational distribution. Compared to whites, Asians have lower rates of high school completion and higher rates of college graduation. The unemployment rates show a similar pattern, with whites and APIs having the lowest rates and with the rates being considerably higher for blacks, American Indians, and Hispanics. The mean household income for Asians is higher than that of whites, but all of the other racial/ethnic groups have average levels of income that are $7,000 to $11,000 less than the white population. The higher rates for Asians reflect larger families with more earners per family than the total population. Thus, whites have a higher per capita income than Asians, and all of the other racial/ethnic groups. The overall poverty rates for Asians, American Indians, and Hispanics are about twice that of whites, while the rate for blacks is three times higher. Most markedly for the black population, poverty rates for children and youth are higher than the overall rates. Within each racial group, rates of poverty for the elderly are about the same or slightly higher than those of the total population for that group.

Data on poverty tells only a part of the story of economic vulnerability. In addition to persons who actually fall below the government's poverty threshold, a large number of persons are only slightly above this level. Many of these persons are at a high risk of becoming poor. Table 6 presents national data on this issue.[26] In addition to those who fall below the poverty line, the table also shows the percent of Americans who are

Table 5

Selected Socioeconomic Characteristics for Kansas, 1990 Census

	White	Black	Asian or Pacific Islander	American Indian, Eskimo, or Aleut	Hispanic Origin of Any Race
Educational attainment (persons 25 yrs. and older), percent					
High school graduate or higher	82.4	71.0	73.6	75.4	58.1
Bachelor's degree or higher	21.7	11.6	39.9	10.8	10.1
Employment status (persons 16 yrs. and older), percent					
Unemployed	4.1	11.7	5.5	9.4	8.3
Not in the labor force	33.2	36.4	36.8	32.2	27.6
Mean household income in 1989, dollars	34,962	23,477	36,865	25,464	27,587
Per capita income in 1989, dollars	13,817	8,445	10,528	8,767	8,007
Below the poverty level by age, percent					
All ages	9.9	30.0	22.2	21.6	19.7
Under 18 years	11.5	40.3	22.2	26.8	23.5
Under 5 years	13.7	45.3	25.5	29.9	25.7
65 years and older	11.4	28.0	23.6	20.9	18.4

Source: reference 25.

Table 6

U.S. Census Percent of Persons Poor and Near Poor, 1995

Race and Hispanic Origin	Poor	Near Poor	% Vulnerable
ALL PERSONS			
All Races	13.8	19.8	33.6
White, Non-Hispanic	8.5	17.2	25.7
Asian or Pacific Islander	14.6	18.4	33.0
Black	29.3	25.0	54.3
Hispanic	30.3	31.4	61.7
CHILDREN UNDER 18 IN FAMILIES			
All Races	20.8	22.5	43.3
White, Non-Hispanic	11.2	19.3	30.5
Asian or Pacific Islander	19.5	21.0	40.5
Black	41.9	26.2	68.1
Hispanic	40.0	32.9	72.9
CHILDREN UNDER 18 IN FEMALE-HEADED HOUSEHOLDS			
All Races	50.3	25.7	76.0
White, Non-Hispanic	33.5	27.8	61.3
Asian or Pacific Islander	42.4	18.8	61.2
Black	61.6	25.2	86.8
Hispanic	65.7	22.6	88.3

Source: reference 26.

near poor (annual income above the poverty threshold but less than twice the poverty level). The combination of the poor and near poor categories shows the percent of persons who are economically vulnerable. These data reveal that substantial proportions of the U.S. population are economically vulnerable. One in every three persons in the U.S. falls into this economically marginal category. This ranges from 26 percent of whites to 62 percent of Hispanics. These numbers are disconcertingly high for children, especially those who reside in female-headed households. These data also shed light on the complex association of race to SES. Although there is a strong relationship between race and SES, they are not equivalent. For example, the rate of poverty is three times higher for blacks than for whites, but two-thirds of blacks are not poor, and two-thirds of all poor Americans are white.

RACE, SES, AND HEALTH

RESEARCH reveals that SES differences between the races account for much of the racial differences in health. Adjusting racial (black/white) disparities in health for SES sometimes eliminates, but always substantially re-duces, these differences.[27-29] However, race often has an effect on health independent of SES. It is frequently found that within each level of SES blacks still have worse health status than whites. Table 7 presents the association between household income and years of formal education with self-assessed health for blacks and whites.[30] Self-assessed health, a subjective evaluation of health status, is a very robust indicator of health and is strongly related to objective measures of health.[31] For example, persons who assess their health as excellent or good live longer than those who report it as fair or poor.

When we consider the distribution of self-reported health by income and education for blacks and whites, three important trends emerge. First, for both racial groups income and education are strongly linked to health status. Consistently, persons of lower levels of income and education report worse health than their more economically favored peers. For example, almost 40 percent of all black persons, who did not complete high school and have incomes of less than $20,000, report their health to be fair or poor, compared to 6 percent of college-educated African Americans with incomes greater than $20,000. Among whites, one-third of those in the lowest income and education category report

their health as fair or poor, compared to 4 percent of those in the highest income and education group. Moreover, for all of the comparisons in the table, for both blacks and whites, the data follows a linear graded pattern with persons at each higher level of SES experiencing better health than those at the level immediately preceding theirs.

A second noteworthy pattern in Table 7 is that SES differences are generally larger than racial ones. For both racial groups, there are large SES ratios when the health status of persons in the lowest SES group is contrasted to that of their counterparts in the highest SES category. For example, for blacks and whites, among house-holds with less than $20,000 annual income, per-sons with less than 12 years of education are more than three times as likely to be in fair or poor health than their peers with more than 12 years of education. An even stronger pattern is evident for households with more than $20,000 income where fair or poor health is four times as com-mon among those with low education compared to those with high education. It is striking that despite these patterns of social inequality, the routine reporting of health data in the U.S. is preoccupied with racial differences in health and gives scant attention to health status variations by SES. Numerous calls have been made for

Table 7

Average Annual Percent of Persons Reporting to Be in Fair or Poor Health by Income and Education, for Blacks and Whites

Education	Income <$20,000		Income >$20,000	
	Whites	Blacks	Whites	Blacks
Less than 12 years	33.1	38.8	16.1	20.5
12 years	15.2	17.9	6.8	9.6
More than 12 years	9.2	13.2	3.7	5.9
Total	16.6	19.0	5.1	7.6

Source: reference 30.

more systematic reporting of U.S. health data by SES.[32-35]

The third pattern that clearly emerges in these data is that race is more than socioeconomic status. For all of the racial comparisons in the table, blacks report worse health status than whites at comparable levels of income and education. Moreover, the black/white gap in health status becomes larger with increasing SES. African Americans in the lowest income and education category are 1.2 times more likely to report being in fair or poor health compared to their white peers. In contrast, blacks in the highest income and education category are 1.6 times more likely to report being in fair or poor health compared to their white counterparts. The power of SES in shaping racial differences in health is clearly evident by comparing the highest SES blacks with the lowest SES whites. At both income levels in the table, whites in the lowest education category are more than twice as likely to report being in fair or poor health than blacks in the highest education category. Thus, the disproportionate concentration of African Americans at the lower SES levels is a major factor behind the overall racial differences in health. A clear implication of this pattern is that studies seeking to understand racial differences in health must always control for SES.

The role of SES in health is evident across multiple health status indicators. Table 8 shows infant mortality rates by mothers' education for the U.S. For all racial populations, there is an inverse relationship between maternal education and infant mortality. A similar pattern is evident for prenatal care. Table 9 indicates that there is a graded stepwise relationship for all racial groups in which increase in formal education is associated with higher levels of prenatal care in the first trimester.[36] At the same time, consideration of race and SES simultaneously reveals a consistent pattern of elevated rates of morbidity, mortality, or poor health behavior for minority populations compared to the white population, at equivalent levels of SES. For example, whites with less than 12 years of education have higher levels of prenatal care than similarly educated women in all of the other racial/ethnic groups.

INSTITUTIONAL RACISM AND RACIAL INEQUALITY

THERE is a growing attention in the literature to the nature of the association between race and SES.[22,23,27,37] This work

Table 8

Infant Mortality for Mothers 20 Years of Age and Older by Mothers' Education

Race/Ethnicity	Maternal Education			
	<12 Years	12 Years	13–15 Years	>15 Years
White, Non-Hispanic	9.9	6.5	5.1	4.2
Black, Non-Hispanic	17.3	14.8	12.3	11.4
Hispanic	6.0	5.9	5.4	4.4
American Indian or Alaska Native	12.7	7.9	5.7	*
Asian or Pacific Islander	5.7	5.5	5.1	4.0

Source: reference 36.
*Number is too small for stable rate calculation.

Table 9

Prenatal Care in First Trimester Among Mothers 20 Years of Age and Older, United States, 1995

Race/Ethnicity	Maternal Education			
	< 12 Years	12 Years	13–15 Years	>15 Years
All Races	66.8	81.6	87.5	93.9
White, Non-Hispanic	71.7	86.0	90.3	95.2
Black, Non-Hispanic	59.6	71.3	79.5	88.6
Hispanic	65.7	75.7	82.4	88.3
American Indian or Alaska Native	56.6	68.6	74.3	86.8
Asian or Pacific Islander	67.4	76.6	83.5	89.1

Source: reference 36.

emphasizes that inequality between the races did not just happen. Race is a social status category that was created by large scale societal factors and racism. Understanding and addressing the health of the African-American population requires attention to the role of racism.[38] By racism, I mean an ideology that categorizes and ranks human groups, with some being inferior to others. This in turn can lead to negative attitudes and beliefs toward defined outgroups, as well as differential treatment of members of these groups by both individuals and societal institutions. The racial attitudes of whites toward blacks have dramatically improved over the last 50 years, although whites' support for the principles of equality is considerably stronger than their commitment to policies that would implement them.[39]

At the same time, substantial proportions of the white population continue to hold negative attitudes toward African Americans. Table 10 presents data on whites' stereotypes of blacks from the 1990 General Social Survey, a highly respected nationally representative social indicators survey.[40] More than half of all whites believe that blacks are prone to violence, prefer to live off welfare, and lack motivation and willpower to pull themselves out of poverty. Only 17 percent of whites believe that blacks are hard working, and only 1 in 5 believe that blacks are intelligent. Substantial numbers of whites opted for the "Neither Agree or Disagree" response category on these questions. The extent to which social desirability concerns underlie this pattern is not known. It is also instructive that almost 4 out of 5 whites rejected a biological explanation (blacks have less inborn ability) for the social situation of African Americans. Instead in these and other data, whites point to motivational and cultural differences as the reasons why blacks have worse jobs, income, and housing than whites. Thus, there appears to be a shift over time from the racism that emphasizes the biological inferiority of blacks to one that focuses on cultural inferiority.

The dominant society's ideology of the inferiority of blacks was actively translated into policies that facilitated the social exclusion of, and truncated economic mobility for, the black population. Many health researchers and policy makers understand that there is an association between race and SES but tend to view SES as a confounder of the relationship between race and health. Instead, SES is part of the causal pathway

Table 10

White Americans' Stereotypes of Blacks

Stereotype	Percent
1. Lazy	
Blacks are lazy	45
Neither	33
Blacks are hardworking	17
2. Violent	
Blacks are prone to violence	51
Neither	28
Blacks are not prone to violence	15
3. Unintelligent	
Blacks are unintelligent	29
Neither	44
Blacks are intelligent	21
4. Welfare	
Blacks prefer to live off welfare	56
Neither	26
Blacks prefer to be self-supporting	12
5. Unpatriotic	
Blacks are unpatriotic	16
Neither	35
Blacks are patriotic	39
6. Blacks have worse jobs, income, and housing than whites because:	
a. Most blacks have less inborn ability to learn	
Yes	18
Don't know	3
No	78
b. Most blacks just don't have the motivation or willpower to pull themselves up out of poverty.	
Yes	60
Don't know	6
No	33

Source: reference 40, p. 37

by which racism affects health. Race is causally prior to SES, and differences between the races in SES reflect, in part, the impact of economic discrimination produced by large-scale societal structures. That is, the black-white differences in SES noted earlier are a direct result of the systematic implementation of institutional policies premised on the inferiority of blacks and the need to avoid social contact with them.

Historically, racial residential segregation is a prime example of a societal structure that importantly restricted socioeconomic opportunity and mobility for blacks.[41] Residential segregation determined housing conditions, educational and unemployment opportunities, and thus truncated economic mobility for African Americans. That is, the lower levels of income and education among African Americans reflect the results of systematic societal policies that excluded African Americans from educational opportunities. This lack of educational training and opportunity combined with systematic discrimination in employment[42,43] are manifested in the current economic fortunes of African-American adults.

NONEQUIVALENCE OF SES INDICATORS FOR BLACKS AND WHITES

ONE consequence of institutional discrimination is that SES indicators are not equivalent across race. For example, racial differences in income do not represent the true extent of racial differences in economic resources between households of different races. Racial differences in wealth are much larger than those for income. Eller[44] shows that while white households have a median net worth of $44,408, the median net worth is $4,604 for black households and $5,345 for Hispanic ones. Moreover, these racial differences in wealth are evident at all levels of income and are largest at the lowest income level. That is, for persons in the lowest quintile of income in the United States, the net worth of whites is 10,000 times larger than that of blacks ($10,257 versus $1), while at the highest quintile of income the net worth of whites is twice as large as that of blacks ($129,394 versus $54,449). A growing number of studies find that measures of assets such as home or car ownership are predictive of health status, independent of traditional

indicators of SES such as income, education and occupational status.[45-47]

Another example of the nonequivalence of economic indicators across race is the differential income returns to investments in education. On average, members of minority groups receive lower levels of income for a given level of education than whites. This is true if one considers persons working full time in the labor force.[48] For example, national data reveal that a white male high school graduate working full time in the labor force has a median annual income of $26,500, compared to $20,300 and $20,900 for his black and Hispanic counterpart, respectively. This pattern of lower income returns for education exists at both high and low levels of education, with blacks and Hispanics, males and females, earning less income than whites. It is also readily evident in Table 11, which presents data on median family income by years of education.[36]

Because of conditions created by residential segregation, the purchasing power of a given level of income is much greater for whites than for blacks. Studies reveal that compared to whites, African Americans pay higher prices for new cars, higher property taxes on homes of similar value, and higher costs for food and mortgages.[49] These racial differences in purchasing power illustrate the nonequivalence of a given level of income across race in terms of its ability to procure goods and services in society.

NON-ECONOMIC DISCRIMINATION

SYSTEMATIC discrimination can also affect the quantity and quality of services received, including medical care. There is a fairly consistent pattern of racial differences in the receipt of a broad range of diagnostic and treatment procedures.[50] Table 12 presents black/white ratios and 30-day post-admission mortality rates per 1,000 enrollees for the most common procedures performed in hospitals for Medicare beneficiaries.[51] In the Medicare Program, for

Table 11

Median Family Income by Education

Sex, Race, and Hispanic Origin	12 Years	16 or More Years
	MEN	
White, Non-Hispanic	$36,703	$63,178
Asian or Pacific Islander	$34,000	$57,338
Black, Non-Hispanic	$28,040	$52,683
Hispanic	$29,020	$50,661
	WOMEN	
White, Non-Hispanic	$33,000	$57,997
Asian or Pacific Islander	$35,050	$54,620
Black, Non-Hispanic	$19,226	$40,141
Hispanic	$25,400	$48,050

Source: reference 36.

example, black inpatients were less likely than their white peers to receive all of the 16 most common procedures received by Medicare beneficiaries. In general, the observed racial differences are largest for the newer, more highly elective and referral sensitive procedures such as the cardiovascular and the orthopedic and back procedures. Moreover, African Americans had higher 30-day post-admission mortality rates than whites for most of the procedures.

Further analysis of the Medicare files revealed that there were four procedures that black beneficiaries of Medicare received more frequently than their white peers. Table 13 presents the black/white ratios and mortality rates for these four nonelective procedures.[51] The amputation of part of the lower limb, usually as a consequence of diabetes, was 3.6 times more likely to be performed on African Americans compared to whites. Excisional debridement, removal of tissue, usually related to decubitus ulcers, was performed 2.7 times more frequently on black than on white patients. Arteriovenostomy, the

implantation of shunts or cannulae for chronic renal dialysis, was 5.2 times more likely to be performed on black patients than white ones. Finally, bilateral orchiectomy, removal of both testes, generally performed for cancer in males, was 2.2 times more likely to be performed on black than white patients. Racial differences in disease prevalence could play some role in the racial difference for the four procedures that were performed more frequently on black than white patients. (Blacks have higher rates of diabetes, prostate cancer, and end-stage renal disease than whites.) At the same time, these four procedures can frequently be averted or delayed if medical care is comprehensive and characterized by continuity. That is, these four procedures reflect delayed diagnosis or initial treatment (in the case of prostate cancer), poor or infrequent medical care (for diabetes and vascular disease leading to amputations and skin infections), and failure in the management of chronic conditions such as diabetes and hypertension.

There are many potential explanations for

Table 12

*Black/White (B/W) Ratios for Procedure Rates and 30-Day Post-Admission Mortality Rates,
Per 1,000 Enrollees, for Selected Major Procedures Performed on Medicare Beneficiaries,
65 Years of Age and Older, 1992*

Procedures	Procedure Rates B/W Ratio	Mortality Rates B/W Ratio
Cardiovascular		
1. Cardiac Catheterization	0.68	—
2. Coronary Angioplasty	0.44	1.05
3. Coronary Bypass Graft	0.39	1.12
4. Carotid Endarterectomy	0.31	1.32
Orthopedic and Back		
5. Total Knee Replacement	0.64	1.47
6. Total Hip Replacement	0.49	1.10
7. Excision of Disc	0.50	2.12
8. Spinal Fusion	0.63	1.56
9. Reduction of Fracture of Femur	0.44	0.83
10. Other Arthroplasty of Hip	0.45	0.84
11. Laminectomy	0.53	2.02
Surgical Procedures		
12. Prostatectomy	0.97	1.27
13. Mastectomy	0.80	1.50
14. Hysterectomy	0.60	2.04
15. Appendectomy	0.76	2.33
16. Repair of Inguinal Hernia	0.85	1.13

Source: reference 51.

these racial differences. A greater percentage of black Medicare beneficiaries make out-of-pocket payments for deductibles and copayments for ambulatory medical care compared to their white counterparts.[51] This higher financial cost could lead to lower utilization of ambulatory care and the postponement and avoidance of treatment. There may also be higher levels of severity of illness among black patients at the time that the procedures are performed. In addition, blacks may be more likely than whites to refuse procedures recommended by their physicians.[52] Alternatively, whites may be more aggressive in pursuing medical care and more likely than blacks to request high technology medical procedures. However, these racial differences among Medicare beneficiaries may also reflect the role of racial discrimination in the delivery of medical care. In a world of limited resources, could race, consciously or unconsciously, be a social criterion that clinicians use to establish the worthiness of patients for the receipt of medical care? Other data reveal that Medicare is not unique. A similar pattern has been found in studies of Veteran Administration hospitals[53] and in the National Hospital Discharge Survey.[54]

Table 13

Black/White (B/W) Ratios for Procedure Rates and 30-Day Post–Admission Rates,
Per 1,000 Enrollees, for Procedures for Which the Rates Are Higher for Black than
White Medicare Beneficiaries, 65 Years of Age and Older, 1992

Procedure		Procedure Rates B/W Ratio	Mortality Rates B/W Ratio
1.	Amputation (lower limb)	3.62	0.79
2.	Excisional Debridement	2.65	1.22
3.	Arteriovenostomy	5.17	0.66
4.	Bilateral Orchiectomy	2.21	0.99

Source: reference 51, p. 47

1 = Usually a consequence of diabetes
2 = Removal of tissue, usually related to decubitus ulcers
3 = Implanting shunts for chronic renal dialysis
4 = Removal of both testes, generally performed because of cancer

BELIEFS ABOUT INFERIORITY

HOW do minority group members cope with the negative societal perceptions of their group? Some may reject and fight the stereotypes, while others may accept and internalize them. Some research suggests that assumptions of inferiority at the societal level have negative consequences for at least some members of stigmatized groups. That is, a stigma of inferiority may create specific expectations, anxieties, and reactions that affect the functioning of marginalized groups. Research in multiple countries (UK, Japan, India, South Africa, and Israel) indicates that groups that are socially unequal have lower scores on standardized tests.[55] Moreover as groups move to political and social parity over time, test scores converge and in some cases the disparities disappear. Similarly, Claude Steele's research indicates that when African-American students are explicitly confronted with the stereotype of black intellectual inferiority, they perform worse on examinations.[56,57] The performance of women on a standardized exam was also adversely affected when told in advance that women usually do worse than men, and white men also performed poorly when they were contrasted to Asians.[55]

Endorsing the dominant society's negative beliefs about one's group also adversely affects health status. Studies of African-American women found that those who scored high on internalized racism—believed that blacks are inferior—had higher levels of psychological distress and alcohol use.[58,59] Similar findings come from the National Study of Black Americans.[60] In these data, African Americans who endorsed stereotypes of blacks as accurate were more likely to report poorer physical and mental health than those who disagreed with the stereotypes. Racism in the larger society can also lead to exposure to personal experiences of discrimination. These experiences of discrimination may be an important part of subjectively experienced stress that can adversely affect health. Several studies have found that self-report measures of discrimination are adversely related to physical and mental health in a broad range of racial/ethnic minority populations.[60-66] A recent study of a large metropolitan area in the U.S. found that SES accounted for most of the black/white differences in physical health. However, exposure to both chronic and acute indicators of discrimination completely accounted for the residual racial differences in self-reported physical health.[37]

SOCIAL STRUCTURE AND HEALTH BEHAVIOR

UNDERSTANDING how the social environment adversely affects health also requires us to attend to the societal forces that initiate, facilitate, and encourage unhealthy behaviors on the part of vulnerable communities. The major risk factors for the burden of chronic disease in our society are preventable.[67] Similarly, the major risk factors for the excess level of disease and death for minority populations are also preventable.[13] For example, cigarette smoking or alcohol use are risk factors for 5 of the 6 causes of death responsible for the excess mortality in the African-American population.

Many researchers view health behaviors as individual characteristics and ignore the larger forces in the social environment that are consequential for the initiation and maintenance of health practices.[68] Alcohol, for example, is a mood-altering drug that is frequently utilized to obtain relief from stressful living and working conditions. Feelings of powerlessness and helplessness are predictors of alcohol use and alcohol problems.[69] Alcohol consumption is positively related to the unemployment rate and increases during economic recessions.[70] There is also a strong positive association between the availability of alcohol and alcohol consumption.[70] Thus, state licensing boards that have permitted more retail outlets for the sale of alcohol in poor and minority neighborhoods than in affluent areas[71] facilitate alcohol abuse in those areas. Vulnerable populations, such as blacks and Hispanics, have also been specially targeted by the alcohol industry. For example, 80 percent of billboards in the

U.S. contain advertisements targeted to African Americans and Hispanics.[72,73] Alcohol ranks second to cigarettes as the most heavily advertised product on this medium. Similarly, levels of tobacco use for the black and Hispanic population reflect the cooperative efforts of a broad range of governmental and commercial interests to initiate and maintain cigarette use within these populations. Thus, efforts to change health behaviors must target not only the individual, but also must move upstream to change the social structures that constrain individual behavior.

There is a need of greater recognition that health behaviors are induced and constrained by the social and material context.[74] Lower SES persons face more stress and have fewer resources to cope with it than their higher SES peers. Preoccupation with daily survival is often foremost in the minds of minority group members. Behaviors that may be detrimental to health outcomes in the long run may provide sustenance and relief from structural impediments in the short term. Cigarettes, for example, are the most important single source of preventable deaths, but they are widely used to alleviate stress and tension. Cigarette smoking appears to be a potent strategy that can break up the drudgery of people's lives and bring diversion and at least temporary relief from the chronic irritations and hassles people face. Higher SES persons may have alternatives to the use of cigarettes, while the structural constraints and truncated options the lower SES persons face may leave them to perceive that cigarette smoking is their only viable stress-reduction option. Williams[74] emphasizes that health behaviors are higher on the hierarchy of need than the more basic needs of food, clothing, and shelter. Accordingly, until these primary needs are met, low SES persons will (appropriately) focus on addressing basic needs and confronting their most immediate dangers before being concerned about health issues that are distant, uncertain, and less relevant to the daily struggles of basic survival.

DIRECTIONS FOR STUDYING RACE
AND HEALTH

HEALTH researchers have been giving increasing attention to the quality of racial data and concern has surfaced regarding the uncritical use of race[75-77] and the reliability and validity problems in the measurement of racial identification.[49,78] First, the distribution of a study population into different racial groups varies by mode of assessment, with respondent reports of racial self-identification differing, substantially for some groups, from observer assessment. Second, racial self-identification depends, at least in part, on the wording of particular questions. Third, for a growing number of persons in our society, racial and especially ethnic identification is not singular and static, but multiple and dynamic. Fourth, the differential census undercount of minority populations by understating the denominators used to calculate health events can erroneously inflate the picture of the rates of health conditions for these groups.

Fifth, given the centrality of racial identity to the self-concept of many, researchers should use terms that are broadly recognized by a wide variety of people and reflect the preferences of respondents. A recent national study of over 60,000 adults found that members of racial groups are divided over preferred terminology.[79] Fifty-eight percent of Hispanics preferred "Hispanic" (12 percent prefer "Latino"), 62 percent of whites preferred "white" (17 percent prefer "Caucasian"), 44 percent of blacks preferred "black" (28 percent prefer "African American"), and 50 percent of American Indians prefer the term "American Indian" (37 percent prefer "Native American"). In an effort to respect individual dignity, researchers should use the most preferred terms for each group interchangeably (e.g., black or African American, Hispanic or Latino).

Sixth, race must be comprehensively assessed. There is considerable ethnic heterogeneity within each of the five OMB categories, and an understanding of health status variations requires that these categories be disaggregated, whenever possible. These subgroups vary across a broad range of sociodemographic characteristics, as well as in access to and utilization of medical care. For example, although most Hispanics have a common language, religion, and various traditions, the timing of immigration and incorporation experiences in the United States have varied for the more than 25 national origin groups that make up the Hispanic group, such that each group is distinctive. An overall health statistic for the Hispanic population is not particularly useful. In general, Cuban Americans have an SES and health profile that is similar to whites, Puerto Ricans have a health profile that tends to be more similar to that of African Americans than whites, and although Mexican Americans are disadvantaged in SES and access to health care, they have a health profile that is similar to and sometimes better than that of whites. However, the American way of life appears to be dangerous to our health, with the health status of Mexican Americans declining with length of stay in the U.S. and adoption of the American lifestyle.

Although the API population in the United States is geographically concentrated, with almost 80 percent of all persons in this category residing in only 10 states, the API category lumps together persons coming from 28 Asian countries and 25 Pacific Island cultures.[9] Each of these subgroups has its own distinctive history, culture, and language. Not surprisingly, an overall value on a health status indicator for the API population hides the considerable heterogeneity that exists for subgroups within that population. For example, the API population in California has death rates of homicide and legal intervention for 15–24 year olds that is 17 per 100,000, but the rates range from 6 for Chinese Americans and 13 for Japanese Americans to 54 for Samoans and 73 for the other Pacific Islander category.[80]

The American Indian (or Native American) population is also characterized by considerable diversity. There are more than 500 federally recognized tribes and entities, and this variation predicts differences in health status. Researchers have also given inadequate attention to the variations within both the black and white population. Although there are important commonalities to the African-American experience in the United States, there is nonetheless considerable heterogeneity within the black population. Some have suggested that there are distinctive "cultural-ecological areas" for the black population that vary across a wide range of social and environmental factors. The black population in the United States includes black immigrants from the Caribbean area and the African mainland. Even these immigrant groups have considerable diversity. The diagnostic and therapeutic utility of racial labels has been exaggerated. That is, although an African American born and raised in the South, a Jamaican, Haitian, Nigerian, and an African American born and raised in the Northeast are all black, they are likely to differ in beliefs, behavior, and even biology.

IMPLICATIONS FOR INTERVENTION

THE evidence reviewed clearly indicates that health-enhancing and pathogenic resources cannot be viewed as autonomous individual factors unrelated to living and working conditions and independent of the broader social and political order. Renewed attention must be given to identifying why populations, as opposed to individuals, vary in their level of risk factors. We must also give more attention to identifying the ways in which the lives of individuals are constrained by broader social, economic, and political forces. Some evidence suggests that the effectiveness of behavioral interventions varies by the social situation in which individuals are embedded. Relaxation techniques, for example, have been shown to be relatively effective in the treatment of mild to moderate hypertension, but the efficacy of those procedures is linked to the social context.[81,82] The amount of stress in an

individual's life affects the effectiveness of stress reduction techniques. The effectiveness of these techniques is enhanced in populations of highly motivated patients in favorable social circumstances.

Some practitioners are intimidated by the prospect of implementing interventions that might make a difference given the power of social structure. However, relatively small changes in the delivery of services can have a dramatic impact in terms of outcome for lower SES persons. Syme's[83] study of 244 hypertensive patients clearly illustrates how addressing underlying social and economic conditions appears to enhance the management of hypertension and improve the effectiveness of anti-hypertensive therapy. The patients in this study were matched on age, race, gender, and blood pressure history and randomly assigned to one of three groups. The first group received routine hypertensive care from a physician. In addition to routine hypertensive care, the second group also attended weekly clinic meetings for 12 weeks that were run by a health educator and nurse practitioner. These didactic sessions provided health education with regard to hypertension. In addition to routine hypertensive care, the third group were visited by community health workers who had been recruited from the immediate community and provided one month of training to address the diverse social and medical needs of persons with hypertension. These lay outreach workers provided information on hypertension, but also discussed family difficulties, financial strain, employment opportunities and, as appropriate, provided support, advice, referral, and direct assistance.

After seven months of follow-up, the hypertensive patients in all groups were evaluated by the clinic medical staff. Patients in the third group were more likely to have their blood pressure controlled than patients in the other two groups. In addition, those in the third group knew twice as much about blood pressure and were more compliant with taking their hypertensive medication than patients in the other two groups. Interestingly, the good compliers in the third group were twice as successful at controlling their blood pressure as good compliers in the health education intervention group. Thus, even the effectiveness of the pharmacological treatment appeared to be enhanced in the group that also addressed the underlying stressful conditions of these hypertensive persons. This study dramatically illustrates that reducing stress and helping patients deal with the challenges of their socioeconomic context can importantly affect the outcomes of interventions.

A study by Buescher and colleagues[84] further illustrates how addressing underlying economic and social issues can improve the impact of medical care. This study compared the effectiveness of two approaches to delivering prenatal care in a population of predominantly black low SES women in Guilford County, North Carolina. One group received prenatal care at the county health department. The other group received prenatal care from private practice physicians. Women who received care from the community-based physicians were twice as likely to have a low birthweight baby, compared to those visiting the health department. The health department's prenatal care program attempted to comprehensively address the medical and social needs of the pregnant mothers. Prenatal care was provided by nurse practitioners, instead of physicians. Time was devoted during prenatal care visits to counseling the women about nutrition and other aspects of personal care. As appropriate, referrals were made to the Women, Infants and Children Program that provides nutritional supplements to poor women. These referrals, as well as missed clinic appointments, were aggressively followed up. James[85] argues that the positive cultural features of this program may have been very important. It appears that the county health department's program offered low-income women an extended network of social support, capable of meeting their needs in much

the same way that older more knowledgeable women have traditionally guided and supported young inexperienced mothers.[85]

CONCLUSION

LIEBERSON'S[86] distinctions between basic causes and surface causes is one with which researchers and practitioners should constantly grapple. Basic causes are those forces responsible for generating a particular outcome. Changes in these factors in turn produce change in the outcome. On the other hand, surface causes are related to the outcome. The changes in these causes do not produce corresponding change in the outcome. That is, as long as the underlying basic causal mechanisms are intact, changes in surface causes will lead to the emergence of new intervening mechanisms to maintain the same outcome. Racial variations in health cannot be simply explained by individual choices, cultural traditions, or biological inheritance. The larger social context in which minority group members live and function is a basic cause of group differences in health status. McKinlay[87] warns that efforts to change the lifestyle of the poor without also altering social structure and life chances not only may be ineffective, but also may do more harm than good. Telling people that they and their treasured practices are somewhat deviant and harmful and not giving them the resources to change the immediate and larger environments which foster such behaviors can be counterproductive. Syme[88] argues that it is difficult to change high risk behaviors even when the targeted social group really wants to and even when every effort is made to help them, if little is being done to alter the societal forces that caused the problem in the first place. The larger social environment plays a large role in the generation of racial disparities in health. Changes in the social environment must be a critical part of any effective strategy to reduce socially induced health inequalities.

NOTES

1. Anderson, M.J. *The American Census: A Social History.* Yale University Press, New Haven, Conn., 1988.

2. Evinger, S. How shall we measure our nation's diversity? *Chance* 8:7–14, 1995.

3. Office of Management and Budget. Statistical Directive No. 15: Race and ethnic standards for federal agencies and administrative reporting. *Federal Register* 43:19269–19270, May 4, 1978.

4. U.S. Bureau of the Census. 1990 Census of Population and Housing, Summary Tape File 1A. Using 1990 Census Lookup 1.4a, <http://venus.census.gov/dcrom/lookup>, July 24, 1998.

5. National Center for Health Statistics. *Vital Statistics of the United States, 1994, Vol. II, Mortality, Part A.* (PHS) 98–1101. Public Health Service, Washington, D.C., 1998.

6. National Center for Health Statistics. *Trends in Indian Health—1993.* U.S. Department of Health and Human Services, Indian Health Service, Rockville, Md., 1993.

7. Sorlie, P. D., Backlund, E., Johnson, N. J., and Rogot, E. Mortality by Hispanic status in the United States. *JAMA* 270:2464–2468, 1993.

8. Vega, W. A., and Amaro, H. Latino outlook: Good health, uncertain prognosis. *Annual Review of Public Health* 15:39–67, 1994.

9. Lin-Fu, J. S. Asian and Pacific Islander Americans: An overview of demographic characteristics and health care issues. *Asian American and Pacific Islander Journal of Health* 1:20–36, 1993.

10. Chen, M. S., A 1993 status report on the health status of Asian Pacific Islander Americans: Comparisons with *Healthy People 2000* objectives. *Asian American and Pacific Islander Journal of Health* 1:37–55, 1993.

11. National Center for Health Statistics. *Vital Statistics of the United States, 1991, Vol. II, Mortality, Part A.* (PHS) 95–1101. Public Health Service, Washington, D.C., 1995.

12. National Center for Health Statistics. *Health, United States, 1992.* (PHS) 93–1232. Public Health Service, Hyattsville, Md., 1993.

13. U.S. Department of Health and Human Services. *Report of the Secretary's Task Force on Black and Minority Health.* U.S. Government Printing Office, Washington, D.C., 1985.

14. National Center for Health Statistics. *Excess Deaths and Other Mortality Measures for the Black Population: 1979–81 and 1991.* Public Health Service, Hyattsville, Md., 1994.

15. National Center for Health Statistics. *Health, United States, 1994.* (PHS) 95–1232. Public Health Service, Hyattsville, Md., 1995.

16. Kochanek, K. D., Maurer, J. D., and Rosenberg, H.M. Why did black life expectancy decline from 1984 through 1989 in the United States? *American Journal of Public Health* 84:938–944, 1994.

17. Lewontin, R. C. The apportionment of human diversity. In *Evolutionary Biology*, vol. 6, edited by T. Dobzhansky, M. K. Hecht, and W. C. Steere, pp. 381–386. Appleton-Century-Crofts, New York, 1972.

18. Gould, S. J. Why we should not name human races: A biological view. In *Ever Since Darwin*, edited by S. J. Gould, pp. 231–236. W. W. Norton, New York, 1977.

19. Latter, B. D. H. Genetic differences within and between populations of the major human subgroups. *American Naturalist* 116:220–237, 1980.

20. Lewontin, R. C. *Human Diversity.* Scientific American Books, New York, 1982.

21. Krieger, N., and Bassett, M. The health of black folk: Disease, class, and ideology in science. *Monthly Review* 38:74–85, 1986.

22. Cooper, R. S., and David, R. The biological concept of race and its application to public health and epidemiology. *Journal of Health and Politics, Policy and Law* 11:97–116, 1986.

23. Williams, D. R. Race and health: Basic questions, emerging directions. *Annals of Epidemiology* 7:322–333, 1997.

24. See, K. O., and Wilson, W. J. Race and ethnicity. In *Handbook of Sociology*, edited by N. J. Smelser, pp. 223–242. Sage Publications, Beverly Hills, Calif., 1988.

25. U. S. Bureau of the Census. 1990 Census of Population and Housing, Summary Tape File 3A. Using 1990 Census Lookup 1.4a, <http://venus.census.gov/cdrom/lookup>, July 30, 1998.

26. National Center for Health Statistics. 1998. *Health, United States, Socio-economic Status and Health Chartbook.* Hyattsville, MD: USDHHS.

27. Krieger, N., Rowley, D. L., Herman, A. A., Avery, B., and Phillips, M. T. Racism, sexism, and social class: Implications for studies of health, disease, and well-being. *American Journal of Preventative Medicine* 9(6 suppl.):82–122, 1993.

28. Williams, D. R., and Collins, C. U.S. socioeconomic and racial differences in health. *Annual Review of Sociology* 21:349–386, 1995.

29. Lillie-Blanton, M., Parsons, P. E., Gayle, H., and Dievler, A. Racial differences in health: Not just black and white, but shades of gray. *Annual Review of Public Health* 17:411-448, 1996.

30. Ries, P. Health of black and white Americans, 1985–1987. *Vital Health Statistics* 10:55, 1990.

31. Idler, E. L., and Benyamini, Y. Self-rated health and mortality: A review of twenty-seven community studies. *Journal of Health and Social Behavior* 38:21–37, 1997.

32. Navarro, V. Race *or* class versus race *and* class: Mortality differentials in the United States. *Lancet* 336:1238–1240, 1990.

33. Moss, N., and Krieger, N. Measuring social inequalities in health. *Public Health Reports* 110:302–305, 1995.

34. Krieger, N., Williams, D. R., and Moss, N. Measuring social class in U.S. public health research: Concepts, methodologies, and guidelines. *Annual Review of Public Health* 18:341–378, 1997.

35. Williams, D. R. Missed opportunities in monitoring socioeconomic status. *Public Health Reports* 112:492–494, 1997.

36. National Center for Health Statistics. *Health, United States, 1998*. (PHS) 98–1232. Public Health Service, Hyattsville, Md., 1998.

37. Williams, D. R., Yu, Y., Jackson, J. S., and Anderson, N. B. Racial differences in physical and mental health: Socioeconomic status, stress, and discrimination. *Journal of Health and Psychology* 2:335–351, 1997.

38. Williams, D. R. Racism and health: A research agenda. *Ethnicity and Disease* 6:1–6, 1996.

39. Schuman, H., Steeh, C., and Bobo, L. *Racial Attitudes in America: Trends and Interpretations*. Harvard University Press, Cambridge, Mass., 1985.

40. Kinder, D. R., and Mendelberg, T. Cracks in American apartheid: The political impact of prejudice among desegregated whites. *The Journal of Politics* 57:402–424, 1995.

41. Massey, D. S., and Denton, N. A. *American Apartheid: Segregation and the Making of the Underclass*. Harvard University Press, Cambridge, Mass., 1993.

42. Jaynes, G. D., and Williams, R. M. *A Common Destiny: Blacks and American Society*. National Academy Press, Washington, D.C., 1989.

43. Kirschenman, J., and Neckerman, K. M. "We'd love to hire them, but . . .": The meaning of race for employers. In *The Urban Underclass*, edited by C. Jencks and P. E. Peter-son, pp. 203–232. The Brookings Institution, Washington, D.C., 1991.

44. Eller, T. J. *Household Wealth and Asset Ownership: 1991*. U.S. Bureau of the Census, Current Population Reports P70–34. U.S. Government Printing Office, Washington, D.C., 1994.

45. Mare, R. D. Socio-economic careers and differential mortality among older men in the United States. In *Measurement and Analysis of Mortality — New Approaches*, edited by J. Vallin and S. D'Souza, pp. 362–387. Clarendon Press, Oxford, 1990.

46. Goldblatt, P. *Longitudinal Study: Mortality and Social Organisation*. HMSO, London, 1990.

47. Robert, S., and House, J. S. SES differentials in health by age and alternative indicators of SES. *Journal of Aging and Health* 8:359–388, 1996.

48. U.S. Bureau of the Census. *Money Income of Households, Families and Persons in the United States*. Current Population Reports P60–174. U.S. Government Printing Office, Washington, D.C., 1991.

49. Williams, D. R. Race/ethnicity and socioeconomic status: Measurement and methodological issues. *International Journal of Health Services* 26:483–505, 1996.

50. Council on Ethical and Judicial Affairs. Black-white disparities in health care. *JAMA* 263:2344–2346, 1990.

51. McBean, A. M., and Gornick, M. Differences by race in the rates of procedures performed in hospitals for Medicare beneficiaries. *Health Care Financing Review* 15:77–90, 1994.

52. Maynard, C., Fisher, L. D., Passamani, E. R., and Pullum, T. Blacks in the Coronary Artery Surgery Study (CASS): Race and decision making. *American Journal of Public Health* 76:1446–1448, 1986.

53. Whittle, J., Conigliaro, J., Good C. B., and Lofgren R. P. Racial differences in the use of invasive cardiovascular procedures in the Department of Veterans Affairs Medical System. *New England Journal of Medicine* 329:621–626, 1993.

54. Giles, A., Anda, R. F., Casper, M. L., Escobedo, L. G., and Taylor, H. A. Race and sex differences in rates of invasive cardiac procedures in U.S. hospitals. *Archives of Internal Medicine* 155:318–324, 1995.

55. Fischer, C. S., Hout, M., Jankowski, M.S., Lucas, S. R., Swidler, A., and Voss, K., eds. *Inequality by Design: Cracking the Bell Curve Myth*. Princeton University Press, Princeton, NJ, 1996.

56. Steele, C. Race and the schooling of black Americans. *Atlantic Monthly* 269:68ff, April 1992.

57. Steele C., and Aronson, J. Contending with a stereotype: African-American intellectually test performance and stereotype vulnerability. Seminar on Meritocracy and Equality. University of Chicago, Chicago, Ill., May 1995.

58. Taylor, J., and Jackson, B. Factors affecting alcohol consumption in black women, part II. *International Journal of Addictions.* 25:1415–1427, 1990.

59. Taylor, D. M., Wright, S. C., and Ruggiero, K. The personal/group discrimination discrepancy: Responses to experimentally induced personal and group discrimination. *Journal of Social Psychology* 131:847–858, 1991.

60. Williams, D. R., and Chung, A. Racism and health. In *Health in Black America*, edited by R. Gibson and J. S. Jackson. Sage, Thousand Oaks, Calif., in press.

61. Amaro, H., Russo, N. F., and Johnson, J. Family and work predictors of psychological well-being among Hispanic women professionals. *Psychology of Women Quarterly* 11:505–521, 1987.

62. Dion, K. L., Dion, K. K., and Pak, A. W. Personality-based hardiness as a buffer for discrimination-related stress in members of Toronto's Chinese community. *Canadian Journal of Behavioral Science* 24:517–536, 1992.

63. Salgado de Snyder, V. N. Factors associated with acculturative stress and depressive symptomatology among married Mexican immigrant women. *Psychology of Women Quarterly* 11:475–488, 1987.

64. Krieger, N. Racial and gender discrimination: Risk factors for high blood pressure? *Social Science and Medicine* 30:1273–1281, 1990.

65. Krieger, N., and Sidney, S. Racial discrimination and blood pressure: The CARDIA study of young black and white adults. *American Journal of Public Health* 86:1370–1378, 1996.

66. Jackson, J. S., Brown, T. N., Williams, D. R., Torres, M., Sellers, S. L., and Brown, K. Racism and the physical and mental health status of African Americans: A thirteen year national panel study. *Ethnicity and Disease* 6:132–147, 1996.

67. U.S. Department of Health, Education and Welfare. *Healthy People: The Surgeon General's Report on Health Promotion and Disease Prevention.* DHEW Pub. No. (PHS) 79-55071. U.S. Government Printing Office, Washington, D.C., 1979.

68. McKinlay, J. B. A case for refocusing upstream: The political economy of illness. In *The Sociology of Health and Illness: Critical Perspectives,* edited by P. Conrad and R. Kern, pp. 502–516. St. Martin's Press, New York, 1990.

69. Seeman, M., and Anderson, C. S. Alienation and alcohol: The role of work, mastery, and community in drinking behavior. *American Sociological Review* 48:60–77, 1983.

70. Singer, M. Toward a political economy of alcoholism. *Social Science and Medicine* 23:113–130, 1986.

71. Rabow, J., and Watt, R. Alcohol availability, alcohol beverage sales, and alcohol-related problems. *Journal of the Study of Alcohol* 43:767–801, 1984.

72. Hacker, A. G., Collins, R., and Jacobson, M. *Marketing Booze to Blacks.* Center for Science in the Public Interest, Washington, D.C., 1987.

73. Maxwell, B., and Jacobson, M. *Marketing Disease to Hispanics: The Selling of Alcohol, Tobacco, and Junk Foods.* Center for Science in the Public Interest, Washington, D.C., 1989.

74. Williams, D. R. Socioeconomic differentials in health: A review and redirection. *Social Psychology Quarterly* 53:31–99, 1990.

75. LaVeist, T. A. Beyond dummy variables and sample selection: What health services researchers ought to know about race as a variable. *Health Services Research* 29:1–16, 1994.

76. Williams, D. R. The concept of race in *Health Services Research,* 1966–1990. *Health Services Research* 29:261–274, 1994.

77. Jones, C. P., LaVeist, T. A., and Lillie-Blanton, M. Race in the epidemiologic literature: An examination of the *American Journal of Epidemiology,* 1921–1990. *American Journal of Epidemiology* 134:1079–1084, 1991.

78. Hahn, R. A. The state of federal health statistics on racial and ethnic groups. *JAMA* 267:168–271, 1992.

79. Tucker, C., McKay, R., Kojetin, B., Harrison, R., de la Puente, M., Stinson, L., and Robison, E. Testing methods of collecting racial and ethnic information: Results of the current population survey supplement on race and ethnicity. *Bureau of Labor Statistical Notes* 40:1–149, 1996.

80. Suh, D. Cooperative agreements to advance the understanding of the health of Asian and Pacific Islander Americans. In *Proceedings of the 1993 Public Health Conference on Records and Statistics,* pp. 352–356. DHHS Pub. No. (PHS) 94-1214. Centers for Disease Control and Prevention, National Center for Health Statistics, Hyattsville, Md., 1993.

81. Williams, D. R. Black-white differences in blood pressure: The role of social factors. *Ethnicity and Disease* 2:126–141, 1992.

82. Patel, C., and Marmot, M. G. Efficacy versus effectiveness of relaxation therapy in hypertension. *Stress Med.* 4:283–289, 1988.

83. Syme, S. L. Drug treatment of mild hypertension: Social and psychological considerations. *Annals of the New York Academy of Sciences* 304:99–111, 1978.

84. Buescher, P. A., Smith, C., Holliday, J. L., and Levine, R. Source of prenatal care and infant birth weight: The case of a North Carolina county. *American Journal of Obstetrics and Gynecology* 53:204–210, 1987.

85. James, S. A. Racial and ethnic differences in infant mortality and low birth weight: A psychosocial critique. *Annals of Epidemiology* 3:130–136, 1993.

86. Lieberson, S. *Making It Count: The Improvement of Social Research and Theory.* University of California Press, Berkeley, 1985.

87. McKinlay, J. B. The help-seeking behavior of the poor. In *Poverty and Health: A Sociological Analysis*, edited by J. Kosa, A. Antonovsky, and I. K. Zola, pp. 224–273. Harvard University Press, Cambridge, Mass., 1975.

88. Syme, S. L. The social environment and health. *Daedalus* 123:79–86, 1994.

Thirteen

SOCIAL NETWORKS AND HEALTH: THE BONDS THAT HEAL

Lisa F. Berkman

INTRODUCTION

AS our nation confronts a health care crisis and as disease, disability, and violence become centered more and more in the poorest, most isolated, and marginal segments of our populations, it is time to consider new paradigms for the prevention and treatment of disease and disability. In considering new preventive efforts, it is important to keep in mind that individuals do not live in a vacuum, rather they are enmeshed in a social environment and in a series of social relationships. There is now a substantial body of evidence that indicates that the extent to which these relationships are strong and supportive and individuals are integrated in their communities is related to the health of the individuals who live within such social contexts.

Almost 20 years ago, epidemiologists who were interested in how social conditions might influence health status began to develop the idea that one of the most important factors that protected people from what seemed to be overwhelming insults, both natural and humanmade, was the extent to which people maintained close personal relationships with others, and the degree to which they were socially integrated into their communities and had deep and abiding social and psychological resources.[1,2,3,4]

Unlike most epidemiologic research, the hallmark of much of this work from the start was its focus, i.e., not on any specific disease but rather on the degree to which these social conditions influence what was rather loosely termed "host resistance." In other words, in contrast to a host of other conditions and exposures, including psychological stressors, that result in classes of *specific* psychosomatic diseases, this class of experiences seemed to make people more vulnerable to a broad range of diseases and disabilities, which ranged from pregnancy complications and infant health in the early parts of life to disability in old age.[1] This idea was defended on the basis of principles articulated in the early 1900's by such scientists as Wade Hampton Frost, who in speaking about declining rates of tuberculosis occurring in the first half of the century wrote: "one of the most important factors in the decline of tuberculosis has been progressively increasing human resistance due to environmental improvements such as better nutrition and relief from physical stress tending to raise what may be called *nonspecific resistance*."[5]

Recent work in the identification of "non-

This work was supported by NHLBI contract U/NO1HC55148 and NIA contract 7RO1AG11042-03. Parts of this chapter are adapted from L. Berkman: The Role of Social Relations in Health, *Psychosomat Med* 57:245–254, 1995.

specific resistance" mechanisms has focused more specifically on neuroendocrine, immune, and metabolic pathways, but the underlying reasoning remains the same in many cases as that expressed by Frost and later by scientists interested in stress responses, such as Selye and Cannon.

In the last twenty years there has been a proliferation of research on the influence of social relationships at both the individual and community level on a broad spectrum of health outcomes. In this chapter, we will demonstrate that the degree to which people are embedded in a web of social relationships that provide intimacy, love and meaning as well as a larger sense of belonging and "fit" with a larger community:

1. influences health outcomes across the life course
2. influences disease prevalence, progression, mortality and physical and cognitive functioning
3. is biologically plausible
4. is amenable to intervention.

The Structure of Networks and Functions of Support

BEFORE each of these points is discussed in more detail, it is helpful to review the definitions of social networks, and social integration, key components of these assessments and how these structural assessments are related to social support.

Social networks are defined as the web of social relationships surrounding an individual. They are often conceptualized as a series of concentric circles, with most intimate ties forming the center or inner circles and more effective, and "weaker" ties moving to circles further out from the center. Most network analysts have postulated that it is not only the intimate ties that perform critical functions in our society but also the more extended ties that play critical roles. Perhaps one of the most classic examples of the role of these extended ties is the work done by Mark Granovetter on the "strength of weak ties" in which he illustrates that jobs are found as a func-

tion of "weak ties," i.e., people known but not intimately by an individual.[6]

In social science research in this area, a great deal of effort is traditionally devoted to the assessment of social networks, usually by asking a respondent to name many individuals, locating them in this series of concentric circles and identifying the social and/or psychologic characteristics of the individuals who are named by the respondent. This questioning leads to a series of network measures that describe the *structure* of an individual's network. It is important to note that the measures usually describe the configuration of the network and are properties of the network, not of the individual. Therefore structural aspects of networks can be examined not only of individuals but of organizations of almost any type.

In an ideal world, those of us in public health would take full advantage of the very sophisticated work done by social scientists in this area. Unfortunately, rarely do epidemiologists have the time to assess social networks in the detail described above. Rather, very crude indicators and summary measures of social networks or ties are developed and folded into studies in which a great deal of time must also be spent on the ascertainment of health outcomes, behaviors, and health care utilization. Over time, the measures of networks and structure have become richer and more complex in epidemiological studies but, in general, they build on the assessment of several types of ties: 1) ties with spouse or partner, 2) ties with family, 3) ties with friends, 4) ties with colleagues at work, 5) membership in voluntary associations, and 6) affiliation with religious organizations. Scales summarizing these types of ties have been called social network measures as well as measures of "social disconnnection" or "social integration" because they weave together aspects of network size, i.e., contacts with friends and relatives, with more general measures of integration, i.e., memberships in religious and voluntary organizations which reflect both access to extended networks as well as community integration. Whatever the social experience these indicators are tapping, whether it is attachment, as some have theorized,[7] or integration and alienation, as Durkheim[8] proposed, they are among the most consistent and powerful predictors of mortality we have.

Over the last twenty years, thirteen large prospective cohort studies across a number of countries, from the U.S. to Scandinavian countries to Japan, show that people who are isolated or dis "connected" from others are at increased risk of dying prematurely. There are dozens of studies focused on particular health outcomes, which are beyond the scope of this review. Each of these major studies will be reviewed briefly below.

In the first of these studies, from Alameda County,[9] men and women who lacked ties to others (in this case, based on an index assessing contacts with friends and relatives, marital status, and church and group membership) were 1.9 to 3.1 times more likely to die in a nine-year follow-up period from 1965 to 1974 than those who had many more contacts.

The relative risks associated with social isolation were *not* centered in one cause of death; rather, those who lacked social ties were at increased risk of dying from ischemic heart disease (IHD), cerebrovascular and circulatory disease, cancer, and a final category including respiratory, gastrointestinal, and all other causes of death. Clearly, this social condition is not associated exclusively with increased risks from, say, coronary heart disease (CHD). The relationship between social isolation and mortality risk was independent of health behaviors such a smoking, alcohol consumption, physical activity, preventive health care and a range of baseline comorbid conditions.

Another study, in Tecumseh, Michigan (n=2754),[10] shows a similar strength of positive association for men, but not for women, between social connectedness/social participation and mortality risk over a 10–12 year period. An additional strength of this study was the ability of the investigators to control for some biomedical pre-

dictors assessed from physical examination (e.g., cholesterol, blood pressure, and respiratory function). In the same year, Blazer[11] reported similar results from a sample of elderly men and women in Durham County, North Carolina. He compared three measures of social support and attachment: 1) self-perceived impaired social support, including feelings of loneliness, 2) impaired social roles and attachments, and 3) low frequency of social interaction. The relative risks for dying associated with these three measures were, respectively, 3.4, 2.0, and 1.9.

In the last few years, results from several more studies have been reported, one from a study in the United States and three from Scandinavia. Using data from Evans County, Georgia, (n=2059),[12] Schoenbach used a measure of social contacts modified from the Alameda County Study and found risks to be significant in older men and women even when controlling for biomedical and sociodemographic risk factors. In Sweden, the Goteborg study[13] shows that in different cohorts of men born in 1913 and 1923, social isolation proved to be a risk factor for dying, independent of age and biomedical risk factors. A recent report by Orth-Gomer and Johnson[14] is the only study besides the Alameda County one to report significantly increased risks for women who have been socially isolated. Finally, in a study of 13,301 men and women in Eastern Finland, Kaplan and associates[15] have shown that an index of social connections almost identical to the Social Network Index used in Alameda County predicts mortality risk for men but not for women, independent of standard cardiovascular risk factors.

Several recent studies of older men and women in the Alameda County study and the Established Populations for the Epidemiologic Study of the Elderly (EPESE) studies confirm the continued importance of these relationships into late life.[16,17] Furthermore, two studies of a large cohort of men and women in a large HMO[18] and 32,000 male health professionals[19] suggest that social networks are in general more strongly related to mortality than to the incidence or onset of disease. Networks in the health professionals study were related to the incidence of stroke. Some other evidence links lack of social support to incidence of CHD in middle-aged Swedish men.[20]

Two very recent studies, in Danish men[21,22] and Japanese men and women,[23] further indicate that aspects of social isolation or social support are related to mortality. Virtually all of these studies find that people who are socially isolated or disconnected to others have between two and five times the risk of dying from all causes compared to those who maintain strong ties to friends, family and community.

SELECTED STUDIES OF HEALTH OUTCOMES ACROSS THE LIFE COURSE

Pregnancy Outcomes

In addition to the studies discussed above, there are a large number of studies focused on particular health outcomes across the lifecourse that indicate that aspects of social networks and supports are important for all age groups. Of particular interest is the work on pregnancy and pregnancy complications. In a massive review of over 144 studies,[24] Hoffman and Hatch concluded that social support from a partner or family member improves fetal growth. In some of the classic earliest studies of social support, emotional support and psychosocial resources predicted complications in childbirth.[25] Several other studies in extremely diverse and heterogeneous groups confirm that mothers that have high support have fewer complications, healthier babies, and better long-term mental health outcomes in terms of postpartum depression.[26,27,28,29]

Survival Post MI

In the last five years, there have been a host of studies suggesting that social ties, especially intimate ties and emotional support provided by those ties influences survival among people post MI or with serious cardiovascular disease. In the first of these, Ruberman et al.[30] explored 2320 male survivors of acute MI who were participants in the Beta-Blocker Heart Attack Trial. Patients who were socially isolated were more than twice as likely to die over a three-year period than those who were less socially isolated. When this measure of social isolation was combined with a general measure of life stress, which included items related to occupational status, divorce, exposure to violent events, retirement, or financial difficulty, the risks associated with high-risk psychosocial status were even greater. Those in the high-risk psychosocial categories were four to five times as likely to die as those in the lowest risk categories. This psychosocial characteristic was associated with death from all causes and sudden deaths. It made large contributions to mortality risk in both the high-arrhythmia and low-arrhythmia groups. In this study (and most of the studies in which subjects are recruited post-event), the investigators were not able to determine the temporal association between the assessment of psychosocial resources and the severity of disease. Nonetheless, it serves as a powerful model for future studies.

In a second Swedish study of 150 cardiac patients and patients with high-risk factor levels for CHD, the finding that lack of support predicts death was further confirmed.[31] Patients who were socially isolated had a three times higher ten-year mortality rate than did those who were socially active and integrated. Because these patients were examined extensively for cardiological prognostic factors at study entry, it was possible to disentangle effects of psychosocial and clinical characteristics.

In a third study, Williams et al.[32] enrolled 1368 patients who were undergoing cardiac catheterization from 1974 through 1980 and found to have significant coronary artery disease. They examined survival time until cardiovascular death through 1989. Men constituted 82% of the sample. In this study, men and women who were unmarried or without a confidant were over three times as likely to die within five years compared with those who had a close confidant or who were married (odds ratio (OR), 3.34; confidence interval (CI), 1.8–6.2). This association was independent of other clinical prognostic indicators and sociodemographic factors, including socioeconomic status.

In another study, Case et al.[33] examined the association between marital status and recurrent major cardiac events among patients post-MI who were enrolled in the placebo arm of a clinical trial, the Multicenter Diliazem Post-Infarction Trial. These investigators reported that living alone was an independent risk factor with a hazard ratio of 1.54 (CI, 1.04-2.29) for recurrent major cardiac events, including both nonfatal infarctions or cardiac deaths.

In a fifth study, we explored the relationship between social networks and support and the mortality rate among men and women hospitalized for an MI between 1982 and 1988 who are participants in the population-based New Haven EPESE.[34] Over the study period, 100 men and 94 women were hospitalized for an MI. Thirty-four percent of women and 44% of men died in the six-month period after MI.

Among both men and women, emotional support, measured prospectively, that is, before the MI, was related to both early in-hospital death and later death over a one-year period. Among those admitted to the hospital, almost 38% of those who reported no source of emotional support died in the hospital, compared with 11.5% of those with two or more sources of support. The patterns remained steady throughout the follow-up period. At six months, the major end point of the study, 52.8% of those with no source of support had died, compared with 36.0% of those with one source and 23.1% of those with two or more sources of support. These figures did not change substantially at one year. As Figure 1 shows, the patterns were remarkably consistent for both men and women, younger and older people, and those with more or less severe cardiovascular disease, as assessed by a Killip classi-

fication system. In multivariate models that control for sociodemographic factors, psychosocial factors, including living arrangements, depressive symptoms, and clinical prognostic indicators, men and women who reported no emotional support had almost three times the mortality risk compared with subjects who reported at least one source of support (OR, 2.9; 95% CI, 1.2–6.9).

In a study of men and women undergoing coronary bypass surgery or aortic valve replacement, Oxman and colleagues[35] found that membership in voluntary organizations, including religious organizations, as well as drawing strength and comfort from religious or spiritual faith were related to survival post surgery. When these two dimensions were combined, people who endorsed neither of these items were over seven times as likely to die as those who belonged to organizations and drew comfort from their faith. Though it is beyond the scope of this chapter to go into detail on the recent research on religiosity, this later study complements and balances the work on the importance of intimacy by illustrating that a sense of belonging and trust in a larger sense play a role in survival as well.

Life Course Issues

By reviewing the data on pregnancy outcomes at the beginning of life and survival post MI among predominantly older men and women, we can see that social relationships are important at all ages. However, some interesting issues remain. For instance, so far we have viewed network relationships at a single point in time, as a somewhat static phenomenon. In fact, of course, relationships are dynamic and everchanging. Furthermore, it is entirely possible that relationships influence the manifestations of disease long before the manifestation of clinical disease. For instance, several studies of college cohorts from Johns Hopkins and Harvard suggest that parental relationships in early childhood characterized by warmth and closeness are related to

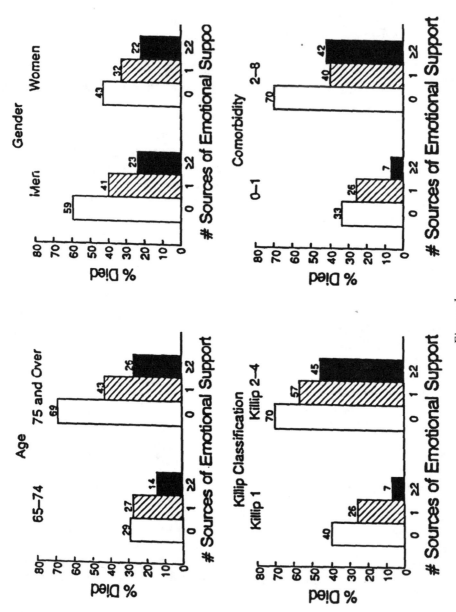

Figure 1

Percentage of patients with MIs who died within 6 months by level of social support. Adjustments were made for age (top left); gender (top right); severity of MI, as defined by Killip class (bottom left); and comorbidity (bottom right). (From Berkman et al. (34) with permission.)

disease thirty-five to fifty years later.[36,37,38] Although the mechanisms or pathways by which such relationships recollected during college might influence disease onset decades later is unclear and likely to be complex, this work highlights the need of investigators to pay close attention to the temporal sequence in which they assume social relationships influence health outcomes.

This work also emphasizes the need to conceptualize social networks in a more dynamic way. For instance, much of the work in social psychology emphasizes that the ability to maintain intimate, enduring, trusting relationships in midlife is learned in early life. Thus, parental closeness may influence health outcomes by setting in motion the opportunity to maintain relationships later in life. It is also important not to oversimplify this association, since much evidence also indicates that cultural, organizational, social, and economic factors influence an individual's ability to maintain enduring social ties. The organization of work and schools, occupational and geographical mobility and patterns of migration, as well as cultural values of types of relationships all exert powerful influences on network development and the receipt and provision of support.

BIOLOGICAL PLAUSIBILITY

SOCIAL networks and the degree to which individuals are embedded in supportive social relationships have pervasive health effects ranging from pregnancy complications to susceptibility to colds, to progression of HIV to mortality and disability. Such pervasive disease consequences are related to multiple mechanisms linking such a social exposure to outcomes. Four major pathways might be defined. First, social networks and support might influence outcomes via access to and quality of health care. Second, socio-environmental conditions have also been tied to aspects of the physical environment, both at work and at home, that might in-

fluence health. Third, social factors in general and networks and support specifically influence health promoting and health damaging behaviors such as cigarette smoking, physical activity, dietary patterns, and alcohol consumption.

Fourth, social networks and social support may have direct effects on health outcomes by influencing a series of biological mechanisms hypothesized to link stressful social experiences to health outcomes.

Evidence indicates that social networks are related to the first three of these pathways, especially to health behaviors as seen in Figure 2. In the Alameda County Study, men and women who lacked social ties were more likely to maintain many risk-related behaviors such as cigarette smoking, heavy alcohol consumption, and lack of physical activity. It is also clear that these pathways do not account for a large part of the relationship between social networks and health.[6] In most instances, relative risks are reduced about 20% when such behaviors are introduced into models. Furthermore, we may most appropriately think of these behaviors as pathways or more proximately factors that are themselves influenced by the social environment.

In either case, let us turn to an examination of potential biological pathways linking social networks and support to health outcomes. One of the common threads running through the studies just reviewed is the broad array of diseases and cause of death associated with social isolation. Thus, we speculate that social networks and support influence mortality and therefore longevity or life expectancy by influencing in general the rate of aging of the organism. In a 1988 review of aging and longevity from a social perspective,[39] we hypothesized that social isolation "was a chronically stressful condition to which the organism responds by aging faster. Isolation would then also be associated with age-related morbidity and functional impairment. Thus, the cumulative conditions that tend to occur in very old age were accelerated."

Characteristic of changes related to aging is

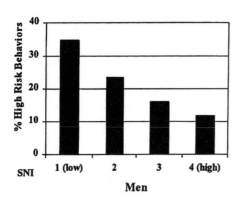
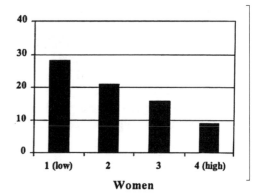

Figure 2
Percent of Men and Women Who Have Several High Risk Behaviors (three of five)
by Level of Social Network Index
(Alameda County Study, n=2229 men, n=2496 women)
Ages 30–69

that peak rises in response to stress or challenge are not as different among young and old as are the fact that old animals have a peak response that is sustained for a longer time following challenge than younger people do. This is illustrated in Figure 3.

For instance, Sapolsky, Krey and McEwen[40] (1983) show that while aging rats have slightly elevated levels of basal corticosterone, by far the most remarkable change with age is the impaired capacity of the older rats to adapt to and recover from stress. In a series of experiments, old and young rats exposed to cold or immobilization stress reacted initially in the same way, with dramatic increases in corticosterone; but after 90 minutes, and even up to 150 minutes after exposure, the young rats had returned to basal levels while the aged rats still maintained very high levels due to continued secretion rates similar to the hypothetical curves in Figure 3. In another set of experiments, Meany and associates[41,42] found that rats handled during the postnatal period also showed faster adrenocortical recovery from stress

than did nonhandled rats. These results look very similar to those comparing young and old rats. Furthermore, the aged rats that were not handled showed an age-related rise in basal glucocorticoid levels that was not apparent among the aged handled rats. The findings suggest that the cumulative exposure to glucocorticoids over the lifespan was greater in the nonhandled compared with the handled rats. Hippocampal cell loss and cognitive impairment were also much more pronounced in the aged nonhandled rats. The results indicate that experiences involving environmental stimulation influence the way rodents react to stress and perhaps account for some of the variability observed among aging animals and humans as well.

The implication for humans of stress research using animals is that age differences in neuroendocrine response in the absence of stress or challenge are minimal compared to those that are manifest under more trying circumstances. The last experiments noted above illustrate how an environmental condition, handling during the early life of the rat, retards a response to stress that is identified with a condition we think of as illustrating "normal aging." The evidence suggests that such response patterns are not entirely intrinsically determined. This finding is of importance because, if we conceive of the way in which an organism recovers from stress as part of biological aging, it illustrates the extent to which patterns of adaptations are environmentally regulated. Importantly, in this case the environmental condition is not a stressor but a behavior that under natural conditions would be related to intimate, nurturant behavior.

This same nurturant behavior of humans toward animals was found to reduce plaque in arteries by 60% in a classic study in which rabbits on a high-cholesterol diet were randomized to handling and attention and "usual care." Again, contact and connectedness are found to be related to important health outcomes.[43]

Recent work by our group from the MacArthur Foundation Research Network on Successful Aging further confirms in observational data on a large cohort of men and women that social networks and emotional support are related to basal levels of several neuroendocrine factors.[44] Social support has also been associated with altered neuroendocrine response in a study of work-related stress.[45]

With regard to cardiovascular reactivity, several recent studies have identified remarkably strong relationships with support and reactivity assessed in terms of blood pressure response to stress or challenge. Among the most elegant of these studies is an experiment conducted by Uchino and Garvey.[46] In this experiment, Uchino and Garvey exposed all subjects to a challenge involving public speaking. They then randomly told half the group that social support was available by telling them before the "challenge" that someone was available for help if they needed it. They would be just outside the room. In fact, no support was actually provided; it was merely available if needed. Figure 4 shows the results of the challenge. People without support

had higher systolic and diastolic pressure both before the actual challenge as well as during the challenge. Thus, support availability protects against the increased blood pressure response often reported during challenges.

Another pathway by which social relationships might influence health involves alteration in immune response. There is a growing body of knowledge in this area. While immune function is a complex and multidimensional phenomenon and not detached from neuroendocrine response, much progress has been made in the last decade or two in understanding how social ties influence immune function. While most of this work focuses on the association between psychosocial exposures and immune response without a further tie to health outcomes, some recent evidence suggests that the structure of ties influences not only immune parameters but also clinical manifestation of the common cold. Since much of our research has focused in social determinants of what are most often thought of as non-infectious disease, this evidence linking social ties to an infectious disease is very important.

In this recent study, Cohen and colleagues[47] exposed 276 healthy volunteers aged 18–55 to nasal drops containing rhinoviruses. Since everyone was exposed to a virus, virtually everyone showed signs of infection. However, the degree to which subjects maintained different kinds of social relationships (e.g., with friends, family voluntary associations, religious affiliation) was strongly related to the development of clinical colds. People who had few types of relationships were over four times as likely to develop a cold as were those with many types of contact (see Figure 5). The relationship was independent of a wide range of health behaviors and was not fully explained by antibody titers.

This study is so impressive because subjects were equally exposed to the viral agent but showed variations in the development of disease. The virus was a necessary but not sufficient factor to cause disease. This model of disease causation may have broad applicability to other infectious

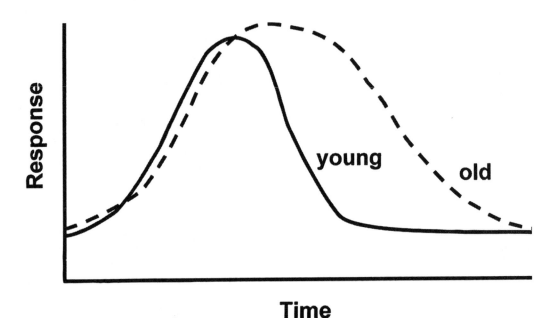

Figure 3
Response to Stress by Age

diseases such as tuberculosis and AIDS, where we know that exposure to the infectious agent does not invariably produce disease, though it may result in subclinical infection.

The largest body of evidence in this area links social support to changes in immune parameters. Early studies showed the pervasive effects of bereavement or living with a severely ill spouse or child in terms of suppressed immune function, particularly cellular immunity.[48,49] Work over the last few years by Kiecolt-Glaser and colleagues and others has found that less devastating aspects of relationships such as the quality of marital relationship or feelings of loneliness among medical students also compromise immunocompetence.[50,51,52,53] The latter studies of

medical students showed that those who were lonely had not only lower levels of natural killer-cell activity but significantly high Epstein-Barr virus (EBV) antibody titers. Thus again, we see provocative evidence that social isolation may regulate immune mechanisms involved in the regulation of latent infections.

Finally, studies of affiliation in nonhuman primates further suggest that such intimate affiliative behaviors are associated with cellular immune response.[54,55] Depending on how we interpret other animal studies in socially stressed groups in which animals lived in socially unstable settings, further evidence for the potent force of social disconnection and isolation may be garnered.

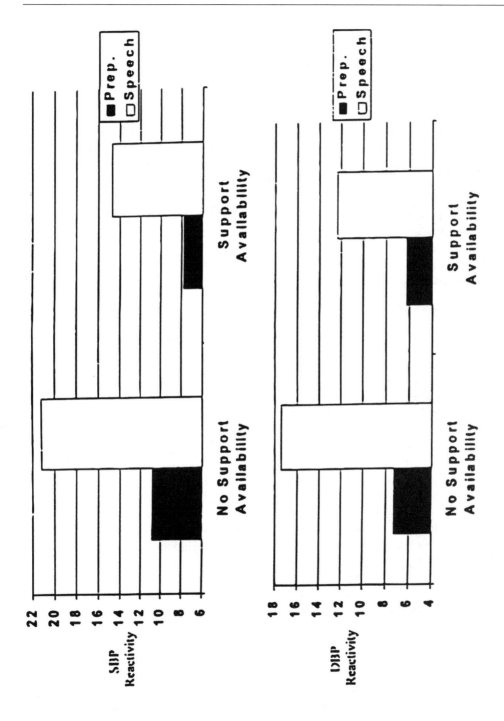

Figure 4

Mean Cardiovascular Reactivity (i.e., Task Minus Pretask Baseline) as a Function of the Availability of Social Support

Allostatic load is a new concept, in which multiple physiologic mechanisms involving blood pressure, neuroendocrine regulation, carbohydrate metabolism and glucose tolerance combine to reflect a noxious response to stress.[56,57] To date, limited evidence has been gathered supporting the specific socioenvironmental conditions that might influence this syndrome, yet it has many attractive features as a plausible biological pathway which should be explored in future studies. First, it is a syndrome that has the capacity to explain many disease outcomes which is a critical feature of many social conditions linked to morbidity and mortality. Secondly, many of the components of allostatic load can be seen as classical aspects of aging whether we view aging as an intrinsic or environmentally driven experience.

The Need to Develop More Informative Animal and Experimental Paradigms

Much of the work in this area in nonhuman primates and nonprimates is developed with the intention of revealing biological responses to stress. This same paradigm is often true to a lesser extent in experimental work in humans. Both the "stressor" and the population randomized (e.g., college students) bear little resemblance to typical at-risk populations or stressful experiences. The biological parameter under investigation, however, often has a direct parallel to human situations. In the early stages of inquiry, the benefits of the approach far outweighed its disadvantages, since classical exposures were developed and standardized (e.g., cold pressor test, biological challenges, rat mazes, enriched environments, etc.) and homogeneous subjects (e.g., genetically similar strains of rodents, monkeys, college students) revealed small variations in response.

I would like to suggest that we are now at a very different stage of scientific inquiry in this area. Having in many cases proven a link between an environmental or "exogenous" exposure

with a biological response, we are often hard pressed to extrapolate from the social experience or stressor in animal studies to something real and meaningful in human populations. Furthermore, we have often either "designed" the variability out of the experimental situations or ignored it in our analysis of results. I would like to relate the findings from one experiment we conducted in the MacArthur Foundation Studies of Successful Aging where we struggled to develop an improved paradigm. We developed two "challenges" in which we were interested in how older people responded in terms of neuroendocrine reactivity.[56] In the first challenge, the standard or classic one, we gave all people a CRF (corticotropin-releasing factor) challenge in the clinical studies unit of a hospital. In the second setting, we developed a driving simulation and subjects were shown different films involving accidents, near misses, and standard driving situations. In both cases, the "challenges" produced substantial neuroendocrine responses. However, of critical importance was the variability in response seen in the second "driving" challenge. In this situation, self-esteem almost completely moderated the response to challenge so that among subjects with high levels of self-esteem there was a great (and significantly dampened) response to the stress of the driving challenge. Self-esteem had no such effect in moderating the biological CRF challenge.

Thus, we see the models of stress we use may not be the most informative when we want to gain more insight into the social experiences and psychological resources that in real life produce biological responses. We need to think carefully about what the handling of animals by humans or rejuggling animals in different cages means in terms of human experience. Also, biological challenges that are in no way cognitively mediated may inhibit the surfacing or moderating of buffering psychological and social conditions that in reality account for a great deal of the variation seen in human responses to challenge or stress. Animal, experimental, and observa-

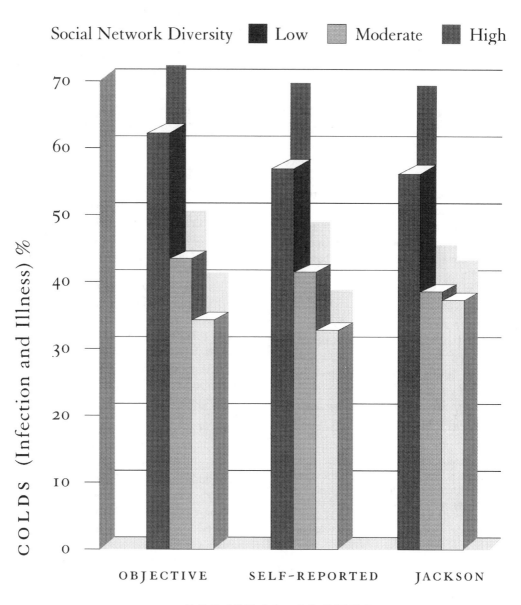

Figure 5
Observed incidence of colds by social network diversity using 3 illness criteria. Low diversity is defined
as 1 to 3 types of social relationships; moderate, 4 to 5; and high, 6 or more. Error bars indicate SEs.

tional studies have the potential to inform each other much better than they currently do. By integrating research across disciplines, progress in this area will advance rapidly.

The Policy Implications of Research on Social Networks and Health: From Individual to Community

THIS conference is designed with the very ambitious but correct agenda of understanding how basic work in public health could lead to improved health for the citizens of Kansas. In order for this goal to be achieved, academics, practitioners, and policy-makers must join forces to develop policies that will promote health. It is apparent that these policies will have little to do with health care policies per se. Rather, we will need to focus attention on those public and private sector social and economic policies that may have a more fundamental impact on health because they influence the determinants of health and well-being and risks of disease and functional decline. With regard to promoting social networks and enhancing support, it is important to keep four key features in focus:

1. The vast amount of evidence accumulated to date suggests that *both* intimate relationships and extended relationships stemming from voluntary and religious affiliations are important and health promoting. While intimate associations build a sense of trust, love and intimacy, extended relationships build a sense of belonging and fit, a sense of community.

2. Networks are comprised of many types of relationships. As a society it is important to acknowledge that today families come in all shapes and sizes—single parent families, dual career marriages, same-sex marriages and communities are created on shared political, religious, cultural and ethnic values. As long as these networks and communities do not devalue other communities, policies that support and value their existence will be health promoting.

3. In a similar vein, support can come from many sources. It is important not to be proscriptive, especially unconsciously, about who provides support. Thus, older people who live alone may not be socially isolated. Aside from daughters and spouses, support for older men and women often comes from peers, siblings, friends, and hopefully, sons. In early life, grandparents, aunts and uncles, and close friends can be key providers to young children whose parents may not be able to meet their needs.

4. Networks are dynamic and are influenced by social and economic forces as well as social skills learned throughout the life course.

What does this mean in terms of policy? Policies may be conceived of in several tiers: Federal and state public policies, private sector policies, and policies within the health care system. It is beyond the scope of this chapter to give a detailed account of policies that influence network structure and support but rather, I will give examples of policies at three levels that might strengthen network structure and bolster support. It is also worthwhile to note that some public and private policies currently in place are actually destructive to the maintenance of family and community ties. Their elimination would de facto support networks and social integration. For instance, corporate policies that move employees geographically, especially in critical times of family growth and development, make it difficult to establish stable relationships. On the public policy side, urban development and renewal policies or even public housing for the elderly that emphasizes the physical or built environment have in the past often been destructive to well-established working class neighborhoods and their tight community functioning.

To turn to a positive side, family-friendly work policies and parental leave are two of the clearest pro-family policies we have initiated. Welfare policies that acknowledge the attainment of work-related skills but *not* at the expense of caring for children or other dependents would bolster social attachment and connectedness not only for welfare mothers and fathers but for young children. In refining these policies, it will be helpful to understand that, as noted earlier, families are constructed in many different ways. Identifying who plays strong functional roles and supporting those links is probably more important than working along more traditional kinship or biological lines.

Urban development and housing policies hold enormous potential to improve the health of the public. Urban planners, economists, and architects are often concerned with patterns of social organization yet lack sufficient interdisciplinary interactions to develop and evaluate complex models of healthy urban development. In Europe, a "healthy cities" project offers a useful way of developing appropriate intersectoral policies yet rarely are these projects evaluated rigorously. As urban areas grow in Kansas over the next decades as they have in the past decades, incorporating intersectoral policies that connect housing, transportation, economic development and public health will be critical.

In the U.S., we have rarely had enlightened policies with regard to the health and well-being of our Native-American population. Nowhere is it more obvious that health is linked to community connectedness, sense of belonging and strong social ties than among Native-American populations. In Native-American communities, attention is now most often focused on health care policies as defined in its narrowest sense. In order to promote health and well-being in these populations, it will be necessary to do more than promote economic development and health care, though these are both important. It will be critical to consider the ways in which family ties and social networks are promoted through schools and educational policies (boarding versus community education), how a sense of belonging is nurtured by a sense of "place," and how traditions are balanced with modern culture to maintain social bonds and integration.

These macro-policies have tremendous potential to improve the health of the public. At the same time, there is great potential to improve health through more micro-social and preventive health strategies. For instance, in spite of a great deal of evidence to the contrary, Americans often assume that formal or institutional provision of support and/or care will reduce or weaken informal (e.g., family or community) support. In fact, in all our interventions, I most often observe that families and communities go to extraordinary lengths to take care of members who need help. Often they do so with very limited resources. For instance, families institutionalize older parents as a last resort after bearing an incredible burden of care for a long time. In the U.S., African Americans and other ethnic minorities rarely institutionalize their parents in spite of very limited economic resources. Our lack of provision of respite care, and limitations of adult day-care and home health care do not strengthen family resources. They place an incredible strain on them. In Kansas, where some communities have experienced out-migration of younger populations with substantial aging of the community, such resources will be critical in enabling older people to maintain not only their health but their independence and sense of worth. These policies are especially needed at a time when the majority of middle-aged women, caretakers of the young and old, are in the work force.

The same U.S. philosophy often guides our policies about child care, day care, and after-school care. That is, we believe we will weaken family bonds by substituting non-family care for family (i.e., mother) care. In fact, in the United States at this moment the majority, 77% of women with school-age children and 62% of women with preschool-age children, are working. To deny children of these parents safe nurturing experiences is to place them at a social disadvantage from which they may never recover and to place parents under enormous physical and mental strain which may also have profound health consequences. Many European countries, France for example, have strong pro-family policies that support day care throughout the country with day-care workers trained and compensated more highly than in the U.S. Whether child care policies emerge from the public or private sector, the need to provide high-quality care to children from all social and economic backgrounds is of the highest priority.

We are at a critical juncture with regard to primary and secondary prevention within the health care system in the United States. As health maintenance organizations grow and fee-for-service systems shrink, it is to the advantage of a new HMO that maintains enrollees over extended periods of time to institute effective primary and secondary prevention strategies. With regard to social support interventions, several models have been shown to be successful and a recent review and meta-analysis[58] suggest that among patients with coronary artery disease, patients who did not receive psychosocial treatment had over 1.7 times the rate of mortality and cardiac recurrences as those who did receive psychosocial treatment.

Among the most promising models of psychosocial intervention is that developed by Spiegal and colleagues at Stanford. In Spiegal's trial,[59] women with metastatic breast cancer were randomly allocated to treatment or usual care. Treatment involved meeting in a group for ninety minutes once a week in a supportive group setting to discuss and express feelings about living with breast cancer and how it affected the women's lives. The women who had the support group lived twice as long as those who were in the usual care group. This study is being replicated in a much larger sample, but it serves as an excellent model for future interventions within an HMO model of health care. As Spiegal writes, "the groups countered the social isolation that often divides cancer patients from their well-meaning but anxious family and friends."

Other support models build more on naturally occurring networks, taking off on the concept that family are often well-meaning but may not be as helpful as they can be in providing effective support. Recent research has documented that not all relationships are supportive and obviously

individuals vary in their ability to elicit social support.[60] Interventions that aim to improve communication among existing networks have great potential. Several interventions, including a large trial of post-myocardial infarction patients, ENRICHD, funded by the National Heart, Lung and Blood Institute and studies among HIV positive men,[61] have incorporated this perspective into their interventions.

CONCLUSION

SOCIAL networks and the support they provide are key determinants of morbidity, mortality and functioning. Social networks are influenced and in turn influence other key social structures. The pathways by which social experiences influence disease are undoubtedly multiple but data suggest it is biologically plausible that there are direct links between social connectedness, support, and disease processes. In order to reduce social inequalities in health stemming from social disintegration and social isolation, we will need to focus on population-based preventive efforts that, at their core, promote social support and develop family and community strengths. Acknowledging that the health of the public rests not on the shoulders of only individuals but also on their families and communities means that we must commit resources over the next decade to developing and implementing policies in this area. This is a critical next step.

NOTES

1. Cassel, J. The contribution of the social environment to host resistance. *Am J Epidemiol* 1976;104:107–123.

2. Cobb, S. Social support as a moderator of life stress. *Psychosom Med* 1976; 38:300–314.

3. Bruhn, J., Wolf, S. *An Anatomy of Health: The Roseto Story.* Oklahoma City, OK, University of Oklahoma Press, 1979.

4. Matsumoto, Y. S. Social stress and coronary heart disease in Japan: A hypothesis. *Milbank Q* 1979; 48:9–36.

5. Frost, W. H. How much control of tuberculosis? *Am J Public Health* 1937; 27:759–766.

6. Granovetter, M. The strength of weak ties. *Am J of Sociol* 1973; 78:1360–1380.

7. Bowlby, J. The nature of the child's tie to his mother. *International J of Psychoanalysis* 1958; 39:350–373.

8. Durkheim, E. *Suicide.* New York, Free Press (1951).

9. Berkman, L. F, Syme, S. L. Social networks, host resistance and mortality: A nine year follow-up study of Alameda County residents. *Am J Epidemiol* 1979; 109:186–204.

10. House, J. S., Robbins, C., and Metzner, H. L. The association of social relationships and activities with mortality: Prospective evidence from the Tecumseh community health study. *Am J Epidemiol* 1982; 116:123–140.

11. Blazer, D. G. Social support and mortality in an elderly community population. *Am J of Epidemiol* 1982; 115(5):684–94.

12. Schoenbach, V. J., Kaplan, B. G., Freedman, L., et al. Social ties and mortality in Evans County, Georgia. *Am J Epidemiol* 1986; 123:577–591.

13. Weblin, L., Tibblin, G., Svardsudd, K., et al. Prospective study of social influences on mortality: The study of men born in 1913 and 1923. *Lancet* 1985; 1:915–918.

14. Orth-Gomer, K., and Johnson. J. Social network interaction and mortality: A six-year follow-up of a random sample of the Swedish population. *J Chronic Dis* 1987; 40:949–957.

15. Kaplan, G. A., Salonen, J. T., Cohen, R.D., et al. Social connections and mortality from all causes and from cardiovascular disease: prospective evidence from eastern Finland. *Am J of Epidemiol* 1988; 128(2):370–80.

16. Seeman, T. E., Berkman, L. F., Kohout, F., et al. Intercommunity variations in the association between social ties and mortality in the elderly: A comparative analysis of three communities. *Ann Epidemiol* 1993; 3:325–335.

17. Seeman, T. E., Kaplan, G., Knudsen, L., Cohen, R., Guralnik, J. Social network ties and mortality among the elderly in the Alameda County Study. *Am J of Epidemiol* 1988; 126:714–723.

18. Vogt, T., Mullooly, J., Ernst, D., Pope, C., and Hollis, J. Social networks as predictors of ischemic heart disease, cancer, stroke and hypertension: incidence, survival and mortality. *J Clin Epidemiol* 1992;45:659–666.

19. Kawachi, I., Colditz, G. A., Ascherio, A., Rimm, E. D., Giovannucci, E., and Stampfer, M. J. A prospective study of social networks in relation to total mortality and cardiovascular disease in men in the USA. *J of Epidemiol and Comm Health* 1996; 50:245–251.

20. Orth-Gomer, K., Rosengren, A., and Wilhelmsen, L. Lack of social support and incidence of coronary heart disease in middle-aged Swedish men. *Psychosom Med* 1993; 55:37–43.

21. Olsen, O. Impact of social networks on cardiovascular mortality in middle-aged Danish men. *J of Epidem and Comm Health* 1993;47:176–180.

22. Penninx, B. W., van Tilburg, T., Kriegsman, D. M., et al. Effects of social support and personal coping resources on mortality in older age: The Longitudinal Aging Study Amsterdam. *Am J of Epidem* 1997; 146(6):510–9.

23. Sugisawa, H., Liang, J., and Liu, X. Social networks, social support and mortality among older people in Japan. *J Gerontol* 1994; 49:S3–13.

24. Hoffman, S., Hatch, M. C. Stress, social support and pregnancy outcomes: a reassessment based on recent research. *Paediatric and Perinatal Epidemiology* 1996; 10(4):380–405.

25. Nuckolls, K. B., Cassel, J. C., and Kaplan, B. H. Psychosocial assets, life crisis, and prognosis of pregnancy. *Am J of Epidem* 1972; 95:431–441.

26. Boyce, W. T., Schaefer, C., and Uitti, C. Permanence and change: psychosocial factors in the outcome of adolescent pregnancy. *Soc Sci and Med* 1985; 21(11):1279–87.

27. Boyce, W. T. Stress and child health: an overview. *Pediatric Annals,* 1985; 14(8):539–42.

28. Collins, N. L., Dunkel-Schetter, C., Lobel, M., et al. Social support in pregnancy: Psychosocial correlates of birth outcomes and postpartum depression. *J of Personality and Soc Psych* 1993; 65:1243–1258.

29. Norbeck, J. S., Anderson, N. J. Psychosocial predictors of pregnancy outcomes in low-income black, Hispanic, and white women. *Nursing Research* 1989;38:204–209.

30. Ruberman, W., Weinblatt, E., Goldberg, J. D., et al. Psychosocial influences on mortality after myocardial infarction. *New Eng J Med* 1984; 311:552–559.

31. Orth-Gomer, K., Unden, A. L., and Edwards, M. E. Social isolation and mortality in ischemic heart disease. *Acta Med Scand* 1988; 224:205–215.

32. Williams, R. B., Barefoot, J. C., Califf, R. M., et al. Prognostic importance of social and economic resources among medically treated patients with angiographically

documented coronary artery disease. *JAMA* 1992; 267:520–524.

33. Case, R. B., Moss, A. J., Case, N., et al. Living alone after myocardial infarction. *JAMA* 1992; 267:515.

34. Berkman, L. F., Leo-Summers, L., and Horwitz, R. I. Emotional support and survival following myocardial infarction: A prospective population-based study of the elderly. *Ann Intern Med* 1992; 117:1003–1009.

35. Oxman, T. E., Freeman, Jr., D. H., and Manheimer, E. D. Lack of social participation or religious strength and comfort as risk factors for death after cardiac surgery in the elderly. *Psychosomatic Med* 1995, 57:5–15.

36. Russek, L. G., Schwartz, G. E. Perceptions of parental caring predict health status in midlife: A 35-year follow-up of the Harvard Mastery of Stress Study. *Psychosom Med* 1997; 59(2):144–9.

37. Funkenstein, D., King, S., and Drolette, M. *Mastery of Stress*. Cambridge, MA Harvard University Press, 1957.

38. Thomas, C. B., Duszynski, K. R. Closeness to parents and the family constellation in a prospective study of five disease states; suicide, mental illness, malignant tumor, hypertension, and coronary heart disease. *Johns Hopkins Medical Journal* 1974;134:251.

39. Berkman, L. F. The changing and heterogeneous nature of aging and longevity: a social and biomedical perspective. *Annual Review of Gerontology and Geriatrics* 1988; 8:37–68.

40. Sapolsky, R. M., Krey, L. C., and McEwen, B. S. The adrenocortical stress-response in the aged male rat: impairment of recovery from stress. *Experimental Gerontology* 1983; 18:55–64.

41. Meany, M., Aitken, D., Bodnoff, S., Iny, L., and Sapolsky, R. The effects of postnatal handling on the development of the glucocorticoid receptor systems and stress recovery in the rat. *Progress in Neuro-Psychopharmacology and Biological Psychiatry* 1985; 9:731–734.

42. Meany, M. J., Aitken, D. H., VanBerkel, C., Bhatnagar, S., and Sapolsky, R. M. Effect of neonatal handling on age-related impairments associated with the hippocampus. *Science* 1988; 239:766–768.

43. Nerem, R. M., Levesque, M. J., and Cornhill, J. F. Social environments as a factor in diet-induced atherosclerosis. *Science* 1980; 208(4451):1475–6.

44. Seeman, T. E., Berkman, L. F., Blazer, D., and Rowe, J. W. Social ties and support and neuroendocrine function: The MacArthur Studies of Successful Aging. *Ann Behav Med* 1994; 16:95–106.

45. Knox, S. S., Theorell, T., Suensson, J., Waller, D. The relation of social support and working environment to medical variances associated with elevated blood pressure in young males—a structural model. *Soc Sci Med* 1985; 21(5):525–531.

46. Uchino, B., Garvey, T. The availability of social support reduces cardiovascular reactivity to acute psychological stress. *J of Behavioral Med* 1997; 20(1):15–27.

47. Cohen, S., Doyle, W. J., Skoner, D. P., Rabin, B. S., and Gwaltney, Jr., J. M. Social ties and susceptibility to the common cold. *JAMA* 1987; 277(24):1940–1944.

48. Schleifer, S. J., Keller, S. E., Camerino, M., et al. Suppression of lymphocyte stimulation following bereavement. *JAMA* 1983; 250:374–377.

49. Bartrop, R. W., Luckhurst, E., Lazarus, L., et al. Depressed lymphocyte function after bereavement. *Lancet* 1977; 1:834–836.

50. Kiecolt-Glaser, J. K., Fisher, L. D., Ogrocki, P., et al. Marital quality, marital disruption and immune function. *Psychosom Med* 1987; 49:13–34.

51. Thomas, P. D., Goodwin, J. M., and Goodwin, J. S. Effect of social support on stress-related changes in cholesterol level, uric acid level and immune function in an elderly sample. *Am J Psychiatry* 1985; 142:735–737.

52. Glaser, R., Kiecolt-Glaser, J. K., Speicher, C. E., et al. Stress, loneliness and changes in herpes virus latency. *J Behav Med* 1985; 8:249–260.

53. Kiecolt-Glaser, J. K., Garner, W., Speicher, C. E., et al. Psychosocial modifiers of immunocompetence in medical students. *Psychosom Med* 1984; 46:7–14.

54. Cohen, S., Kaplan, J. R., Cunnick, J., et al. Chronic social stress, affiliation and cellular immune response in nonhuman primates. *Psychol Sci* 1992; 4:301–310.

55. Kaplan, J. R., Manuck, S. B., Heise, E. B., et al. The relationship of agonistic and affiliative behavior patterns to cellular-mediated immune function among cynomolgus monkeys *Macaca fascicularis* living in unstable social groups. *Am J Primatology* 1991; 25:157–173.

56. McEwen, B. S. Protective and damaging effects of stress mediators. *NEJM* 1998.

57. Seeman, T. E., Singer, B. H., Rowe, J. H., Horwitz, R. I., and McEwen, B. S. The price of adaption—allostatic lead and its health consequences. *Archives of Internal Medicine* 1997; 157:2259–2268.

58. Linden, W., Stossel, C., and Maurice, J. Psychosocial interventions for patients with coronary artery disease: A meta-analysis. *Arch Intern Med* 1996; 156(7):745–752.

59. Spiegel, D., Bloom, J. R., Kraemer, H. C., and Gottheil, E. Effect of psychosocial treatment on survival of patients with metastatic breast cancer. *Lancet* 1989; ii:888–891.

60. Wortman, C. B., Conway, T. L. The role of social support in adaptation and recovery from physical illness. In Cohen, S., Syme, S. L. (eds), *Social Support and Health*. New York, Academic Press 1985; 281–302.

61. Lutgendorf, S. K., Antoni, M. H., Ironson, G., Starr, K., et al. Changes in Cognitive Coping Skills and Social Support During Cognitive Behavioral Stress Management Intervention and Distress Outcomes in Symptomatic Human Immunodeficiency Virus (HIV)-Seropositive Gay Men. *Psychosom Med* 1998; 60:204–214.

Fourteen

SOCIAL STATUS, STRESS, AND HEALTH IN FEMALE MONKEYS

Carol A. Shively

INTRODUCTION

THE relationship between the stresses associated with low social status and disease susceptibility is apparent in human and nonhuman primates. We have studied this relationship in female cynomolgus monkeys for many years. Like human beings, low social status (subordinate) female monkeys are more susceptible than their dominant counterparts to a number of pathological processes that result in disease. There are several themes in Kansas health to which our observations in cynomolgus monkeys seem especially pertinent. First, among Kansans, as well as all Americans, low socioeconomic status is associated with increased susceptibility to disease. Higher rates of depression, suicide, and death from atherosclerosis-induced disease are found among Kansans than in the U.S. population. While all depression does not result in suicide, most suicides are preceded by depression. Depression is twice as prevalent among women than men in Kansas as in most western societies, and it is on the rise. Atherosclerosis causes coronary heart disease which is the leading killer of men and women in this country, as well as in Kansas. Low socioeconomic status is associated

with increased CHD morbidity and mortality, and with increased rates of depression in human beings. For these reasons this chapter will focus on the relationship between social status and two disease endpoints in adult female cynomolgus monkeys: atherosclerosis and depression.

A NONHUMAN PRIMATE MODEL OF CORONARY ARTERY ATHEROSCLEROSIS AND CORONARY HEART DISEASE RISK

EPIDEMIOLOGICAL and clinical studies of the factors that influence CHD risk invariably raise questions that cannot be answered in studies of human beings because such studies are either unethical, not feasible, or unaffordable. In such cases, experiments using appropriate animal models have traditionally been used to supplement scientific knowledge. Atherosclerosis (an accumulation of fatty, connective, and necrotic tissue) of the coronary arteries is the principal pathological process that causes coronary heart disease (CHD). Cynomolgus monkeys (*Macaca fascicularis*) are currently the only animal model of gender differences in susceptibility to diet-induced atherogenesis. Among Caucasians in western society, men have

Acknowledgments: research was supported by NIH grants HL-39789 and HL-14164 from the National Heart, Lung, and Blood Institute, and a grant from Wyeth Ayerst Research.

about twice the incidence of CHD and twice as extensive coronary artery atherosclerosis as women.[1-3] The male-to-female ratio of coronary artery atherosclerosis extent in cynomolgus monkeys is also about 2:1. Like women, female cynomolgus monkeys are protected against atherosclerosis relative to their male counterparts.[4]

Female cynomolgus monkeys have menstrual cycles that are similar to those of women in terms of length and cyclic hormone fluctuations.[5,6] Following bilateral ovariectomy, extensive coronary artery atherosclerosis develops in females in amounts that are indistinguishable from those of males.[7] CHD risk is also increased in oophorectomized and postmenopausal women.[8] Subcutaneous replacement of estradiol, or estradiol and progesterone in physiological doses, protects against atherosclerosis in female monkeys,[9] and hormone replacement therapy (HRT) is associated with decreased CHD risk in postmenopausal women.[10] Thus, ovarian function, and in particular estradiol, is implicated in the phenomenon of female protection, both in women and female cynomolgus macaques.

Psychosocial Factors that Influence Coronary Artery Atherosclerosis and CHD Risk in Female Monkeys: Social Status

CYNOMOLGUS monkeys typically live in large social groups that are characterized by complex social relationships. Complex social living includes the possibility of social stress effects on health. A major social organizing mechanism of monkey society is the social status hierarchy.[11] Female monkeys with low social status, or subordinates, are behaviorally and physiologically different from dominants.

The distinguishing behavioral characteristics of subordinates are depicted in Figure 1. Subordinate females are the recipients of about three times the hostility or aggression of their dominant counterparts. They are groomed less, that is, they spend less time in positive affiliative be-

havior. They spend more time vigilantly scanning their social group than dominants. The purpose of the vigilant scanning appears to be to track and avoid dominants in order to avoid aggressive interactions. Subordinates also spend significantly more time alone than dominant females.[12-14] Primates typically communicate nonverbally by touch, facial expressions, and body language or postures. Although human primates also are able to communicate with language, they still rely heavily on nonverbal communication. When a female monkey spends time alone, it means that the monkey is not in physical contact or within touching distance of another monkey. Rather, the monkey is socially isolated. This is intriguing given the observations in human beings that suggest that social support is associated with reduced CHD risk.[15] Thus, it seems that subordinates are subject to hostility and have very little social support.

Physiological characteristics of subordinates that distinguish them from dominants include adrenal function. Following dexamethasone suppression, the adrenal glands of subordinate females hypersecrete cortisol in response to an adrenocorticotropic hormone challenge.[16] Since the hypersecretion of cortisol is typically viewed as indicative of a stressed individual, this finding implies that, in general, subordinate females are stressed females.

Subordinate females also have more abnormal menstrual cycles than dominant females.[7] Progesterone concentrations are lower during the luteal phase, and estradiol concentrations are lower in the follicular phase of subordinate females. Moderately low luteal-phase progesterone concentrations indicate that although ovulation may have occurred, the luteal phase was hormonally deficient. Very low luteal-phase progesterone concentrations indicate an anovulatory cycle.[17,18] Thus, stressed subordinate females have poor ovarian function compared to dominants.

Subordinate females with poor ovarian function have more coronary artery atherosclerosis

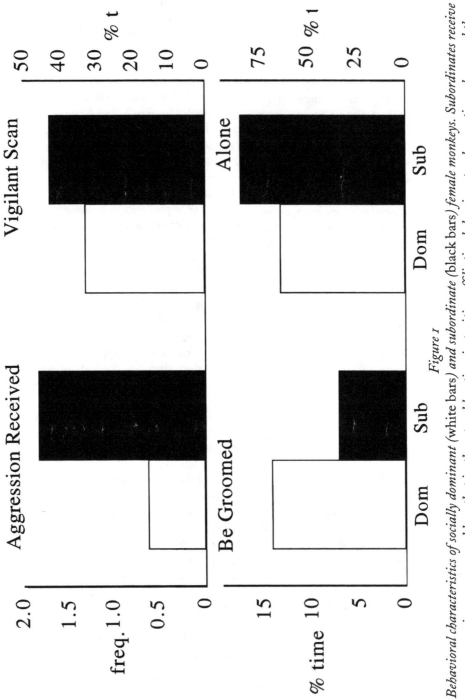

Figure 1

Behavioral characteristics of socially dominant (white bars) and subordinate (black bars) female monkeys. Subordinates receive more aggression, are groomed less, that is, they spend less time in positive affiliative behavior, spend more time alone, and they spend more time vigilantly scanning their social group than dominants. Freq/hr=frequency per hour; % time=percentage of time spent. (Adapted from Shively et al. 1986; 1990.[12,13])

than their dominant counterparts (Figure 2). Indeed, the coronary artery atherosclerosis extent in these subordinate, stressed females is comparable to that found in both ovariectomized females and males.[4,7]

The effects of stress on ovarian function in women are difficult to evaluate because of the difficulties in characterizing menstrual cycle quality over long periods of time. However, the results of several studies are consistent with the hypothesis that stress can have a deleterious effect on ovarian function in women.[19-21] Furthermore, mechanistic pathways relating stress to impaired reproductive function in female primates have been identified, suggesting that the stress-ovarian function impairment hypothesis is plausible from a physiological perspective.[22-27] Intriguingly, women with hypothalamic amenorrhea also have increased hypothalamic-pituitary-adrenal activity similar to that observed in subordinate female cynomolgus monkeys.[28] The relationship between poor ovarian function during the premenopausal years and CHD risk is also difficult to ascertain due to the double challenge of characterizing ovarian function and detecting an adequate number of clinical CHD events in women. However, there is one report that women with a history of irregular menstrual cycles are at increased risk for CHD.[29]

Ovarian hormones (particularly estradiol) are also associated with the *function* of the coronary arteries. In response to neuroendocrine signals, coronary arteries either dilate or constrict to modulate the flow of blood to the heart. Inappropriate coronary artery constriction, or vasospasm, early in life may change flow dynamics, injuring the epithelium and exacerbating atherosclerosis. Coronary vasospasm later in life in the presence of exacerbated atherosclerosis may increase the likelihood of myocardial infarction. The coronary arteries of normal cycling females dilate in response to acetylcholine infused directly into the coronary artery, whereas those of ovariectomized females constrict in response to acetylcholine. The dilation response can be restored in ovariectomized females by administering estradiol, i.e. estrogen replacement therapy.[30,31] Furthermore, preliminary data from our laboratory suggest that the coronary arteries of dominant females with good ovarian function dilate in response to an infusion of acetylcholine, whereas those of subordinate females with poor ovarian function constrict in response to acetylcholine (Figure 3).[32] These data suggest that some chest pain in women may be due to coronary vasospasm caused by estrogen deficiency. Thus, female primates with poor ovarian function may be at increased CHD risk for two reasons: 1) impaired coronary artery function, and 2) increased atherogenesis.

Ovarian function declines at menopause, particularly the production of estradiol and progesterone. Importantly, clinically detectable events occur most frequently during and after the menopausal decline in ovarian function. Thus, the impact of premenopausal ovarian function on CHD risk may be temporally separate from the clinical manifestation of CHD. However, atherogenesis is a dynamic process that occurs over a lifetime. We hypothesize that atherogenesis during young and middle adulthood may be accelerated among socially stressed women. These women enter the menopausal years with exacerbated atherosclerosis. During the estrogen-deficient menopausal years, the combined effect of a more atherogenic lipid profile, exacerbated atherosclerosis, and increased likelihood of coronary vasospasm result in increased CHD among women who experienced excessive premenopausal social stress.

PSYCHOSOCIAL FACTORS THAT
INFLUENCE CORONARY ARTERY
ATHEROSCLEROSIS AND CHD RISK IN
FEMALE MONKEYS: SOCIAL ISOLATION

WE hypothesized that social isolation was associated with exacerbated coronary artery atherosclerosis in female monkeys. To test this hypothesis, we compared the outcomes of

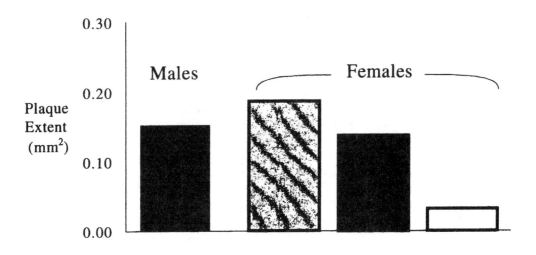

Figure 2
*Coronary artery atherosclerosis (measured as plaque extent) in males and in females in
different reproductive conditions. Among females:* Gray bar=ovariectomized females;
black bars=*intact socially subordinate females with poor ovarian function;*
white bar =*intact socially dominant females with good ovarian function.*
(Adapted from Hamm et al. 1983; Adams et al. 1985.[4,7])

two experiments in which females in each experiment consumed the same atherogenic diet for approximately two years. In one experiment, they were housed in social groups with other females, and in the other they were housed individually in single cages. Socially housed females formed social status hierarchies. Single caged females could see, hear, and smell other monkeys, but they could not touch them. Females that were socially isolated in single cages had four times the coronary artery atherosclerosis of socially housed females.[33]

Since subordinate females spend more time alone than dominants, we compared atherosclerosis extent among socially dominant, socially subordinate, and single caged monkeys. Dominants had the least coronary artery atherosclerosis, single caged females had the most, and socially housed subordinate females fell in between these two groups (Figure 4). Thus, the most socially isolated females had the most coronary artery atherosclerosis, the least socially isolated females had the least atherosclerosis, and those that spent intermediate amounts of time alone (socially housed subordinates) had intermediate amounts of coronary artery atherosclerosis. These data suggest that social isolation may be a behavioral risk factor for coronary artery atherosclerosis in female primates.[33]

PSYCHOSOCIAL FACTORS THAT
INFLUENCE CORONARY ARTERY
ATHEROSCLEROSIS AND CHD RISK
IN FEMALE MONKEYS:
SOCIAL STATUS INCONGRUITY

AN interesting aspect of the nature of social status in cynomolgus monkeys is that females that are dominant in one social group are likely to be dominant in multiple subsequent so-

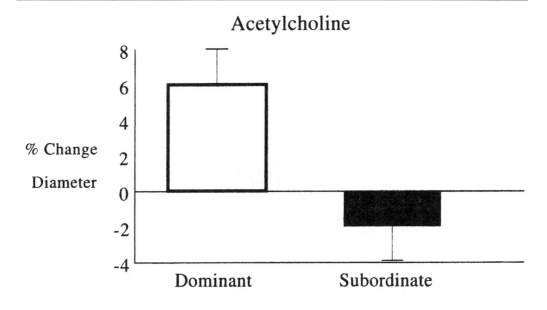

Figure 3
Coronary artery responsivity to intracoronary infusion of acetylcholine (measured as % change
from artery diameter at baseline infusion of saline) in socially dominant (dom) or subordinate (sub)
female cynomolgus monkeys with diet-induced atherosclerosis.
(Adapted from Williams et al. 1994.[32])

cial groups. Likewise, females that are socially subordinate in one group are likely to be subordinate in multiple subsequent social groups. This observation suggests that social status is a reliable characteristic of the individual.[34]

It has been appreciated for some years that health quality of life depends to a large extent on individual-environment congruity or "fit."[35,36] Levi suggested that the fit between the individual and the environment included the satisfaction of needs and congruency between abilities and demands and between expectations and the perception of reality, and suggested that the quality of life was dependent upon it.[35,36] The purpose of the next experiment was to study the effects of the modification of a psychosocial risk factor, social status, on coronary artery atherosclerosis.

Since changing the social status of an individual appears to be equivalent to alteration of a characteristic of the individual, the individual-environment "fit" may be affected.

Forty-eight adult female monkeys were fed an atherogenic diet, housed in small social groups, and social status was altered in half of the animals (subordinates became dominant, and dominants became subordinate). Thus, half of the animals occupied incongruous social positions throughout the majority of the experiment (Figure 5). The manipulation of social status significantly affected coronary artery atherosclerosis, while having minimal effects on risk factors, providing further support for the hypothesis that social status has direct effects on atherogenesis in these females. Additionally, the psychosocial effects

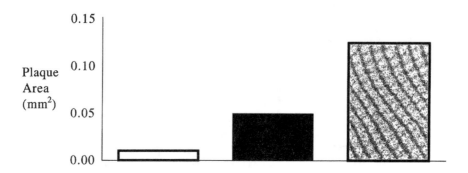

Figure 4
*Coronary artery atherosclerosis extent expressed as plaque area (mm^2) of socially housed dominant
(white bar) and subordinate (black bar) female monkeys, and female monkeys housed alone in
single cages (gray bar).
(Adapted from Shively et al. 1989.[33])*

on coronary artery atherosclerosis were independent of ovarian function. All animals that occupied incongruous social positions had worsened coronary artery atherosclerosis. The modification of this psychosocial risk factor may have resulted in individual-environment incongruity, and exacerbated coronary artery atherosclerosis.[37]

SOCIAL STATUS, SOCIAL STRESS, AND DEPRESSION

SOCIAL stress is believed to precipitate depression; however, the relationship is difficult to demonstrate.[38-41] A recent series of reports suggests that loss and threatening experiences increase risk of anxiety and depression.[42-46] Unfortunately, depressive disorders are prevalent and the rate of occurrence is increasing.[47] It is estimated that 20% of first onset major depressive episodes will be unresponsive to any available treatment, and another 30% will be only

partially responsive.[48] The results of several studies suggest that low social status is associated with increased risk of depression, although the nature of the relationship is unclear.[49,50] In one prospective study in which low social status predicted first onset of major depressive disorder, a lack of social support (social isolation) appeared to mediate this relationship, at least in part.[51] Thus, social support may reduce risk of depression following stressful life events.[52,53]

The hypothesis that social subordination is stressful, and results in a depressive response in some individuals, was examined in the experiment mentioned above in which social status was manipulated, resulting in previously subordinate females becoming dominant and previously dominant females becoming subordinate. Current subordinates hypersecreted cortisol, were insensitive to negative feedback, and had suppressed reproductive function. They also received more aggression, engaged in less affiliation, and spent more time alone than domi-

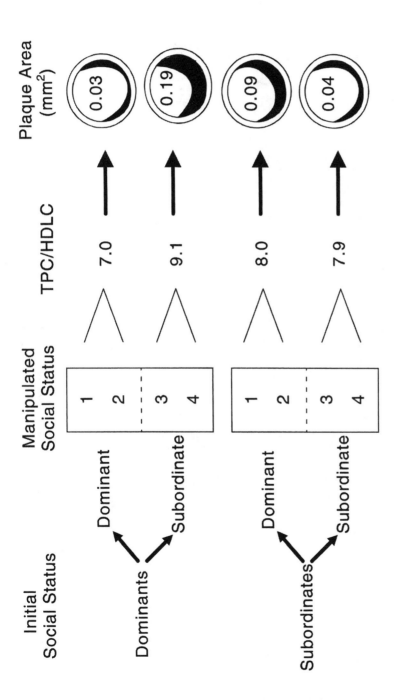

Figure 5

The effects of changing social status on diet–induced coronary artery atherosclerosis extent in female monkeys.
Shown are mean values of coronary artery plaque area adjusted for pre-experimental predictors of atherosclerosis extent.
(Adapted from Shively and Clarkson 1994.[37]*)*

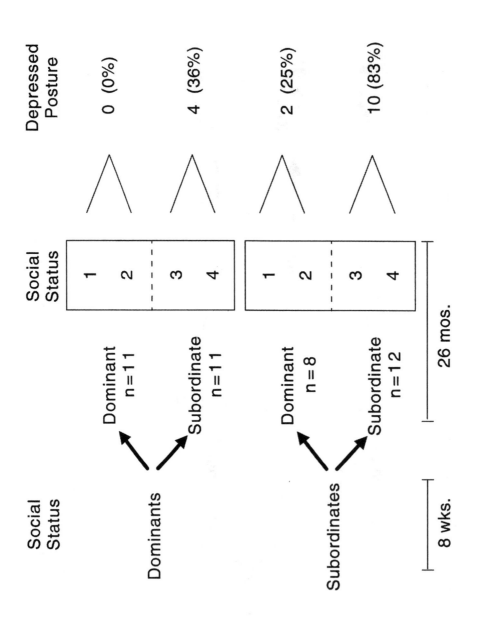

Figure 6
The effects of low social status on the prevalence of behavioral depression in female monkeys.
(Adapted from Shively et al. 1997.[54])

nants. Furthermore, they spent more time fearfully scanning the social environment and displayed more behavioral depression than dominants. Current subordinates with a history of social subordination were preferentially susceptible to a behavioral depression response (Figure 6). The results of this experiment suggest that the stress of social subordination causes hypothalamic-pituitary-adrenal and ovarian dysfunction, and support the hypothesis that chronic, low-intensity social stress may result in depression in susceptible individuals.[14,54]

In this experiment, subordinates who became dominant acted like dominants. They were more aggressive, less submissive, etc. Likewise, dominants that became subordinate adopted a much more submissive behavior pattern in their second social groups. This observation suggests that all individuals have the capacity for high or low levels of aggression, and whether they express a lot or little aggression in these small monkey social groups depends on their social position. Subordinate monkeys have as great a capacity to behave aggressively as dominants, but this aggressive behavior is socially suppressed. Thus, subordinates are subject to hostility, have little social support, are preferentially susceptible to behavioral depression, and have suppressed aggression. Childhood aggression has been observed to be associated with adult aggression in men and women. But childhood aggression is positively associated with adult depression in women only.[55] Depression has often been described as aggression turned inward. We hypothesize that in these female monkeys it is the social suppression of the expression of aggression that may result in behavioral depression.[56]

Summary and Conclusions

IN summary, low social status in female primates is associated with worsened coronary artery atherosclerosis. These females are the recipients of hostility/aggression, and they are also relatively socially isolated. Among female pri-

mates three psychosocial risk factors for coronary artery atherosclerosis have been identified: low social status, social isolation, and social status incongruity. Females with low social status are also preferentially susceptible to a depressive response to social stress, particularly if they have a history of social subordination. Subordinate social status is characterized by suppressed aggression, which may contribute to the likelihood of depression in these individuals.

Social stress increases the risk of CHD and precipitates bouts of depression in human beings. Low socioeconomic status is associated with increased risk of depression and CHD. The relationship between socioeconomic status and health in human beings is linear, there is no apparent threshold. The upper class has better health than the upper middle class, and so on down the hierarchy. Risk of disease is increased even among employed individuals with adequate health care, nutrition, and shelter. Perhaps the reason low social status is associated with increased risk of disease in human beings is that low social status is stressful. Like the monkeys, human primates with low social status have relatively little control over their lives, and low control is a source of chronic stress that could engender physiological responses that are deleterious to health.

NOTES

1. Wingard, DL, Suarez, L, and Barrett-Connor, E: The sex differential in mortality from all causes and ischemic heart disease. *Am J Epidemiol* 117;19–26, 1983.

2. Vanecek, R: Atherosclerosis of the coronary arteries in five towns. *Bull WHO* 53;509–518, 1976.

3. Tejada, C, Strong, JP, Montenegro, MR, Restropo, C, and Solberg, LA: Distribution of coronary and aortic atherosclerosis by geographic location, race, and sex. *Lab Invest* 18;509–526, 1968.

4. Hamm, TE Jr, Kaplan, JR, Clarkson, TB, and Bullock, BC: Effects of gender and social behavior on the development of coronary artery atherosclerosis in cynomolgus macaques. *Atherosclerosis* 48;221–233, 1983.

5. Jewett, DA, Dukelow, WR: Cyclicity and gestation length of *Macaca fascicularis*. *Primates* 13;327–330, 1972.

6. Mahoney, CJ: A study of the menstrual cycle in *Macaca irus* with special reference to the detection of ovulation. *J Reprod Fertil* 21;153–163, 1970.

7. Adams, MR, Kaplan, JR, Clarkson, TB, and Koritnik, DR: Ovariectomy, social status, and atherosclerosis in cynomolgus monkeys. *Arteriosclerosis* 5;192–200, 1985.

8. Kannel, WB, Hjortland, MC, McNamara, PM, and Gordon, T: Menopause and risk of cardiovascular disease: the Framingham study. *Ann Intern Med* 85:447–452, 1976.

9. Adams, MR, Kaplan, JR, Manuck, SR, Koritnik, DR, Parks, JS, Wolfe, MS, and Clarkson, TB: Inhibition of coronary artery atherosclerosis by 17–beta estradiol in ovariectomized monkeys. *Arteriosclerosis* 10:1051–1057, 1990.

10. Bush, TL, Barrett-Connor, E, Cowan, LD, Criqui, MH, Wallace, RB, Suchindran, CM, Tyroler, HA, and Rifkind, BM: Cardiovascular mortality and noncontraceptive use of estrogen in women: results from the Lipid Research Clinics Program Follow-up Study. *Circulation* 75:1102–1109, 1987.

11. Shively, CA: The evolution of dominance hierarchies in nonhuman primate society, in Ellyson, SL, Dovidio, JF (eds.): *Power, Dominance, and Nonverbal Behavior*. New York, Springer-Verlag, 1985, pp. 67–88.

12. Shively, CA, Kaplan, JR, and Adams, MR: Effects of ovariectomy, social instability and social status on female *Macaca fascicularis* social behavior. *Physiol Behav* 36: 1147–1153, 1986.

13. Shively, CA, Manuck, SB, Kaplan, JR, and Koritnik, DR: Oral contraceptive administration, interfemale relationships, and sexual behavior in *Macaca fascicularis*. *Archives of Sexual Behavior* 19:101–117, 1990.

14. Shively, CA: Social subordination stress, behavior and central monoaminergic function in female cynomolgus monkeys. *Biol Psychiatry*, in press.

15. Shumaker, SA, Hill, DR: Gender differences in social support and physical health. *Health Psychol* 10:102–111,1991.

16. Kaplan, JR, Adams, MR, Koritnik, DR, Rose, JC, and Manuck, SB: Adrenal responsiveness and social status in intact and ovariectomized *Macaca fascicularis*. *Am J Primatol* 11:181–193, 1986.

17. Wilks, JW, Hodgen, GD, and Ross, GT: Luteal phase defects in the rhesus monkey: The significance of serum FSH:LH ratios. *J Clin Endocrinol Metab* 43:1261–1267, 1976.

18. Wilks, JW, Hodgen, GD, and Ross, GT: Endocrine characteristics of ovulatory and anovulatory menstrual cycles in the rhesus monkey, in Hafez, ESE (ed.): *Human Ovulation*. Amsterdam, Elsevier/North-Holland Biomedical Press, 1979, pp. 205–218.

19. Matteo, S: The effect of job stress and job interdependency on menstrual cycle length, regularity and synchrony. *Psychoneuroendocrinology* 12:467–476, 1987.

20. Barnea, ER, Tal, J: Stress-related reproductive failure. *J in Vitro Fertil and Embryo Transfer* 8:15–23, 1991.

21. Gindoff, PR: Menstrual function and its relationship to stress, exercise, and body weight. *Bull NY Acad Med* 65:774–786, 1989.

22. Hayashi, KT, Moberg, GP: Influence of the hypothalamic-pituitary-adrenal axis on the menstrual cycle and the pituitary responsiveness to estradiol in the female rhesus monkey (*Macaca fascicularis*). *Biol Reprod* 42:260–265, 1990.

23. Abbott, DH, O'Byrne, KT, Sheffield, JW, et al: Neuroendocrine suppression of LH secretion in subordinate female marmoset monkeys (*Callithrix jacchus*), in Eley, RH (ed): *Comparative Reproduction in Mammals and Man*. Proceedings of the Conference of the National Center for Research in Reproduction. Nairobi, Institute of Primate Research, National Museums of Kenya, 1989, pp. 63–67.

24. Abbott, DH, Saltman, W, and Schultz-Darken, NJ: Hypothalamic switches regulating fertility in primates. Paper presented at the XIVth Congress of the International Society of Primatology, Strasbourg, France, 1992.

25. Gindoff, PR, Ferin, M: Endogenous opioid peptides modulate the effect of corticotropin-releasing factor on gonadotropin release in the primate. *Endocrinology* 121:837–842, 1989.

26. Ferin, M: Two instances of impaired GnRH activity in the adult primate: The luteal phase and 'stress', in Delemarre-van de Waal, HA, et al. (eds.): *Control of the Onset of Puberty III*. Amsterdam, Elsevier Science Publishers B.V., 1989, pp. 265–273.

27. Biller, BM, Federoff, HJ, Koenig, JI, and Klibanski, A: Abnormal cortisol secretion and responses to corticotropin-releasing hormone in women with hypothalamic amenorrhea. *J Clin Endocrinol Metab* 70:311–317, 1990.

28. Nappi, RE, Petraglia, F, Genazzini, AD, D'Ambrogio, G, Zarta, C, and Genazzani, AR: Hypothalamic amenorrhea: evidence for a central derangement of hypothalamic-pituitary-adrenal cortex axis activity. *Fertil Steril* 59:571–576, 1993.

29. La Vecchia, C, Decarli, A, Franceschi, S, Gentile, A, Negri, E, and Parazzini, F: Menstrual and reproductive factors and the risk of myocardial infarction in women under fifty-five years of age. *Am J Obstet Gynecol* 157:1108–1112, 1987.

30. Williams, JK, Adams, MR, and Klopfenstein, HS: Estrogen modulates responses of atherosclerotic coronary arteries. *Circulation* 81:1680–1687, 1990.

31. Williams, JK, Adams, MR, Herrington, DM, and Clarkson, TB: Short-term administration of estrogen and vascular responses of atherosclerotic coronary arteries. *J Am Coll Cardiol* 20:452–457, 1992.

32. Williams, JK, Shively, CA, and Clarkson, TB: Vascular responses of atherosclerotic coronary arteries among premenopausal female monkeys. *Circulation* 90:983–987, 1994.

33. Shively, CA, Clarkson, TB, and Kaplan, JR: Social deprivation and coronary artery atherosclerosis in female cynomolgus monkeys. *Atherosclerosis* 77:69–76, 1989.

34. Shively, CA, Kaplan, JR: Stability of social status rankings of female cynomolgus monkeys, of varying reproductive condition, in different social groups. *Am J Primatol* 23:239–245, 1991.

35. Levi, L: *Society, stress and disease.* Oxford University Press, New York, 1981.

36. Levi, L: Work, stress and health. *Scand J Work Environ Health* 10:495–500, 1984.

37. Shively, CA, Clarkson, TB: Social status incongruity and coronary artery atherosclerosis in female monkeys. *Arterioscler Thromb* 14:721–726, 1994.

38. Breslau, N, Davis, GC: Chronic stress and major depression. *Arch Gen Psychiatry* 43:309–314, 1986.

39. Richardson, JS: Animal models of depression reflect changing views on the essence and etiology of depressive disorders in humans. *Prog Neuro-Psychopharmacol Biol Psychiatry* 15, 199–204, 1991.

40. Vilhjalmsson, R: Life stress, social support and clinical depression: a reanalysis of the literature. *Soc Sci Med* 37:331–342, 1993.

41. Brown, GW, Harris, TO, and Hepworth, C: Life events and endogenous depression. A puzzle reexamined. *Arch Gen Psychiatry* 51:523–534, 1994.

42. Brown, GW, Harris, TO: Aetiology of anxiety and depressive disorders in an inner-city population. 1. Early adversity. *Psychol Med* 23:143–154, 1993.

43. Brown, GW: Life events and affective disorder: Replications and limitations. *Psychosom Med* 55:248–259, 1993.

44. Brown, GW, Harris, TO, and Eales, MJ: Aetiology of anxiety and depressive disorders in an inner-city population. 2. Comorbidity and adversity. *Psychol Med* 23:155–165, 1993.

45. Brown, GW, Moran, P: Clinical and psychosocial origins of chronic depressive episodes. I: A community survey. *Br J Psychiatry* 165:447–456, 1994.

46. Brown, GW, Harris, TO, and Hepworth, C: Loss, humiliation and entrapment among women developing depression: a patient and non-patient comparison. *Psychol Med* 25:7–21, 1995.

47. Fombonne, E: Increased rates of depression: update of epidemiological findings and analytical problems. *Acta Psychiatr Scand* 90:145–156, 1994.

48. Fawcett, J: Progress in treatment-resistant and treatment-refractory depression: we still have a long way to go. *Psychiatric Ann* 24:214–216, 1994.

49. Murphy, JM, Olivier, DC, Monson, RR, Sobol, AM, Federman, EB, and Leighton, AH: Depression and anxiety in relation to social status. *Arch Gen Psychiatry* 48:223–229, 1991.

50. Cole, DA, Carpentieri, S: Social status and the comorbidity of child depression and conduct disorder. *J Consult Clin Psychology* 58:748–757, 1990.

51. Bruce, ML, Hoff, RA: Social and physical health risk factors for first-onset major depressive disorder in a community sample. *Soc Psychiatry Psychiatr Epidemiol* 29: 165–171, 1994.

52. Aneshensel, CS, Stone, JD: Stress and depression: A test of the buffering model of social support. *Arch Gen Psychiatry* 39:1392–1396, 1982.

53. Serban, G: Stress in affective disorders. *Methods Achieve Exp Pathol* 15:200–220, 1991.

54. Shively, CA, Laber-Laird, K, and Anton, RF: The behavior and physiology of social stress and depression in female cynomolgus monkeys. *Biol Psychiatry* 41:871–882, 1997.

55. Podolski, CL, Huesmann, LR: Outcomes of childhood aggression in women. *Ann New York Acad Sci* 794:394–8, 1996.

56. Shively, CA: Environmental influences and neurobiological correlates of aggression in cynomolgus monkey social groups. In press.

Part Four

PERSPECTIVES

Fifteen

INEQUALITIES IN HEALTH:
CAUSES AND POLICY IMPLICATIONS

Michael Marmot

INTRODUCTION

RESEARCHERS interested in inequalities in health are wont to quote data from the Titanic disaster. The fatality rates from drowning were comparatively low amongst first-class passengers, were higher among second-class passengers, and higher still among passengers in the third class.[1] Perhaps it is not too fanciful to use these data on inequalities in rates of drowning to illustrate different approaches to dealing with the problem of inequalities in health. A typical medical response might be better treatment for hypothermia and more rapid response units. The holistic primary care response might be to deal with the feelings of unhappiness induced by the experience. An orientation that emphasizes the individualistic approach to prevention, namely that individuals have it within their own power to choose healthy ways of living, might focus on swimming lessons. An approach that emphasized the environmental causes of illness might focus on safe navigation. In this instance, whatever power individuals may have had over their own ability to survive the catastrophe, had the catastrophe not occurred no-one would have drowned. This would have been of great advantage, but it is a reasonable prediction that there still would have been inequalities in health. The third-class passengers would have died at a younger age than the first-class passengers but of other causes.

This is the theme of my contribution. There is a gradient in health outcome running from the most to the least advantaged members of society; these health outcomes are not specific to any particular cause; a medical response will not solve the problem; nor will a response that emphasizes individual choices over lifestyle. Inequalities in health are a manifestation of the social determinants of health. While it does not follow automatically that if the causes are social in origin, the solutions need necessarily to be social—aspirin can relieve headache, even if the cause is poverty—it is likely that an understanding of causes of inequality has the possibility to lead to policies that can make a fundamental contribution to improving health in society.

THE PROBLEM OF INEQUALITIES
IN HEALTH

Social Inequalities within Countries

My approach to this problem starts with the Whitehall study.[2-4] Figure 1, from the 25 year follow-up of British civil servants in the original Whitehall study, shows the social gradient in all-cause mortality. These men were all in stable employment and none was in poverty in any

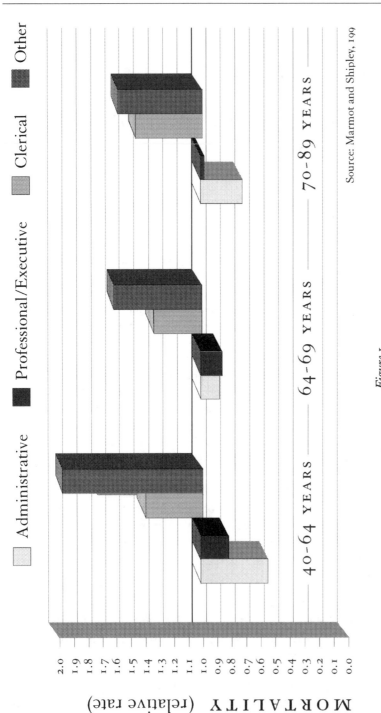

Figure 1
All-Cause Mortality by Grade of Employment
Whitehall Men 25-yr Follow-Up

Source: Marmot and Shipley, 199

absolute sense of that word, yet there is a gradient in mortality. Each grade in the civil service has higher mortality rates than the grade above it in the hierarchy. This figure shows the data for all-cause mortality, but there are similar gradients for all the major causes of death.

The gradient is relevant to the later policy discussion. Poverty is a major public health problem and policies to reduce poverty are likely to have an impact on the health consequences of poverty. These data illustrate a different problem: that of inequality. Inequality is likely to relate to relative, rather than absolute, deprivation. This is likely to require a different policy response.

The magnitude of the social gradient in mortality is not constant but has been changing over time. Figures 2 and 2a show national data for England and Wales over the time period 1970 to 1993. Both for ischaemic heart disease and suicide the social gradient became considerably steeper over the last 20 years.[5]

These social gradients are not confined to the UK. The Panel Study of Income Dynamics in the USA showed a similar gradient in mortality with respondents classified according to household income.[6] This study, too, illustrates that inequalities in health run across the whole of society. People in the lowest income category, less than $15,000 average household income in 1993, had 3.9 times the risk of dying of people in the highest income category (greater than $70,000). But, only about 7% of the population fell into this poverty category. Nearly 25% of the population were in the second highest income bracket and they had 34% higher mortality than the top group. Nearly 30% fell into the third income bracket and they had 59% higher mortality. The implication is clear: poverty is potentially fatal for the worst off members of society, but inequality has a major impact on mortality even among those who are relatively well off but still not amongst the most fortunate.

Inequalities Between Countries

We have been concerned with East West differences in mortality in Europe,[7] as Figure 3 illus-

trates. It shows life expectancy at age 15, thereby removing the effect of infant and child mortality. In 1970 the differences in life expectancy between the Nordic and European Union countries on the one hand and the communist countries of Central and Eastern Europe on the other, were relatively small. The Soviet Union lagged behind the other countries and the difference in life expectancy for men at age 15 was 4 years compared with the European Union. Over the next 25 years life expectancy improved steadily in the Nordic and European Union countries and stagnated or declined in the countries of Central and Eastern Europe. By 1994 the gap in life expectancy at age 15 between Russia and the European Union was about 10 years—a dramatic widening of inequalities across Europe in a relatively short time. The causes of death that contribute most to the East West difference in mortality are cardiovascular disease and external causes of death.[8] Interestingly, these particular causes make a major contribution to inequalities in mortality within the UK and the USA. This has led us to speculate that the causes of inequalities in health within countries may be similar to the causes of international differences.[7] This is similar to the implication of Wilkinson's work summarized in another chapter in this volume.

The worsening mortality pattern has not affected all groups equally within Central and Eastern European countries. In general, there has been a widening social gradient within those countries.[9]

The fact that, in addition to poverty, other more general social factors may also be operating is illustrated by the comparison of three countries that all had an equivalent Gross National Product in the early 1990s of around $2000 (Table 1). The high infant mortality in South Africa is related to poverty, as is the high probability of death between the ages of 15 and 60, given that ischaemic heart disease mortality is low. The relatively favorable infant mortality in Hungary and Costa Rica is, in a sense, better than one would have predicted from their GNP. The

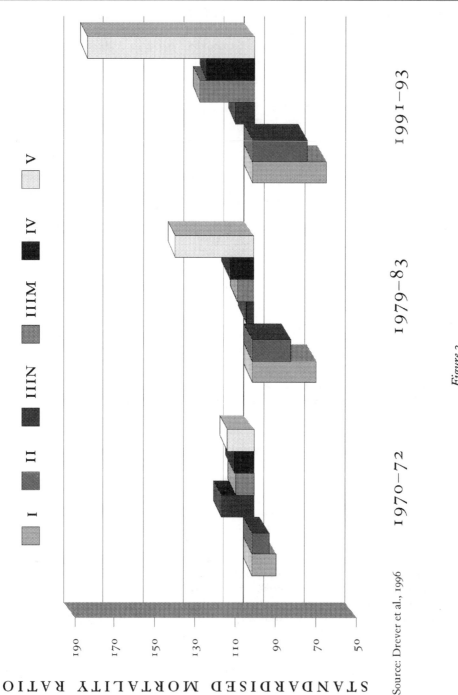

Figure 2
IHD by Social Class in England and Wales. Males 1970–93

Source: Drever et al., 1996

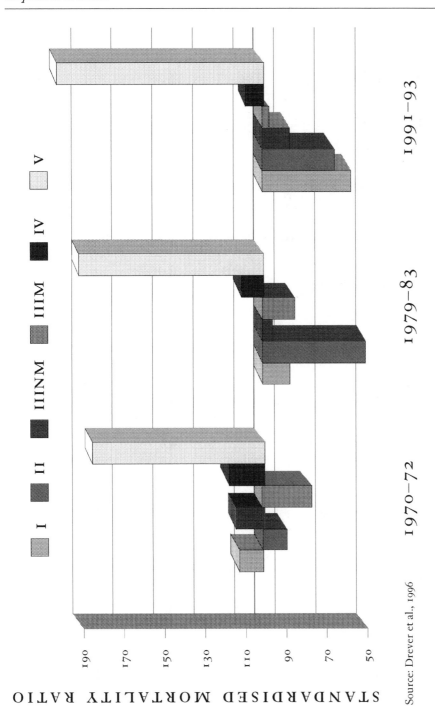

STANDARDISED MORTALITY RATIO

Source: Drever et al., 1996

Figure 2a
Suicide by Social Class in England and Wales. Males 1970–93

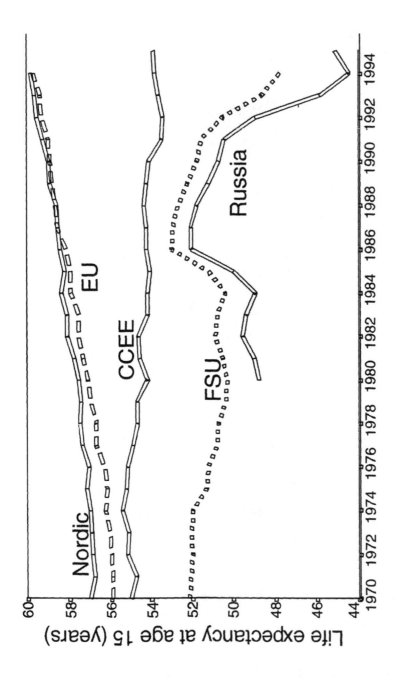

Figure 3
Life Expectancy at Age 15 in Europe, Men

Table 1

Structure of mortality in middle income countries

	Infant Mort/ 1000	Prob of Death 15–60 M	IHD	LE Birth Males
South Africa	53	30.8	Low	60
Hungary	15	27.7	High	65
Costa Rica	14	14.5	Low	74

difference between these two countries is in the mortality among middle aged men, high in Hungary, largely due to ischaemic heart disease, which results in a dramatic difference in life expectancy. There is something about society in Hungary, that cannot be summed up under the rubric "poverty," that relates to the high mortality among middle aged men. If the above speculation is correct, an understanding of what this factor(s) might be, might help us understand the causes of inequalities in health within our own societies.

EXPLANATIONS FOR INEQUALITIES IN HEALTH

Social Causes of Disease Rates in Society

In paying a tribute to the work of Geoffrey Rose,[10] I illustrated his insight, along with Durkheim, that the causes of disease rates of a population may be different from the causes of individual differences in disease occurrence.[11] Table 2 illustrates. We tend to think of accidental deaths as accidents, but the relative constancy of their rate of occurrence suggests that each population has a characteristic accident rate. The figures on suicide are quite remarkable. The number of suicide deaths appears to be relatively constant year on year. There are, of course, long-term secular trends, but not wide fluctuations from one year to the next. This suggests, following Durkheim and Rose, that populations have a characteristic rate of occurrence of causes of death. As the characteristics of populations change, so the death rates may change. We will not, however, necessarily discover the causes of the population rate of occurrence by studying the differences among individuals within a population.

Table 2

"Accidental" Deaths
England and Wales

	Male		Female	
	1993	1994	1993	1994
Motor vehicle traffic accidents	2,395	2,287	1,039	998
Accidental falls	1,517	1,481	2,400	2,189
Suicide and self-inflicted injury	2,875	2,838	866	803

Source: *Mortality Statistics, ONS 1996*

A Causal Model

We have been working with a simplified causal model of inequalities in health (Figure 4). At the right-hand end of this figure it shows the health outcomes that have been the focus of much of our research: diabetes mellitus (DM), coronary heart disease, and measures of well-being; and at the upper left, aspects of the social structure that manifest themselves as social inequalities. The boxes in between are an oversimplified way of representing the causal pathways. This could be made impossibly complex, but in this simple version, it allows us to study how, for example, individual risk factors might relate to circumstances from early life or the conditions in adulthood in which people live and work, and hence the potential role of these individual factors in mediating the relation between social factors and disease outcome.

Figure 5 illustrates that individual risk factors do not help greatly in understanding the Whitehall gradient in mortality. It shows that within each employment grade plasma total cholesterol is a predictor of CHD mortality. Within each quintile of cholesterol level the social gradient in mortality is evident. Plasma cholesterol is a predictor of coronary heart disease mortality but it does not account for the social gradient. Smoking shows a clear social gradient, but the social gradient in CHD mortality was similar in non-smokers to that in smokers.[3]

However much of the social gradient is explained by risk factors, we must bear in mind that individual behaviors are affected by the environment. In the case of alcohol, for example, the evidence shows that the higher the mean consumption of a population, the greater the prevalence of heavy drinkers.[11,12] The clear implication is that a societal intervention might be more effective in reducing the harm associated with alcohol than targeting individual heavy drinkers.

Psychosocial or Material Causes of Inequalities

In Britain, there has been lively debate as to how much of the causes of inequalities in health are material or psychosocial. There is a good case to be made that material deprivation in one way or another accounts for the link between poverty and ill health. Even here, material deprivation may have an important psychosocial component. The ways of doing without in Britain, at least, have changed (Alan Marsh, personal communication). Whereas in the past, material deprivation meant inadequate housing, under-nutrition, inadequate clothing, and risky work places, now the definition of what it means to be on the "bread line" has broadened. It also means inability to entertain children's friends, buy children new clothes, go on holiday, and pursue a hobby or leisure activity. In other words, material deprivation in a modern context may mean inability to participate fully in society and to control one's life.

Thus, there is a link with the concept of relative deprivation that may underlie the social gradient. The mechanisms linking social position to health, across the whole social gradient, are likely to involve psychosocial factors. Among the psychosocial factors with the strongest evidence to support their role in generating inequalities in health are: social supports/social integration, the psychosocial work environment, control/mastery, hostility, and parenting.

Social Supports/Integration

Lisa Berkman has reviewed the evidence, elsewhere in this volume, for the strong and consistent protective effect of participation in social networks and of social supports. Evidence from the Whitehall II study shows that the lower the position on the hierarchy, the less participation in social networks outside the family, and the more negative the degree of social support.[13]

Data from Central and Eastern European countries show that the adverse trend in mortality has affected particularly men who were single, widowed or divorced.[14,15] The adverse effect was not seen in women. One possible explanation for

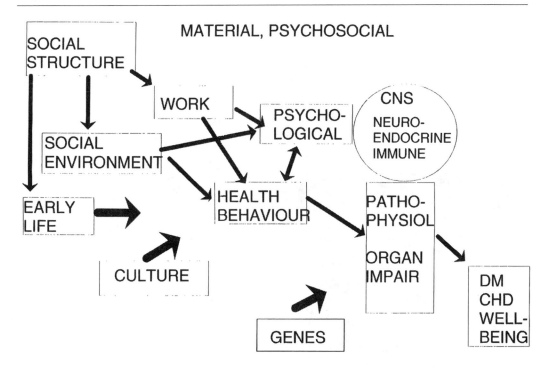

Figure 4

this is that marriage provided the main source of support for men in societies where other forms of social participation were weak.[16] Women on the other hand were more likely to participate in informal social networks, at least in part, because barter and other forms of informal exchange were mechanisms that allowed families to function.

There is a clear potential link between social ties and social capital as reviewed in this volume by Kawachi.

Psychosocial Work Environment

The two dominant models in the field of the psychosocial work environment are the demand/control model[17] and that of effort reward imbalance.[18]

In the Whitehall II study, along with a number of other studies,[19] the demand dimension did not predict coronary heart disease. Low control in the workplace was an important predictor of CHD incidence rates.[20] Figure 6, from the Whitehall II study, shows the social gradient in the occurrence of incident CHD events[21] and the contribution of three sets of factors, taken one at a time to explaining this social gradient. Short height, as a measure of early life effects, is a predictor of coronary heart disease incidence and makes a small contribution to explaining the social gradient. As in Whitehall I, the standard coronary risk factors, serum cholesterol, blood pressure, smoking, body mass index, and physical activity accounted for between a quarter and a third of the social gradient. More than half the gradient appeared to be accounted for by low control in the workplace. Figure 7 shows that, in multivariate analysis, the combination of height, coronary risk factors, and low control in the

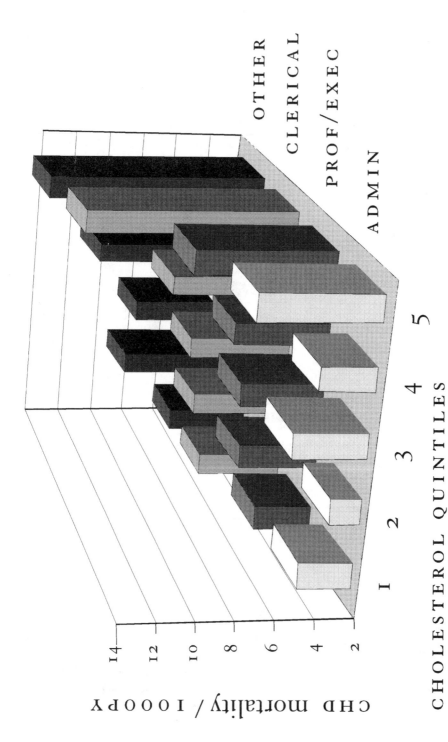

Figure 5
25-yr CHD Mortality by Grade and Plasma Cholesterol Level in Whitehall Men

workplace appear to provide a complete explanation for the social gradient in occurrence of CHD.

Using the same methods, but in a very different population in the Czech Republic, we had remarkably similar findings. A combination of coronary risk factors and low control in the workplace provided an explanation for the association between low education and risk of myocardial infarction.[22]

In discussing these findings we noted that there are, of course, social gradients in the occurrence of coronary heart disease among people who are not working. However, if low control is important, it does not derive only from the workplace. It may be a feature of the social conditions under which people live, as well as work.

Control/Mastery

There is a large literature on this subject.[23] It tends to view low control as a characteristic of individuals. Indeed, our work from Central and Eastern Europe would confirm that individuals who report low control have worse health.[24] It may be possible to characterize whole societies on degree of control. Figure 8 plots mean control for population subgroups against coronary heart disease rates for whole populations in an "ecological" analysis. It shows that the higher the mean level of control of a society, the lower the coronary heart disease rates.

Hostility

Redford Williams has produced similar findings for hostility.[25] He and others have shown that hostile people have higher risk of coronary heart disease than those who are not hostile. If hostility is viewed as a stable trait of individuals, there is no particular reason why it should be related to the environment. Williams did a Gallup survey of ten American cities and showed that they differed in mean hostility levels. He showed further

that there was a direct correlation between mean hostility of a city and that city's mortality from coronary heart disease (Figure 9).

Parenting

Barker's group in the UK have provided strong evidence for the programming hypothesis.[26] The in-utero environment programs organ systems of the developing fetus that change the individual's likelihood of developing chronic disease later in life. The British Birth Cohorts confirm that there are substantial effects of early life that continue to influence disease risk later in life.[27-29] Working with data from the 1958 Birth Cohort, Power shows that it is accumulation of advantage and disadvantage throughout the life course that accounts for inequalities in health in adulthood.[30]

Nevertheless, what happens in early life is likely to be crucial. The review by Fonagy in this volume shows the substantial effect that quality of parenting and relationships within families has on the health and well-being of children. Putting this together with Hertzman's and Mustard's reviews (this volume) of what happens to children from disordered families when they enter the school system, and evidence from the longitudinal studies, one can build a case for the impact of parenting on the health of adults.

Biological Pathways

It could be argued, that we did not need to know what the biological effects were of smoking to reach conclusions about its health effects. However, the criteria for assessing causation developed by Bradford-Hill and the U.S. Surgeon General had much to do with the controversy around smoking and health. One of these criteria is biological plausibility. The argument was that without a biologically plausible mechanism, the causal nature of epidemiological association remains suspect.

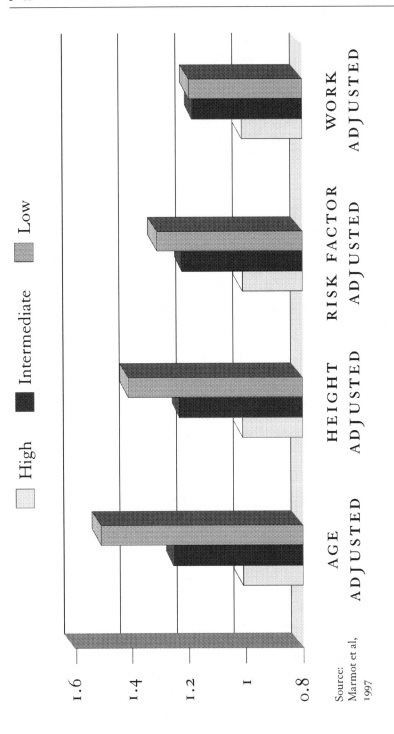

Figure 6
Odds Ratio for New CHD in Whitehall II by Employment Grade—Men
(contribution to explaining the gradient of short height, coronary risk factors and low control at work)

Source:
Marmot et al,
1997

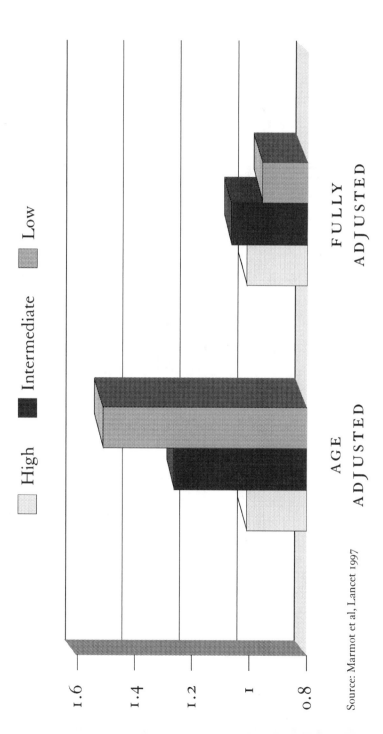

Source: Marmot et al, Lancet 1997

Figure 7
Odds Ratio for New CHD in Whitehall II by Employment Grade—Men
Combined contribution of height, risk factors and low control at work.

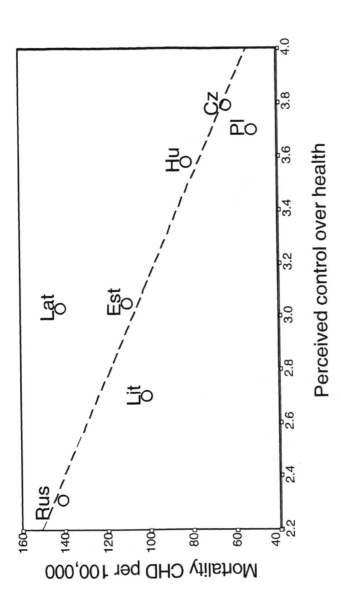

Figure 8
Standardized mortality from CHD, 0–64 yrs in the populations shown, plotted against mean levels of control in population samples.
The analysis is "ecological."

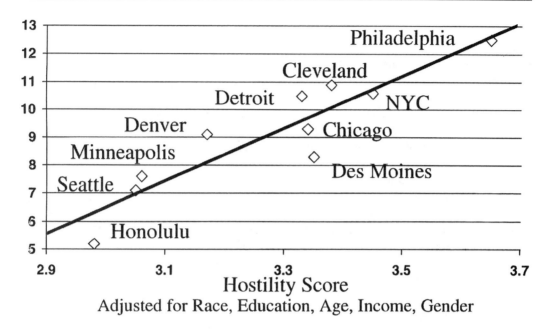

Figure 9
Hostility and Mortality by City

When we reported our findings suggesting that low control in the workplace was an important contributor to the social gradient in coronary heart disease, we asked ourselves, why pick on low control in the workplace?[21] After all, a number of factors showed a social gradient, why incriminate this particular feature of the workplace? Part of our answer was that low control was related to levels of plasma fibrinogen[31] and that plasma fibrinogen in turn is a predictor of coronary heart disease. We do not think that plasma fibrinogen is necessarily "the answer" to the question of biological mechanisms. Plasma fibrinogen is an acute-phase protein and is correlated with the metabolic syndrome of insulin resistance.[32] This is an active area of research and it is important for those of us concerned with social and psychological causes of illness not to be ignorant of modern biology.

Insights as to biological pathways linking social status to cardiovascular risk come from the animal work. Shively (this volume) reviews the work on nonhuman primates showing the importance of the hypothalamic pituitary and sympatho-adrenal medullary axis.

IMPLICATIONS FOR POLICY

THERE is a view that observational evidence is an inadequate basis for formulation of health policies. The only reliable guide, in this view, is the evidence that an intervention works. The best evidence for this is likely to come from a randomized controlled trial. For years, critics of the dietary fat/plasma cholesterol theory of the etiology of coronary heart disease claimed that a) there was no evidence that lowering plasma cholesterol would produce benefit, and b) there was concern that it might produce harm. This was in the face of a wealth of evidence from observational studies that argued for the safety and efficacy of lowering plasma cholesterol. With the advent of the 4S and WOSCOPS studies showing that lowering plasma cholesterol by treatment with statins produced a predictable reduction in primary and secondary occurrence of CHD, most critics of cholesterol converted. In passing, it might be noted that much of this conversion was not to a public health approach to reducing coronary heart disease but to a medical approach that relied on choosing which individuals should receive prescriptions for cholesterol-lowering drugs.

The randomized controlled trial is the best tool we have for evaluating medical interventions on individual patients. The further upstream we go in our search for causes (see Figure 4), the less applicable is the randomized controlled trial. A randomized controlled trial to improve social capital and evaluate its effect on mortality is difficult to conceive of, and perhaps impossible to execute.

We must therefore rely on observational evidence and judgment in formulating policies to reduce inequalities in health. In this process, the best should not be the enemy of the good. While we should not formulate policies in the absence of evidence to support them, we must not be paralyzed into inaction while we wait for the evidence to be absolutely unimpeachable. The evidence in this volume provides ample basis for formulating policies to address the social determinants of health.

ACKNOWLEDGMENTS

Michael Marmot is supported by an MRC Research Professorship and by the John D. and Catherine T. MacArthur Foundation Research Networks on Socioeconomic Status and Health and Successful Midlife Development.

NOTES

1. Broom, L., Selznick, P. *Sociology. Harper International Edition.* Tokyo: Harper & Row and John Weatherhill, Inc, 1968;–562.

2. Marmot, M. G., Rose, G., Shipley, M., and Hamilton, P. J. S. Employment grade and coronary heart disease in British civil servants. *J Epidemiol Community Health* 1978;32:244–249.

3. Marmot, M. G., Shipley, M. J., and Rose G. Inequalities in death—specific explanations of a general pattern. *Lancet* 1984;i:1003–6.

4. Marmot, M. G., Shipley, M. J. Do socioeconomic differences in mortality persist after retirement? 25 year follow up of civil servants from the first Whitehall study. *Br Med J* 1996;313:1177–1180.

5. Drever, F., Whitehead, M., and Roden, M. Current patterns and trends in male mortality by social class (based on occupation). *Population Trends* 1996;86:15–20.

6. McDonough, P., Duncan, G. J., Williams, D., and House, J. S. Income dynamics and adult mortality in the United States, 1972 through 1989. *Am J Public Health* 1997;87:1476–1483.

7. Bobak, M., Marmot, M. G. East-West mortality divide and its potential explanations: proposed research agenda. *Br Med J* 1996;312:421–425.

8. Bobak, M., Marmot, M. East-west health divide and potential explanations. In: Hertzman, C., Kelly, S., Bobak, M., eds. *East-West life expectancy gap in Europe. Environmental and non-environmental determinants.* Dordrecht: Kluwer Academic Publishers, 1996;17–44.

9. Marmot, M., Bobak, M. Psychosocial and biological mechanisms behind the recent mortality crisis in central and eastern Europe. In: Cornia A, ed. submitted, 1997.

10. Rose, G. *The strategy of preventive medicine.* Oxford: Oxford University Press, 1992.

11. Marmot, M. G. Improvement of social environment to improve health. *Lancet* 1998;351:57–60.

12. Colhoun, H., Ben-Shlomo, Y., Dong, W., Bost, L., and Marmot, M. Ecological analysis of collectivity of alcohol consumption in England: importance of average drinker. *Br Med J* 1997;314:1164–1168.

13. Stansfeld, S. A., Marmot, M. G. Deriving a survey measure of social support: the reliability and validity of the Close Persons Questionnaire. *Soc Sci Med* 1992;35:1027–1035.

14. Hajdu, P., McKee, M., and Bojan, F. Changes in premature mortality differentials by marital status in Hungary and in England and Wales. *Eur J Pub Health* 1995;5:259–264.

15. Watson, P. Explaining rising mortality among men in Eastern Europe. *Soc Sci Med* 1995;41:923–934.

16. Rose, R. Russia as an hour-glass society: a constitution without citizens. *East European Constitutional Review* 1995;4:34–42.

17. Karasek, R., Theorell, T. *Healthy work: stress, productivity, and the reconstruction of working life.* New York: Basic Books, 1990.

18. Siegrist, J. Adverse health effects of high-effort/low-reward conditions. *J Occup Health Psychol* 1996;1:27–41.

19. Hemingway, H., Marmot, M. Psychosocial factors in the aetiology and prognosis of coronary heart disease: a systematic review of prospective cohort studies. *Br Med J* 1998;in press.

20. Bosma, H., Marmot, M. G., Hemingway, H., Nicholson, A., Brunner, E. J., and Stansfeld, S. Low job control and risk of coronary heart disease in the Whitehall II (prospective cohort) study. *Br Med J* 1997;314:558–565.

21. Marmot, M., Bosma, H., Hemingway, H., Brunner, E. J., and Stansfeld, S. A. Contribution of job control and other risk factors to social variations in coronary heart disease incidence. *Lancet* 1997;350:235–239.

22. Bobak, M., Hertzman, C., Skodova, Z., and Marmot, M. Association between psychosocial factors at work and non-fatal myocardial infarction in a population based case-control study in Czech men. *Epidemiol* 1998;9:43–47.

23. Skinner, E. A. A guide to constructs of control. *J Pers Soc Psychol* 1996;71:549–570.

24. Bobak, M., Pikhart, H., Hertzman, C., Rose, R., and Marmot, M. Socioeconomic factors, perceived control and self-reported health in Russia. A cross-sectional survey. *Soc Sci Med* 1998;in press.

25. Williams, R., Haney, T., Lee, K., Kong, Y., Blumenthal, J., and Whalen, R. Type A behavior, hostility and coronary heart disease. *Psychosom Med* 1980;42:539–549.

26. Barker, D. J. The fetal and infant origins of adult disease. *Br Med J* 1990;301:1111.

27. Wadsworth, M. E. J. *The Imprint of Time:Childhood, History and Adult Life.* Oxford: Clarendon Press, 1991.

28. Wadsworth, M. E. J. Changing social factors and their long term implications for health. *Br Med Bull* 1997;53.

29. Power, C., Manor, O., and Fox, J. *Health and class: the early years.* London: Chapman & Hall, 1991.

30. Power, C., Matthews, S., and Manor, O. Inequalities in self-rated health: explanations from different stages of life. *Lancet* 1998;351:1009–1014.

31. Brunner, E., Davey Smith, G, Marmot M, Canner R, Beksinska M, and O'Brien J. Childhood social circumstances and psychosocial and behavioural factors as determinants of plasma fibrinogen. *Lancet* 1996;34:1008-1013.

32. Brunner, E. J., Marmot, M. G., Nanchahal, K., et al. Social inequality in coronary risk: central obesity and the metabolic syndrome. Evidence from the Whitehall II study. *Diabetologia* 1997;40:1341–1349.

❧

Sixteen

PUBLIC POLICY FRAMEWORKS
FOR IMPROVING POPULATION HEALTH*

Alvin R. Tarlov

INTRODUCTION

COPIOUS data, confirmed in practically every study and society examined, have identified with sufficient confidence many of the key social and societal factors that, if improved, would elevate population health. Further research undoubtedly will broaden, add important insights to, and refine the texture of our understanding. Nonetheless, the knowledge base that exists in 1999 is sufficiently comprehensive and robust to support the beginning of selected aspects of a population health improvement program.

The improvement of certain societal features would at a minimum improve the general quality of living, but would likely improve population health as well. These features include improved opportunities for successful child development, strengthened community cohesion, enhanced self-fulfillment, increased socioeconomic well-being, and modulated hierarchical structuring.

Multipronged actions initiated by multiple sectors are likely to be most effective. The sectors include nonprofit community and national organizations; faith organizations; philanthropies; schools; the recreational, entertainment, and media groups; business; political parties; public policy interests; and local, regional, and national governments. This chapter will be limited to public policies to improve population health, but the public policies are unlikely to be effective, or even adopted, unless there is in parallel an activation of the other sectors and synergism is achieved. Social currents, directions, and norms become embedded in expectations, behaviors, operations, and accepted paradigms and are ultimately encoded in laws and regulations. Even relatively modest shifts in social norms, say five degrees out of a whole circumference, will be difficult to achieve. Movement toward more healthful societal circumstances will require multiple approaches and the mobilization of understanding, concern, and commitment of multiple sectors. Public policy development usually does not lead, but rather follows broad public concern.

Four conceptual frameworks, when integrated, can provide guidance for constructing public policy ideas and developing strategies for improving population health within developed nations. These are *1*) Determinants of Population Health, *2*) Complex System Modeling, *3*) Intervention Framework, and *4*) Public Policy Development Process. The four conceptual frameworks will be described briefly, and the In-

* This manuscript, slightly modified, has also been published in *Annals of the New York Academy of Sciences*, 896, 281–293, 1999.

tervention and Public Policy Development frameworks will be applied to an assessment of the 39 recommendations made in *Independent Inquiry into Inequalities in Health*,[1] the 1998 Sir Donald Acheson Report from the United Kingdom—the most ambitious research-based attempt to date to formulate a comprehensive plan to improve population health. Although many chapters in this book advance policy recommendations, the comprehensiveness and coherency of the *Independent Inquiry* provide advantages for illustration of the conceptual frameworks for policy that have been developed for this chapter.

DETERMINANTS OF POPULATION HEALTH

THERE are five major categories of influence on health: genes and associated biology; health behaviors such as dietary habits, tobacco use, alcohol and drug use, and physical fitness; medical care and public health services; the ecology of all living things; and social and societal characteristics. This topic is dealt with in some detail in the book's introduction and will not be repeated here. To summarize, the relative proportional influence of each of the five categories is unknown in precise quantitative terms. Genes, health behaviors, medical care, total ecology, and social/societal characteristics make up a big, complex, and dynamic network of interactive variables that is understood in a general sense but not in a precise quantitative way. Research has indicated that social/societal factors exert a major influence on population health (as do health behaviors and medical care). Efforts to improve population health that leave social/societal characteristics unchanged are unlikely to be successful.

COMPLEX SYSTEM MODELING

MOST of the factors that influence population health are highly interactive. Changes in one induce responses in the others.

Positive and negative feedbacks and cancellation and synergistic effects are predominant features of hugely complex systems, as exemplified by the influence of surrounding factors on population health. Add to the surrounding factors the physiological systems within the human being that mediate the social effects with uncountable numbers and kinds of adaptations and adjustments, and the health production system reveals itself as almost incomprehensibly complex. Linear-affects models, multiple independent-affects models, and other multivariate analytic methods that have driven the social-determinants-of-health field up to this time fail to yield results that satisfactorily explain the dynamics of population health production. Population health production is unlikely to be understood from analyses of individual components. Sociobiologic system complexity cannot be explained mechanistically or predictably, as can the internal combustion engine or chemical equations. The social-determinants-of-health field, and most particularly the ability to predict with greater certainty the multitudinous consequences of interventions, requires that the concepts and measures of complex systems be applied. It is noteworthy that 30 pages of a recent issue of *Science*[2] were devoted to exploring complex systems related not only to chemistry and the nervous system but also to social systems, such as the grouping behavior of animals, and the economy.

Yet despite quantitative shortcomings—being unable to assign precise numerical causal roles to each class of population health determinant, and being unable to isolate with precision the impact on population health of each variable in the complex social-health system—there are several broad categories of interventions that could beneficially be applied now. Improved child development, community cohesion, self-fulfillment, total ecology, and socioeconomic mobility would result generally in improved quality of life; at the same time, these improvements would likely be salutary to population health. Reasonable evidence, not certainty of knowledge, permitted tobacco control to move forward 40 years ago. Existing data are adequate for formulating policies and other actions that could affect population health importantly. Awaiting new analytic methods and quantitatively more precise information will delay by decades or longer attempts to improve population health.

AN INTERVENTION FRAMEWORK FOR POPULATION HEALTH IMPROVEMENT

THE Intervention Framework (Table 1) identifies five broad intervention objectives that are likely to be salutary for population health. The five are improved child develop-

ment, strengthened community cohesion, enhanced opportunities for self-fulfillment, increased socioeconomic well-being, and modulated hierarchical structuring—that is, aimed at children, the community, adults, the economy, and arrangements for social positioning. Each intervention can be classified as either ameliorative or fundamentally corrective. For example, ameliorative interventions to improve child development might include approval of a city ordinance that allows surplus space in public school buildings to be used for day care while parents are working, or to reinvigorate YMCAs and YWCAs so that after-school supervised recreational activities for children and youths become generally available. Fundamentally corrective programs to improve child development might

Table 1

INTERVENTION FRAMEWORK
Population Health Improvement

	Ameliorative	Fundamentally Corrective
• improve <u>child</u> development		
• strengthen <u>community cohesion</u>		
• enhance opportunities for <u>self-fulfillment</u>		
• increase <u>socioeconomic</u> well-being		
• modulate <u>hierarchical</u> structuring		

Conceptual framework for five broad objectives to improve population health, each categorized as either ameliorative or fundamentally corrective innovations.

include programs to train fathers and mothers in parenting skills and to establish home environments conducive to positive cognitive, emotional, and behavioral development, and the development of day-care programs having high standards, well-trained and culturally diverse professionals who earn professional wages, transportation that places the programs within practical reach of families, and financial foundations to make the programs affordable to all. The Intervention Framework could help a community or organization develop short-range and long-range planning and identify a combination of ameliorative and fundamentally corrective strategies to provide some near-term accomplishments as well as long-term restructuring to address the population health problem at its roots.

Other examples can be chosen for strengthening community cohesion, enhancing opportunities for self-fulfillment, increasing socioeconomic mobility, or modulating the effects of hierarchical structuring. The examples are likely to include combinations of public policies, private sector actions, community programs, and the active involvement of multiple sectors as presented earlier in this chapter. We will return to this Intervention Framework in reference to the *Independent Inquiry into Inequalities in Health*.

PUBLIC POLICY DEVELOPMENT PROCESS

THIS framework separates policy development into two phases (Figure 1), an initial phase leading to the development of a public consensus, and a later political phase when specific policy actions are taken. Prior to political action, a broad public understanding needs to be acquired that population health problems have origins in real issues that can be addressed remedially to everyone's advantage. Once that understanding has been assimilated, an evident desire at a high-enough priority must develop among a

sufficient proportion of the population to create a national agenda, or an authorizing environment and momentum for action. When sufficient momentum has developed, the political process will be authorized to pursue policies to address the problem. This framework helps decide where to apply energy in implementing strategies for population health improvement.

In the example of improved child development used above, all aspects of the initial phase have already been accomplished. That is, a public consensus has formed, a national agenda has been developed, and an authorizing environment has developed that will make it natural and acceptable to engage the political process in thinking through alternative proposals to improve opportunities for successful child development. However, although early childhood experiences are commonly known to be related to cognitive, emotional, and behavioral development, it is not well known that the quality of early children development is tied to adult health. Americans also place a high value on adult health. Therefore, while the issue of child development is ready for political engagement, the policy action phase can be advanced with greater force if the adult health issue is joined.

On the other hand, a plan to improve socioeconomic well-being that includes a component of income redistribution should acknowledge that the startling rise in income inequality in the U.S. has been well documented in books and reports from universities, research organizations, some nonprofit organizations, and journalists. Yet the relationship of income inequality to gross inequalities in health has so far not stimulated a broad and sustained dialogue in the U.S. media and on the political campaign trails. Nor has the problem risen to occupy a position on the national agenda, as has been achieved for issues in education, social security, Medicare, patient bill of health care rights, and international finance and trade. In contrast to the child development issue, which is ripe for political action, the in-

PUBLIC POLICY DEVELOPMENT PROCESS

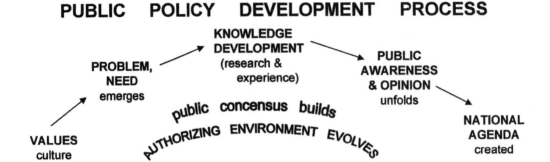

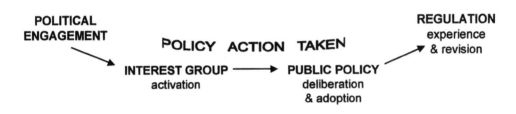

Figure 1
Conceptual framework for the two phases of the public policy development process: public consensus/national agenda building, and political/public policy actions taken.

come distribution issue should start in the public awareness and public consensus arena. Political productivity is the endgame of social transformation.

Interventions related to the four conceptual frameworks mentioned earlier should be integrated into a coherent strategy for improving population health. Although the emphasis in this chapter is on public policies, surely corporate policies, community programs, medical care, and health behaviors have important roles to play in child development and adult health. Important potential allies will be lost if the corporate, community, health care, and behavior-change sectors are ignored. Likewise, an understanding of complex systems, even at a low level of sophistication,

will be important in anticipating the likelihood of multiple effects of interventions, and in maintaining an early alertness and watchful eye for unintended and undesired consequences of interventions. Further, desired outcomes in complex systems can be accomplished through several routes, allowing the selection of an alternate public policy initiative that has a greater public and political chance of being adopted and sustained. The Intervention Framework provides the key choices in relatively neutral terms for specific objective setting and intervention concentration, while the Public Policy Development Framework can help design the strategy and select the target in which to initiate and focus the strategy.

INDEPENDENT INQUIRY
INTO INEQUALITIES IN HEALTH

IN July 1997 the new Labor Party government of British prime minister Tony Blair requested Sir Donald Acheson, former chief medical officer of the National Health Service, to review and summarize inequalities in health in the United Kingdom and to identify priority areas for future policy development likely to offer opportunities for government to develop beneficial, cost-effective, and affordable interventions to reduce health inequalities.

The charge of the inquiry instructed that the policy proposals were to be based on "scientific and expert evidence" and "within the broad framework of Government's financial strategy."[3] The report was to be completed in about a year and was indeed submitted to the government in September 1998.

Several limitations were imposed at the outset. The report was to be focused on government opportunities, as opposed to private sector initiatives. The recommendations were to be framed in the context of the new government's financial plans for the country. Only one year was allowed for a project that many of us would have regarded as an undertaking of three or more years.

A salient feature of the inquiry is its consistent insistence that the summarization of knowledge be based on science and that the recommendations be supportable by the scientific evidence and by peer review by scientists expert in this field. The process followed in preparing the report and preparation of the report itself were overseen by a five-member Scientific Advisory Group.

The inquiry was guided by a socioeconomic model of health initially proposed by Dahlgren and Whitehead in 1991.[4] The model emphasizes the context in which we live and by which health or disease is generated. The context is depicted by concentric rings with people at the center, enveloped successively by the influences of lifestyle, social and community characteristics, and finally an array of macro-socioeconomic, cultural, and environmental conditions. The influence of this contextual conceptualization, sometimes referred to as socioecologic, is evident in the report.

The report is in two parts. Part 1 contains a summary of research data on inequalities in health. Part 2 consists of reviews of the evidence, amplified from the data cited in Part 1, upon which the policy formulations are discussed. A list of 39 policy recommendations is given at the end of Part 2.

Readers might tend to turn directly to the list of recommendations, but it would be a mistake to end one's analysis of the report there. Out of context, the recommendations can be interpreted as a war on poverty or as a welfare program for disadvantaged mothers and children. A reading of the entire Part 2, however, adds background, content, depth, and texture to the recommendations. They become a comprehensive, integrated, and plausible set of recommendations for government policies designed to reduce inequalities in population health. The recommendations address population health inequalities induced by health behaviors, deficiencies in medical care planning and delivery, and the pervasive influence of social and societal characteristics. Although the principal emphasis is on social and societal factors, the argument is well made that inequalities in medical services often sustain or amplify inequalities in health.

The Recommendations. Most of the 39 recommendations have multiple subrecommendations, and many recommendations are cross-listed under several of the 13 recommendation categories listed in Table 2. For simplicity in this chapter, the recommendation categories can usefully be collected into four "groupings" (Table 3). The groupings will only be scanned briefly here.

Group A, Scope and emphasis (recommendations 1 and 2), sets a comprehensive tone by indicating that *all* government policies should be examined for their possible impact on health inequalities and indicates that the report gives special emphasis to the less well off, with the highest

Table 2

INDEPENDENT INQUIRY
RECOMMENDATION CATEGORIES

1. GENERAL	8. MOTHERS, CHILDREN, FAMILIES
	9. YOUNG PEOPLE & WORKERS
2. POVERTY, INCOME, BENEFITS	10. OLDER PEOPLE
	11. ETHNIC MINORITIES
3. EDUCATION	12. GENDER
4. EMPLOYMENT	
5. HOUSING	
6. MOBILITY, TRANSPORT, POLLUTION	13. NATIONAL HEALTH SERVICES
7. NUTRITION & AGRICULTURE POLICY	

Thirteen categories used for the 39 recommendations of the Independent Inquiry into Inequalities in Health, United Kingdom, 1998.

(but not exclusive) priority accorded to women of childbearing age, expectant mothers, and children.

Group B, Sociostructural improvements (recommendations 3 through 20), perhaps will be of greatest interest to this book's readers. The recommendations are summarized in Table 4. Recommendation number one that all public policies be assessed for their impact on health inequalities is exemplified in Table 4, with specific attention to employment and nutrition policies. Income transfers are invoked to lift the bottom out of poverty, to ameliorate the effects of unemployment, and to assure the affordability of wholesome foods for all. Benefits strategies are

advanced by the report with respect to expanding preschool opportunities, improving job training, increasing the availability and quality of public housing, and increasing public transport. Again, a full understanding of the sweep of the report should be achieved by reading the texts of both Parts 1 and 2.

Group C, Disadvantaged emphasis (recommendations 21 through 36), specifies the report's emphasis on mothers, children, and families; young people and workers; older people; ethnic minorities; and young men and young women separately. To cite just a few examples, for families the report recommends elimination of poverty by income transfers, the elimination of food

Table 3

INDEPENDENT INQUIRY
RECOMMENDATION GROUPS

	Number of Recommendations
A. Scope & Emphasis	(2)
B. Sociostructural Improvements	(18)
C. Disadvantaged Emphasis	(16)
D. Health Services	(3)

Four groupings (by the authors of this chapter) for the 39 recommendations in the Independent Inquiry into Inequalities in Health, United Kingdom, 1998.

poverty, greater opportunities for day care and preschool education, and social and emotional support services for parents by increasing the role of "health visitors." The issue of material inequality is addressed for older people through income transfers and benefits, and for ethnic minorities the report recommends that socioeconomic inequalities be reduced. The span of the recommendations for the disadvantaged can be appreciated by reading the full report. A large fraction of the specific recommendations under Groups, A, B, and D would also be beneficial to the disadvantaged.

Group D, Health services (recommendations 37 through 39), seeks to promote equity in access to and quality of services. The report recommends that resource allocation for health services be differentially determined by needs, weighed for each specific population. Monitoring of improved equity should be achieved by data systems and triennial audits.

A brief summary of the report does not do justice to its expanse. Its objective is to reduce inequalities in health through a reassessment of all government policies that might have a direct or indirect effect on health inequality. It uses all avenues, including medical care, preventive public

health measures, encouragement of more salutary health behaviors, and a large measure of sociostructural remodeling. The latter includes direct actions for diminishing income inequality (income transfers) and recommends a wide range of expanded benefits intended to reduce inequalities in health. The comprehensiveness of the report's attention to a wide panoply of structurally embedded societal features commands attention from everyone concerned about the recalcitrant problem of health inequalities within societies.

A U.S. PERSPECTIVE:
THE INTERVENTION FRAMEWORK
APPLIED TO THE INDEPENDENT
INQUIRY'S RECOMMENDATIONS

THE cultural, social, and political contexts of the United Kingdom and the United States are sufficiently dissimilar to justify skepticism that conceptual frameworks for actions are cross-applicable. Nonetheless, as scientists and others working in the field of society and population health turn attention to the practical work of fostering the development of actual programs and social policies to improve population health, concepts and theories will be needed to guide the

Table 4

INDEPENDENT INQUIRY
SOCIOSTRUCTURAL IMPROVEMENTTS

NEEDING IMPROVEMENT	RECOMMENDATIONS
• POVERTY & INCOME INEQUALITY	• income transfers • benefits
• EDUCATION	• increase funds for preschools & less well off schools, and expand health-promotive schools
• EMPLOYMENT	• improve training & job quality • study impact all employment policies • ameliorate effects of unemployment
• HOUSING	• increase availability and quality of public housing
• MOBILITY, TRANSPORT, POLLUTION	• increase public transport • decrease motor vehicle use • lower speed limits • increase cycling & walking
• NUTRITION	• study impact agricultural policies • improve distribution surplus • wholesome foods in groceries • assure affordability of foods

Recommendations for sociostructural improvements, Group B (18 recommendations), in the Independent Inquiry into Inequalities in Health, United Kingdom, 1998.

formulations and to ground our imaginations in reality. Two of the conceptual frameworks offered in this presentation are works in progress (Interventions, and Public Policy Development). There is no empiric evidence of their validity or practical usefulness. These works in progress might be sharpened and made more useful by applying them to the *Independent Inquiry*'s recommendations in a test, more or less, of the validity of the concepts within the frameworks. Table 5 is an attempt to do that.

In this depiction we have placed each of the report's recommendations on sociostructural remodeling into the grid of intervention objectives and assigned them as most likely to be in the ameliorative or fundamentally corrective category. Using child development as an example, expanding preschool opportunities for children aged 0–5 and using formulas for allocating financial support that are weighted according to the needs of the particular students of each school are both fundamentally corrective. For

Table 5

INTERVENTION FRAMEWORK
Population Health Improvement

	Ameliorative	Fundamentally Corrective
• improve child development		EDU: preschools, weighted funding NUT: agric. policies, affordability
• strengthen community cohesion		MOB: ↑ public transport ↓ motor vehicles ↑ cycling, walking
• enhance opportunities for self-fulfillment	EMP: unemployment effects HOU: public housing NUT: distribute surplus grocery stores	EMP: training/skills, policies review
• increase socioeconomic well-being		PII: income transfers, benefits
• modulate hierarchical structuring		

EDU = Education
EMP = Employment
HOU = Housing

MOB = Mobility
NUT = Nutrition
PII = Poverty, Income Inequality

Recommendations for sociostructural improvements made by the Independent Inquiry into Inequalities in Health (U.K.), placed by this chapter's author into the conceptual Intervention Framework.

increasing socioeconomic well-being, income transfers and benefits programs are fundamentally corrective. For enhancing opportunities for self-fulfillment using employment policies, assessing and responding supportively to the effects of unemployment can be ameliorative when a problem already exists, whereas elevating skill levels of workers by institutionalizing training and undertaking a comprehensive assessment of all employment policies regarding their direct and indirect effects on health inequalities could be fundamentally corrective actions.

What does the Intervention Framework reveal about the recommendations of the report? Our interpretations should be regarded as tentative, and perhaps even foolhardy, because of our ignorance of the British value structure, politics, present and long-range currents in social transformation, and the present state of laws and regulations. With reservations, and in the spirit of a desire to understand whether the framework has any utility, two interpretations are offered. First, the report advances relatively few recommendations that are ameliorative, at least with respect to sociostructural modifications. Ameliorative actions respond to the present population's needs and sufferings and in many ways are reflections of a society's empathy and humanitarianism toward its fellow citizens. The empty spaces in the ameliorative column can possibly be explained by the fact that the charge to the inquiry specifically directed the attention to "government interventions to reduce health inequalities." Private sector organizations and communities are more likely to take ameliorative actions. Perhaps the report's relatively greater emphasis on fundamentally corrective policies should be lauded, especially in light of its recommendation No. 1—that *all* policies be reviewed for their possible impact on health inequalities.

Second, the report offers no recommendations to modulate hierarchical structuring. This might be the most difficult target area to restructure. Most of the research and published attention on social inequality has concentrated on the most

easily measured social variable—that is, per capita or household income. But other elements of hierarchical social structures might be fundamentally and more profoundly causative of health inequalities. Some of these include hierarchically graded distributions within the social structure of status, opportunity, privilege, power, and authority. These variables have not been addressed in the research and have been absent from the public discourse, little as there has been, on social characteristics and population health inequalities.

How do the *Independent Inquiry*'s recommendations on sociostructural improvements fit into the framework of the Public Policy Development Process? To reiterate, the conceptualization of the process for the U.S. is likely not to be transferable to the U.K. But perhaps something can be learned from doing so.

To begin, all the recommendations of the report are framed as recommendations for government action because the inquiry was conceived of and framed by the government elected to office at that time. As a result, all recommendations enter a late phase of the Public Policy Development Process—at the public policy deliberation stage.

I would think that in the hypothetical exercise of applying the inquiry's report to America, a preferred strategy would enter the process at an earlier phase, as depicted in Figure 2. Political, media, and public awareness of the causative connection of social position to inequalities in health does not exist in the U.S. The national popular agenda does not include the relation of health to hierarchical structuring except as an issue of poverty. A public consensus on this subject does not exist. An authorizing environment has not been created. Social-health inequalities cannot be effectively engaged as a political issue in the U.S. at this time.

In the U.S., political engagement has begun for certain of the inquiry's recommendations. For example, expanding preschool availability receives consistent attention in policy discussions related both to working mothers and to children

FRAMEWORK

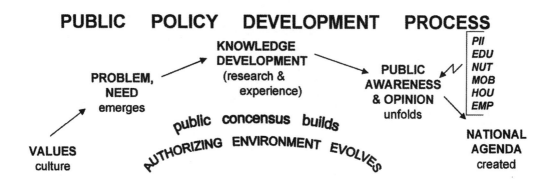

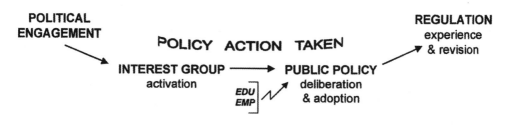

Figure 2

Recommendations for sociostructural improvements made by the Independent Inquiry into Inequalities in Health (U.K.) inserted into the Public Policy Development Process in places that the author of this chapter believes would be appropriate for the circumstances of the U.S.

being raised in poverty. Several large and influential nonprofit advocacy organizations promote and sustain these issues. Consistent media attention is directed. The environment has evolved, a national agenda has developed, political engagement and interest groups have been activated, and public policy deliberations are taking place.

But the larger agenda, acquisition by the U.S. society of an understanding of the dynamics of health production through sociostructural influences, has not even begun. Therefore, a strategy more likely to succeed in the U.S., according to the framework depicted in Figure 2, would start

with a national public information program to create public awareness at a level of concern that will elevate the issue to the national agenda. The strategy for the U.S. would begin with research to understand just what the American public, by subpopulations, already knows about the relationship of social features to population health. It is probably little, except as related to poverty. Knowledge would also have to be gained about specific values and beliefs already held by the public that might be sparked into reverberation with the social-health gradient subject. This would provide focus for a national public information program using multiple channels of communication and education.

The British report *Independent Inquiry into Inequalities in Health*, given its purpose, is a highly valuable and progressive source of information and recommendations. It sets out a comprehensive policy agenda to improve population health at least for developed nations. Other nations, with knowledge of the public attitude development process in their country, and with approaches that activate public sector, private sector, and community action, will find that the *Independent Inquiry* provides a treasure of summarized knowledge and comprehensive approaches that can be useful to them in building their own conceptual frameworks to select social restructuring targets for intervention.

The conceptual frameworks developed in this chapter, with some modifications, might be of use for health improvement planning at the individual state level or in smaller geopolitical units. The *Independent Inquiry* from the United Kingdom could be useful at the state level, at least for the example it sets for comprehensiveness and probably for more.

NOTES

1. *Independent Inquiry into Inequalities in Health: Report.* (London: Her Majesty's Stationery Office, with the permission of the Department of Health, 1998).

2. "Complex Systems." *Science* 284, no. 5411. (2 April 1999): 79–109.

3. *Independent Inquiry into Inequalities in Health: Report.* (London: Her Majesty's Stationery Office, with the permission of the Department of Health, 1998): pp. 155–157.

4. *Independent Inquiry into Inequalities in Health: Report.* (London: Her Majesty's Stationery Office, with the permission of the Department of Health, 1998): pp. 5–6.

❦

Appendix

WHAT KANSANS RECOMMEND
TO IMPROVE HEALTH AND WELL-BEING

Leonard E. Bloomquist, Stephen B. Fawcett, and Arnold Kaluzny

O NE objective of the Kansas Conference on Health and Its Determinants was to actively engage participants in a process of formulating programs and policies to improve health in the state and local communities. The audience of 250 invited Kansans was selected from a variety of sectors including educational institutions, social service agencies, community organizations, local government, public health agencies, professionals in health care, business, labor, farming, and state government.

Each attendee was assigned to a group of 15 persons, with individuals assigned to groups to assure diverse representation by sector. Fifteen groups were formed. Facilitators and recorders were briefed on goals and facilitation techniques, and then a pair was attached to each group. Each group convened in a breakout session immediately following each of the first three general sessions. The subject matter of each dialogue session was as follows:

Part I.   Building Healthy Communities
Part II.   Promoting Child Development and Health
Part III. Influencing the Health of Adults

At the beginning of the breakout sessions, group members were asked to generate a list of programs and policies to improve health in the respective subject area (e.g., Building Healthy Communities; Promoting Child Development and Health). The lists were to be derived from the participants' experience with the subject theme and the presentations and manuscripts distributed at the conference. Groups were also requested to try to achieve consensus on the top ten recommendations for improving health related to the subject theme (i.e., healthy communities, children, adults). Each group deliberated approximately 60–90 minutes. The membership of each group, including its assigned facilitator and recorder, was the same throughout the three breakout sessions. Group discussions were lively, with participants demonstrating an impressive understanding of the themes and research findings that had been presented. Moreover, individuals contributed perspectives and insights based on their own experiences in state government and/or local communities. All told, approximately 450 recommendations were made by the 15 groups in their three breakout sessions. The recommendations are printed in their entirety below:

Part I:
Building Healthy Communities

Group #1

1. Massive TV approach to increase understanding among all people of the importance of early childhood development and how to positively impact it.

2. Recognize that there are many illiterate people and make connection to poor health. Use community agencies and coalitions to help make this connection.

3. Make prenatal care available with transportation and other supports to access service.

4. Encourage community initiatives to develop youth for future leadership roles.

5. Statewide initiative to encourage health habits and the value of a healthy routine to preschool and school-age children.

6. Statewide health promotion Internet site that would outline changes in policies and health issues, interactive for communities. "Knowledge bank" for different ideas in the state.

7. Methodology for a joint effort to have education at all levels (state-community-school-parents) and among funding agencies.

8. Encourage business to have family friendly policies:
> —child care
> —health care
> —wellness
> —flex time so *both* parents can take part in child rearing
> —wage/salary

9. Reduce economic inequalities through strengthening policies in employment, education, taxes and benefits, reducing hierarchy and less social exclusion.

10. Make early childhood education available to all. Partnership at federal, state and local level.

Group #2

1. Encourage volunteerism:
> —mobilize older volunteers (to fill gaps in previous vol. populations)
> —provide opportunities for young (grade school-university age) to volunteer— *build commitment* at young age to social involvement
> —provide information and incentives to business community concerning needs for volunteers, resources—solicit opportunities for working folks to volunteer

2. Develop community commitment to community planning political/programmatic strategy to ensure duration and intensity of long-term commitment.

3. Culturally and socially relevant clearing house for interests, resources, needs, skills, activities in community—matching function.

4. Design government and corporate policy intervention to promote "shopkeeper" and small community and family environment—strengthens connection and trust in communities.

5. Bridging mechanism to bring vertical and horizontal integration (bring leaders together).

6. Commitment, trust built on sense of productive use of input and progress (measure outcome and process).

7. Expand definition of community (faith, culture, etc.) to allow strategies to expand.

8. Use birth as a way of identifying families, moms and children to provide information on resources available.

9. Build on Kansans' sense of place to improve community connectedness.

Group #3

1. Educate parents as to critical timing in child mental development.

2. Business leaders awareness of importance of first five years in child development.

3. Make available information that is in existence for use by responsible parties.

4. Better utilize media in distributing information.

5. Develop coordinating strategies to better unify activities of service agencies.

6. Identify marketplace and how to best deliver service.

7. Support flex-time programs for parent/child, prof/child time needs.

8. Develop user-friendly marketing research.

9. Encourage programs for adult/child contacts and interactions.

10. Include an integrated Health Education component in the school system.

Group #4

1. Social marketing campaign targeting children 0–3 and their families in their communities. Building consensus around priorities and formulating action plan on an individual and collective basis.

2. Utilize grass roots/individual citizens in formulating action plans complete with desired outcomes.

3. Develop strategies to get "Kansas Health" information and stats into community.

4. Personalize information.

5. Build collaboration/partnership to minimize fragmentation, overlap and duplication.

6. Deliver services/commodities in non-traditional ways/settings.

7. Correlate public spending with brain development opportunities.

8. Target parents/caregivers in providing education.

9. Teach young children about their societal roles as it relates to health (reestablish social contract).

10. Blend education/training into welfare reform.

Group #5

1. School districts take responsibility for early childhood development (0–5).

2. Work to increase community participation and interaction.

3. Multi-faceted approach to health promo-

tion—health and other settings—outreach—media—health promoters, other sectors.

4. Engage citizens from different sectors in long range planning.

5. Fund universal coverage for all ages (up to 200% of poverty).

6. Educate the public about the cost effectiveness of early childhood intervention and infant stimulation.

7. Maximize decision-making power and control at the local level to enhance buy-in.

8. Utilize mentoring (cross sectors and generations) to build the "big web."

9. Maximize media as a partner.

10. Maximize potential of older persons to contribute to communities.

Group #6

1. Develop a social marketing campaign that will operationalize a collective vision for the future.

2. We need to increase social capital—but this is an active process, e.g., Kauffman's "Social contracts" with youth and their educational opportunities.

3. Take two counties as models—one rural, e.g., Bourbon, and one urban, e.g., Wyandotte—then use centralized resources (from SRS, KDHE, Foundation and other granting agencies), then let the members of the community make the decisions as to how to allocate the resources as the community knows its problems best.

4. Restore social civility—get rid of the loud voices (the bullies) so that we can be heard.

5. We tend to forget the commonalities that may underlie many health and social problems—as a result our focus is too narrow.

6. We need state or county level institutions that are not top-down and exclusive as this may have led a loss of community spirit.

7. Define the community, create neighborhood associations.

8. Take "concepts" that come from research that can be used in the community.

9. Celebrate our successes.

Group #7

1. Making informed decisions using data involving all of the community.

2. Building trust around the right issues (Community's agenda).

3. More collaboration, less turf-guarding at state and local level.

4. Clearly defined vision at state and local level.

5. Qualitative vs. Quantative (Outcome vs. Process).

6. Changing social norms at organizational, individual and community level.

7. Funders need to understand that the process takes time.

8. Training for community leaders.

9. Coordination between groups with common interest.

10. Children first (i.e. Parents As Teachers).

Group #8

1. Public education of citizens and leaders for a broader definition of health.

2. Integration of community groups to have greater linkages between them and fewer barriers.

3. Leadership training in a broader definition of health.

4. Combined and integrated community resources that encompass all community groups.

5. Promoting a cultural acceptance of being healthy.

6. Fostering interagency agreement.

7. Expanding health insurance industry to encompass health promotion and disease prevention.

8. Change medical school curriculum to expand its focus on prevention and health promotion.

9. Building integrated programs at existing community institutions—"one-stop shopping."

10. Improving the image of public health to make it more positive—not to be identified with only poor people.

11. Identify the informal leaders in a community and involve them in the promotion of community health.

Group #9

1. Build strategy to assess and understand problems locally to broadly inform and educate community.

2. Umbrella organization to coordinate allocation of categorical $$.

3. Strategy to bring critical MASS together (i.e. business/industry).

4. New role for government as *facilitator.*

5. Universal role as change agent to build trust and local intermediary.

6. Embrace cultural differences.

7. Help communities define an evaluation process.

8. Identify commodities among public/private partners.

9. Identify strategies to reduce barriers—e.g., volunteering, mentoring.

Group #10

1. Convince policy makers to use data.

2. Parent education.

3. At the state level, organize governmental functions for better efficiency and coordination toward local community need.

4. Develop and implement community health plan.

5. Address the erosion of the public health infrastructure.

6. Opportunities for exercise in the community.

7. Encourage volunteerism:

   a) businesses develop workplace policy for employee volunteers,

b) tax breaks (state, federal, local) to businesses and individuals for volunteer activity,

c) recruit retired, older as volunteer work force, and

d) encourage/create role model volunteers.

8. Healthy families 0–3 for high risk.

9. Partnership with businesses to hire people at decent wage.

10. Coordinate, integrate, form community/civic events, services and resources.

Group #11

1. Transportation.

2. More money for infant and preschool education/home visits restructured.

3. Adequately fund public education, reduce class size.

4. Holistic way to deal with families/program and location integration.

5. Involve the local community across cultural lines.

6. Invest in health information systems.

7. Enhancing the quality and amount of child care.

8. Community health council—create new leaders/be inclusive.

9. Telemedicine—school health.

10. Why cut taxes, but rather effectively help people. Reinvest tax surpluses to effectively help people.

Group #12

1. Health care appropriation should be divided equally between treatment and prevention.

2. Mandate a % of global capitation rate to prevention.

3. Mandates for no TV in day care.

4. New mandates into early education from new research.

5. Involving people we are targeting to plan and follow through on innovations.

6. Education, education, education.

7. Grants targeted to multi issues.

8. Fortify private and public partnerships starting with libraries and schools.

9. Mandate pre-birth parenting classes and mentoring.

10. Build in incentives in prenatal care.

11. Encourage neighborhood associations.

Group #13

1. Tax credits to individuals and businesses who spend time serving their communities, using new and established volunteer programs (e.g., BB/BS, Girl Scouts, animal clubs).

2. "One-stop shopping" networks across services and resources that address multiple needs of clients. The "shopping centers" should recognize cultural differences. The type and number of shops should be determined by clients.

3. Affordable group rates (e.g., insurance) for small businesses (e.g., farmers, including co-ops).

4. Create employer initiatives (e.g., incentives, rewards, permissive policies) that allow people to care for their children, elders and community-at-large.

5. Parent education: make it a priority for funding and resources, such as Parents As Teachers, Even Start, child resource centers, parent information lines and other successful programs.

6. Create programs that connect moms-to-be to natural support systems (e.g., other moms) in close proximity in their neighborhood.

7. Identify and create mechanism to measure the success of community programs, policies and practices.

8. Whether in a business setting or the larger community setting, get broad-based input from clients/residents on health objectives and outcomes. This could be community forums, listening sessions or town meetings.

9. Create funding mechanisms to support reaching short-term and long-term outcomes.

10. Educate the populace how to and benefits

of getting involved in the community (e.g., build civic involvement in High School classes).

Group #14

1. Promote the "publics' health" as everyone's business—educate the taxpayers.

2. Focus on the long-term *process* of health promotion vs. products/outcomes.

3. Improve the awareness of funding, best practices and programs among community workers.

4. Assure funding flexibility with accountable outcomes.

5. Increase integration of health across SRS/Education/KDHE/APAs/Aging/Insurance Commissioner.

6. Work on asking and involving community citizens beyond the usual suspects—"key leaders."

7. Improve the use of data for prioritizing and funding—also to provide increased accountability for both public and private providers.

8. Work to increase the status of the public health system so that it is not stigmatized—not seen as "health welfare."

9. Convene an annual "think tank" bringing policy makers and experts, citizens, etc., together. "Expose ourselves to something different."

10. Increase public health's link with non-traditional partners, e.g., link economic development with health promotion locally.

Group #15

1. Regulatory, corporate legislative policy incentives to support education about health and wellness with respect to social determinants of health.

2. Integrate single issue coalitions.

3. More community events that bring diverse communities.

4. Educating providers on wellness/change financial incentives to support wellness care.

5. Businesses promote/provide incentives to their employees for civic engagement.

6. Identify *community* (and its many interests).

7. Inclusion from bottom-up—engage in community activity.

8. More businesses become part of the partnerships.

9. Disseminate what we know about the issues and social determinants and what we learn from evaluation.

10. Promote the integration of communication between all health-related research with application.

PART II:
PROMOTING CHILD DEVELOPMENT AND HEALTH
Group #1

1. Increase role of nurse practitioners in child assessment and services.

2. Must change stereotypes to be able to address changes in the systems.

3. Access to health care.

4. Support and increase availability of Head Start and Early Intervention programs (0–3), i.e., home visits, Parents As Teachers, Healthy Start, Healthy Start Plus and Early Learning Center.

5. Assure availability of high quality childcare.

6. Parent training, particularly for first-time parents. Education for parents regarding what children need to develop.

7. Smaller classes for K–3 grades.

8. Monitoring and measurement of domestic conflict and maternal depression.

9. Bring back therapeutic foster care for children.

10. Monitor social-attachment in home and school to understand trends.

11. Assessment of juvenile court outcomes to develop system to meet needs.

Group #2

1. Family planning—to promote readiness for parenting.

2. Provide a secure home setting/environment for young/teen moms/kids
    —promote self esteem
    —support systems

3. *Early* sex education for a long-term approach to more secure settings in childbearing years. Introduce family parenting skills into extra-curricular education for both boys/girls (grades 1–6) (parenting centers).

4. Develop consensus and commitment to outcome measure(s) to test strategies and programs.

5. Parenting skills to both moms/dads training/education
    —hospitals at birth
    —employer incentives to provide/allow education

6. Home follow-up for families. Training older adult to support new mothers and families in learning parenting skills. Train moms who were visited to provide same service to other moms.

7. Develop family support initiatives that are relevant to the family structure.

8. Blending daycare and parenting (flow of information and training).

9. Support for families in divorce (prevent acrimony during divorce process).

10. Increase Head Start funding (dramatic increase for proven program).

Group #3

1. Start education of new parents during prenatal period.

2. Utilize seniors in child development process.

3. Develop public policy to support parents and other childcare providers.

4. Engage development of childhood development curricula in educational institutions.

5. Enhance economic and social status of those providing childcare services.

6. Emphasize importance of extended family.

7. Expand existing quality-proven programs.

8. Recognize cultural differences in child rearing strategies.

9. Develop strategies to engage fathers irrespective of relationship.

10. Differential subsidies for accredited childcare centers.

11. Match businesses with childcare providers who seek to upgrade their services.

Group #4

1. Determine what all children (but focusing on children 0–5) and their families need, at least minimally, moving towards the development of optimal model standards.

2. Develop education for families, legislators, general public, etc., relative to the importance of these standards.

3. Develop strategies to accomplish them.

4. Develop mechanism to evaluate where individual children, communities and the state are relative to the standards.

5. Develop report card for *programs* serving children 0–5 for public dissemination.

6. Develop report card relative to the status of *children* for public dissemination.

7. Develop family impact statement (like a fiscal impact statement) for all legislative bills being considered by governors and legislators.

8. Recommend appropriate salary for providers of service to children 0–5 and their families because of the high regard we have for this age group.

9. Develop mechanism to solicit broad and varied input to any of the decisions, ideas, etc., coming from this meeting.

10. Recommend a broad educational program targeting business as to the importance of the development of children 0–5 and their families.

Group #5

1. Fund 0–5 (at same rate as K–12) for communities with comprehensive child development plan.

2. Educate parents to improve parenting skills early—link to childbirth classes.

3. Create informal networks to provide parenting support, e.g., block mothers.

4. Improve community resources for local childcare providers.

5. Require private companies requesting public funds to provide childcare for their employees.

6. Provide access to abortion.

7. Provide more support for pregnant moms to maximize beneficial conditions.

8. Provide human development education at middle school (or younger).

9. Mandate parent education with condom vending.

10. Fund information technology for schools to increase access for health and human development education.

Group #6

1. Look at programs that have worked for decades, such as Head Start, and figure out how to successfully replicate them in a given community.

2. Develop strategies to ensure child readiness to learn, e.g., through summer reading programs.

3. Model good parenting skills.

4. Develop early interventions that also focus on maladaptive behaviors—for both children and parents.

5. Converge what people want with what people do.

6. Extend maternity and paternity leave to enable parents to be the primary care giver (restructure where and when necessary).

7. On-site daycare center to provide opportunities for parents and their children to interact during day including child-care for ¹/₂ day.

8. Don't solely focus on deviance—be more universal in the approach and promote wellness.

9. Encourage social scientists and medical scientists to work together to develop research continuity.

10. Develop expectations and foster social norms that empower parents as parents (rather than passively allowing institutions to function as parents).

Group #7

1. Mentoring programs for mothering and fathering. *Professional* home visits to assist parents (assess of need).

2. Parent/teacher conferences at the work site. Home visits by teacher.

3. Child placement (in school) by development, not chronological age:
   a. develop better identification program for mental and physical aspects
   b. develop better tools for implementing education programs
   c. lower teacher/child ratio

4. Alternative schools for children.

5. Require license to be parent.

6. Provide free health services (e.g., delivery) if parenting classes taken to 24 months.

7. Utilize faith community more.

8. Enforce school discipline.

9. More interaction between schools and parents.

10. Equalize opportunities for all children 0–3, regardless of S-E status.

Group #8

1. Establish a state-wide dialogue on public policy focus on early childhood.

2. Coordination of school hours and calendar to match usual work hours of parents, i.e., instituting 8 hours a day, 5 days a week school program.

3. Expand and improve parenting education including enriching the content of prenatal care. Parenting education for all, not just single parents or high risk families.

4. Improve preschool educational opportunities by moving from a custodial to education focus, instituting accreditation program for

childcare facilities, offering more opportunities for preschool education to all families.

5. Improve nutrition of children including greater participation in Kansas of federally funded programs and encourage breast feeding and employee policies to facilitate breast feeding.

6. Improved support of families and parenting by businesses, public services, and employers by flex time, on-site day care, expanded hours of operation of post office and other services.

7. Reduce the disconnect between what we know works to improve children's health, resource expended and public priorities.

8. Promoting a cultural acceptance of parenting as a challenge that benefits from community involvement and investment.

9. Increase early health promotion in the schools and include parents, i.e., nutrition, smoking.

Group #9

1. Strategy for "healthy home"
   —home visits/mentoring
   —*coordinated* strategy

2. Strengthen sense of neighborhood and community (e.g., sidewalks).

3. Increase support for Head Start and Early Head Start.

4. Engage children in decision-making.

5. Volunteerism in support of children
   —encourage/reward
   —in schools also

6. Universal hearing assessments by local hospitals for newborns.

7. Increased support for people who care for children (KACCRRA).

8. Make communities aware of gang symbols.

9. Partner with schools to identify kids "in trouble."

10. TV; lobby for better content, reduced consumption.

11. Develop reward system for "good"/ appropriate behavior.

Group #10

1. Affordable, available, high quality childcare on a sliding scale for kids 0–12.

2. Allowing choices to enable parents to stay home during baby's first year of life.

3. Designate reliable, stable funding source for children's programs.

4. Expand parent support and visitation programs such as Perry preschool with required parenting classes.

5. Consider MH and dental health as integral to public health with preventive dentistry (sealants, fluoride).

6. Use public health data to inform public and to lobby for funding.

7. Provide quality training for counselors and more responsive counseling for teens including parenting.

8. Free access to quality healthcare for every child.

9. Create environmental parent support
   a) family support centers in every community/neighborhood
   b) partnership with business—for childcare
   c) after school programs
   d) mentoring

10. Create fiscal incentives to reward early childhood prevention programs.

Group #11

1. D-5 funding uses: Healthy Start, All day K, subsidize childcare, parents as teachers, home visitation, mother to mother.

2. Better utilize schools as community centers, i.e., preschool-adult activities.

3. Mandate parenting classes for H.S. graduation.

4. Accreditation of childcare centers and providers.

5. Subsidize childcare even on a sliding fee scale.

6. Incentives for corporate involvements:

with tax abatements/incentives require corporate businesses to give back to the community.

7. Create mechanisms for collaboration across service providers.

8. Corporate America gets involved by utilizing flex time, other family friendly policies, and time to take care of your child or other children.

9. Three meals a day at school.

Group #12

1. Collaborate with business in need for early interventions.

2. More responsible media toward well-being of children.

3. Social equivalent of wrap around services for kids.

4. Quality interactions between parent and children.

5. Best practices available to communities.

6. Better data for decision making and making it readily available to communities.

7. Business giving youth scholarships for volunteering.

8. Business offering flex time for parents.

9. Mentors for parents.

10. Sliding scale for childcare.

Group #13

1. "Positive" not penalty driven/status driven training for childcare workers who have decent wages and benefits.

2. Redistribution of income—redress income gradient—(social inequality).

3. Livable wage, universal access to healthcare, free prenatal care.

4. On-site daycare (working with incentive to business).

5. Involving parents in daycare policy setting (especially *young* parents).

6. Encourage and support more stable home environments—foster care, etc.—increase incentives for this "saintly work."

7. Identify individual community agency suc-

cesses and connect with those who would like to benefit from their experience.

8. Create standards (quality) for daycare.

9. *Even*—parent and kids together at workshops—start to compliment Head Start.

10. Home sharing—older adults who open home to younger individuals/families who share some responsibilities.

Group #14

1. Cultural competency and diversity are critical to both individual programs and to community level strategies.

2. Wide-spread adoption of programs "that work" such as Parents As Teachers and Early Head Start.

3. Raise the dialogue on children's well-being to that equal to "infrastructure investment" (e.g., spend as much on children as highways).

4. De-politicize children's development and well-being—it's all our kids.

5. Work toward adequate funding of programs.

6. Use schools as "health" providers—e.g., supportive.

7. Establish criteria for "quality daycare."

8. Develop statewide methodologies for data collection and indicators of child well-being. Need data system enhancements so that we can follow long-term cohorts.

9. Work for "mental health" parity in the field of "public health."

10. Good children's health includes prenatal care.

11. Wide spread adoption of pregnancy prevention programs that emphasize greater access to family planning services/products and peer-to-peer interventions.

Group #15

1. Provide financial incentives for a parent to stay at home.

2. Prenatal support program (comprehensive—parents, too), i.e., case management—

public health advising—longitudinal, i.e., mother to mother.

3. Comprehensive parenting education across the life span (in schools) as children libraries, faith communities, etc.

4. Childcare—increase quality improvement, increase regulation—beyond KBI check.

5. Teenage pregnancy prevention (preventing pregnant children).

6. Multi-level mass media parenting promotion—schools—age appropriate.

7. Elementary—???—partner with business, grandparents as teachers.

8. Increase investment in early childhood pre-schools, research, etc.

PART III:
INFLUENCING THE HEALTH OF ADULTS
Group #1

1. Conduct seminars for CEO's and Union Leaders regarding the social determinants of health in the workplace and how increased employee control, reduced hierarchy and increased social support positively impact productivity and profitability within the company.

2. Conduct public information campaign regarding social determinants of health on the population.

3. Encourage MD's in western Kansas to form networks to allow for time away. Continue to use KUMC telemedicine for support of rural MD networks.

4. Increase programs like RSVP [not targeted just for the elderly] as an example of network creation.

5. Begin studying the well adult population for insights rather than studying disease.

6. Make available information about community resource book.

7. Publicize to all potential of returning control to employees.

8. Have employee assistance programs available to all.

9. Re-establish agenda for employers for what

is needed regarding what employers can do individually and collectively for improving health.

10. Change policy to change from categorical funds to direct funds to what communities need.

11. Increase community workers that come from the neighborhood.

12. Make health delivery system less necessary with more emphasis put on health consequences (social determinants).

13. Navigator Program (example UKMC, Cancer Society, Truman Medical Center, Rogers Comprehensive Health Care) outreach to assist people with navigating health system and health education components.

14. Tackle health risk behaviors through the socio-economic structure that created them.

Group #2

1. Revise data collection to accurately reflect what is going on in people/families lives.

2. Urban planning—what kind of family structure do we live in? More integration of lower income housing. Improve housing standards and consistent implementation of beautification efforts.

3. Flex family time for employees—more healthful activities to increase wellness—flexible benefits.

4. Increase education of adults on health care issues (men: PSA levels, women: Pap smears, all pop: diabetes).

5. Incentive program to increase volunteerism for people and not necessarily programs. Need to address interpersonal needs.

6. Look at what legislative action is needed to look at transportation inaccessibility.

7. Investigate alternatives to the socioeconomic inequalities.

8. Develop neighborhood associations.

9. Integration of schools, social groups and churches across socioeconomic lines.

10. Implement intergenerational networks.

Group #3

1. Encourage private sector to help build community partnerships involving all cultures, net-

works. Find strategies to "think globally but act locally" for business.

2. People are our competitive advantage.

3. The gradient is everyone's health problem.

4. Develop incentives and strategies for people to work together to solve problems.

5. Develop programs to get communities to use "chartbook."

6. Work with existing institutions "relevant" to particular communities to transfer knowledge (e.g., train the trainer).

7. Working with CEO to build culture of support involving all races and culture.

8. Create an index of good corporate citizenship in helping build healthy communities (top 100 employees in state) publish and awards dinner.

9. Develop a society and health curriculum for high school and integrate into curriculum. Focus on inequality. Also develop curriculum for teachers.

10. Recognize youth who make a difference in communities (provide scholarships).

11. Integrate society and health perspectives into ongoing youth leadership forums.

Group #4

1. Assure equal access to "alternative forms of medicine" that incorporate all social support. e.g., lay home visitor concept.

2. Provide resource network so those at the grass root level can have access to self-help services.

3. State should take leadership to encourage businesses, civic groups and faith groups to provide opportunities for employees and members to participate in volunteerism; physical fitness opportunities, and in obtaining education.

4. Business should provide for on-site opportunities for physical fitness and education. (Example: UAW provide on-site education (from GED to Ph.D.) for employees and family members.)

5. Tax incentives to promote such things as

volunteerism for individuals and reductions of stress in the workplace for employers.

6. Develop a way to role model concept of volunteerism to youth.

7. Kansans should be more neighborly, willing to help out, volunteer, etc., this can including concept of a sharing co-op or having sidewalks (sidewalks can promote socialization, diminish isolations and promote physical fitness).

8. System for identification of depression in individuals in the work place or in their participation in public programs.

9. Look for model neighborhoods, identify ways to measure them and analyze what makes them good for replication.

10. Promotion of a living wage.

Group #5

1. Redistribute earned leave throughout the life span as opposed to retirement (e.g., parental leave).

2. Enable non-professional workers to have more flexible hours.

3. Educate ourselves about what it means to be part of an equalitarian work place—benefits.

4. Encourage volunteerism within our businesses and communities.

5. Promote experiential exposure to other cultures, races, within our communities and businesses to reduce prejudice.

6. Teach benefits of new and different management styles—enhance respect and value for support staff.

7. Turn this conference into a NOVA or Bill Moyers program—educate the public and also use for human resource training.

8. Link economic development, health, and social capital in the public mind—educate regarding benefits of social capital.

9. Promote activities to eliminate bias at an early age.

10. Productive aging—retirees as resources.

Group #6

1. Enable employees to practice a healthy lifestyle within the work context.

2. Don't ignore our diversity, embrace it.

3. Develop strategies to address and change the social disparities—create equality.

4. Develop values such that all workers feel valued and are valued.

5. Promote health and healthy behaviors as the norm, don't focus on illness.

6. Natural support should be identified by health providers, professionals and should be included and promoted in the health plans, e.g., give us sidewalks. How can we engage in an active lifestyle if our social environment prevents it, e.g., build houses with porches so that neighbors can talk to each other.

7. Teach people the value of support to prevent social isolation and the ensuing problems.

8. Adulthood covers many years. The life tasks of a 21-year-old are different from those for a 40-year-old.

9. Develop trust between employers and employees so as to assist both to accept loyalty as the reward and reduce stress in the work place.

Group #7

1. Redesign work settings: More space—task sensitive design.

2. More autonomy in decision making at work.

3. Inform decision-makers about the issues discussed in the conference.

4. Increase volunteerism in the work place setting.

5. Increase social network in the community.

6. Decrease government intervention (spending) on social issues and force increase involvement of charitable organizations in community.

7. Fair recognition and gratification for work accomplished.

8. Increase awareness of tax credits/deductions for charity.

9. Promote neighborhood association.

10. Promote community foundations.

Group #8

1. Public policy changes that allow flexibility and local discretion.

2. Incentives to businesses to better serve their communities and individuals in their communities.

3. Incentives to commercial media—(TV/Radio) to deliver more effectively public service programs.

4. Recognize potential for libraries to be a vehicle for greater involvement in health promotion.

5. Promoting job policies that support families and religious traditions.

6. Churches and religious organizations link beliefs to health benefits.

7. Identify and reduce racial/ethnic housing segregation.

8. Promote volunteerism through public policies, in-kind support (Capital and Human) from business and government.

9. Promote opportunities for increased physical activity in daily living, work place with incentives, gym or showers on site.

10. Using the "PRIDE" program as a vehicle for extending local community planning to create greater opportunities for healthy behaviors.

11. Mentoring Programs.

Group #9

1. Change the business culture to foster greater worker control. Encourage total quality management.

2. Greater focus on family. Need to improve supports; respite care; adult day care; home health.

3. Encourage community empowerment. Improve needs assessment and trust building. Establish community and inter-community networks.

4. Educate citizens on the relationship of health to social inequalities. Help communities place greater value on socialization.

Group #10

1. Create environments that offer easy access to physical exercise.

2. For all public health and mental health agencies to hire outreach workers for the communities that suffer the most from health problems within the community.

3. City/community partnerships for interdisciplinary planning related to health concerns.

4. Unplug TV/TV-free nights/tax breaks for no TV in house/tax breaks for non-violent programming.

5. Faith communities adopt high risk families.

6. De-stigmatize social services and de-categorize funding.

7. Re-invent public health work that encompasses changing demographic needs: aging, population migration.

8. Fund research to show relationship of biology to social determinants.

9. Reduce work week to 30 hours, guarantee livable wages, flatten hierarchy work structures.

Group #11

1. Increase access to medical care.

2. Fund more research taking results to community.

3. Partnering with faith community for transportation.

4. Linking community organizations.

5. Tax breaks for high education.

6. Education programs for chronically unemployed.

7. Day care funding for education.

8. Suggestion program team based and used in the work place.

9. Involve ethnic community leaders in decision making and defining needs.

10. Increasing awareness within the community to educate the people outside the community, encourage more integration.

Group #12

Group #13

1. Create community plans/zoning so that access to community resources/services is im-

proved and opportunity to connect and serve others is increased social networks such as inter-generational activities.

2. Identify and resolve contradictory policies.

3. Create opportunities such as this conference and less formal ones for business leaders and powerful social and health advocate groups to communicate and set common population wellness objectives.

4. Support and recognize organizations who help our community.

5. Empowerment: increase training of professionals on how to help empower those they serve and increase programs that empower clients to participate in their care and policies that affect them.

6. Pool strengths/talents/expertise of adults, business leaders, and others in order to help their peers.

7. Make legislators/policy influences aware of how social determinants, stress, social inequalities effect the "bottom line" of their constituents and make them stand behind their pro-family stance.

8. Educate (through media, etc.) individuals on the root cause of stress and ways to take actions to remove those root causes. Don't take "daily stress" as a given or necessary condition.

9. Include health challenged youth, the poor, or other minority or neglected groups in meeting/conferences like this one by KHI.

10. Create/support flexible schedules by employers and by service providers to help clients access resources and services.

Group #14

1. Identify the intervention models that address social determinants—especially home-grown "Kansan success" and seriously examine the broader system changes needed to make these interventions more likely.

2. We must reframe the health issue before we can expect broad progress—move away from health as commodity.

3. Create local task forces of employers/business leaders to examine health and economics. The scarce labor market is an opportunity and there are strong national business leaders who model and train on these issues.

4. Look for interventions that increase social cohesion in all areas—work/school/community—spaces that foster connections.

5. Re-examine health education programs to expand beyond biomedical risk factor education.

6. Focus on leadership development locally to implement this better understanding of health promotion.

7. Maintain a continuum perspective—the social determinants affect all of us differently.

8. Focus on inter-ethnic social interaction and promoting bridge building.

9. Understand the interactive/transactional nature of social determinants when implementing new approaches.

10. Take on alcohol like we have tobacco.

Group #15

1. Broad calculation with regard to social determinants of health.

2. Reduce poverty toward raising income floor through legislative action.

3. Community-based programs to support social network development.

4. Report cards on businesses, new and old.

5. Create incentive in business/employment to encourage utilization of wellness/health promotion employee benefits.

6. Enhance the profile of environmental health issues with regards to adult health.

7. Consider impact on business on community health and human services.

8. Maximize people's employability.

9. Government policy more sensitive to issues relevant to employability.

The dialogue process and its products suggest: 1) the potential effectiveness of a conference as a forum for critical reflection and learning about social determinants of health and how to address them; 2) the understandability of the concept of social determinants and people's related experiential knowledge; 3) the value of using locally-relevant health and socioeconomic data in promoting high levels of participant engagement; and 4) participants' capacity to identify creative and promising ways to improve health and well-being of communities, children, and adults.

A model for other ongoing efforts to improve population health in states and communities, the dialogue aspect of the Kansas Conference on Health and Its Determinants provided an effective forum for representatives of diverse sectors to discuss the social determinants of health and to suggest specific interventions that might improve the health of the community and its citizens.

❧

ABOUT THE CONTRIBUTORS

Manuella Adrian, Kansas Health Institute.

Benjamin C. Amick III, Behavioral Sciences, University of Texas, Houston School of Public Health.

Lisa F. Berkman, Harvard School of Public Health.

Paul Evensen, Human Development and Family Life, University of Kansas.

Stephen B. Fawcett, Human Development and Family Life, University of Kansas.

Jacqueline L. Fisher, Bureau of Child Research, University of Kansas.

Peter Fonagy, Menninger, Topeka, Kansas.

Vincent T. Francisco, Bureau of Child Research, University of Kansas.

Clyde Hertzman, Department of Health Care and Epidemiology, University of British Columbia, Vancouver, Canada.

Anna Higgitt, Menninger, Topeka, Kansas.

Derek Hyra, Human Development and Family Life, University of Kansas.

Ichiro Kawachi, Harvard School of Public Health.

John N. Lavis, Center for Health Economics and Policy Analysis, Department of Clinical Epidemiology and Biostatistics, McMaster University, Hamilton, Ontario, Canada; Institute for Work & Health, Toronto, Ontario, Canada; The Canadian Institute for Advanced Research, Toronto, Ontario, Canada.

Michael Marmot, Department of Epidemiology and Public Health, University College London, London, England.

J. Fraser Mustard, The Founders Network, Toronto, Ontario, Canada.

Adrienne Paine-Andrews, Bureau of Child Research, University of Kansas.

Thanne Rose, Kansas Health Institute.

Stergios Russos, Human Development, University of Kansas.

Robert F. St. Peter, Kansas Health Institute.

Jerry A. Schultz, Bureau of Child Research, University of Kansas.

Carol A. Shively, Department of Psychology, Wake Forest University Baptist Medical Center.

Gopal K. Singh, National Cancer Institute.

Frank Song, Virginia Health Quality Center.

Stephen J. Suomi, Laboratory of Comparative Ethology, The National Institute on Child Health and Human Development.

Alvin R. Tarlov, Baker Institute for Public Policy, Rice University.

Anna Wilkinson, Baker Institute for Public Policy, Rice University.

Richard G. Wilkinson, T.C.M.R., University of Sussex, Brighton, England.

David R. Williams, Sociology Department, University of Michigan.

ABOUT THE EDITORS

Alvin R. Tarlov is currently director of the Texas Program in Society and Health, a collaboration between the University of Texas, Houston Health Science Center; Baylor College of Medicine; University of Texas MD Anderson Cancer Center; University of Houston; and Rice University. The Texas Program organizes research, public policy formulation, and action programs that concentrate on the influence of social and societal factors on population health. At the time of this book's genesis he served as interim president of the Kansas Health Institute in Topeka. He was formerly the chairman of the Department of Medicine at the University of Chicago (1969–1983), president of the Henry J. Kaiser Family Foundation in Menlo Park, California (1984–1990), and executive director of the Health Institute in Boston, Massachusetts (1990–1999).

Robert F. St. Peter, M.D., is president of the Kansas Health Institute, a non-profit, independent health policy and research organization based in Topeka, Kansas, as well as a research associate professor in the department of preventive medicine at the University of Kansas School of Medicine. He has authored several scientific articles on health care and health policy. Dr. St. Peter is a board certified pediatrician with experience in health policy development and health services research. He has been a Robert Wood Johnson Foundation Clinical Scholar, a senior medical researcher at Mathematica Policy Research and the Center for Studying Health System Change in Washington, D.C., a health policy adviser on the U.S. Senate Committee on Labor and Human Resources, the Luther Terry Senior Fellow in Preventive Medicine and coordinator of child and school health programs in the office of disease prevention and health promotion, Office of the Assistant Secretary for Health, U.S. Department of Health and Human Services, and an International Health Fellow in Zaria, Nigeria.

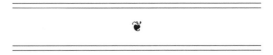